Occupational Therapy Manual for Evaluation of Range of Motion and Muscle Strength

DONNA LATELLA, MA, OTR/L
Assistant Professor
Department of Occupational Therapy
Quinnipiac University
Hamden, Connecticut

CATHERINE MERIANO, JD, MHS, OTR/L
Associate Professor
Department of Occupational Therapy
Quinnipiac University
Hamden, Connecticut

THOMSON
DELMAR LEARNING™

Australia Canada Mexico Singapore Spain United Kingdom United States

THOMSON
™
DELMAR LEARNING

Occupational Therapy Manual for Evaluation of Range of Motion and Muscle Strength
by
Donna Latella, MA, OTR/L and Catherine Meriano, JD, MHS, OTR/L

Executive Director, Health Care Business Unit:
William Brottmiller

Executive Editor:
Cathy L. Esperti

Development Editor:
Maria D'Angelico

Editorial Assistant:
Chris Manion

Executive Marketing Manager:
Dawn F. Gerrain

Channel Manager:
Jennifer McAvey

Production Editor:
Mary Colleen Liburdi

Printed in the United States of America
2 3 4 5 XXX 07 06 05 04 03

For more information contact
Delmar Learning,
Executive Woods, 5 Maxwell Drive,
Clifton Park, NY 12065-2919
Or find us on the World Wide Web at
http://www.delmarlearning.com

Library of Congress Cataloging-in-Publication Data

Latella, Donna.
Occupational therapy manual for evaluation of range of motion & muscle strength / Donna Latella, Catherine Meriano.
p. ; cm.
Includes bibliographical references and index.
ISBN 0-7668-3627-4
1. Muscle strength--Testing. 2. Joints--Range of motion. 3. Occupational therapy. I. Meriano, Catherine. II. Title.
[DNLM: 1. Joints--physiology. 2. Muscle Contraction. 3. Muscles--physiology. 4. Occupational Therapy--methods. 5. Range of Motion, Articular. WE 300 L351o 2003]
RC925.7.L38 2003
612.7'4'0287--dc21

2002041394

NOTICE TO THE READER

Publisher does not warrant or guarantee any of the products described herein or perform any independent analysis in connection with any of the product information contained herein. Publisher does not assume, and expressly disclaims, any obligation to obtain and include information other than that provided to it by the manufacturer.

The reader is expressly warned to consider and adopt all safety precautions that might be indicated by the activities herein and to avoid all potential hazards. By following the instructions contained herein, the reader willingly assumes all risks in connection with such instructions.

The publisher makes no representation or warranties of any kind, including but not limited to, the warranties of fitness for particular purpose or merchantability, nor are any such representations implied with respect to the material set forth herein, and the publisher takes no responsibility with respect to such material. The publisher shall not be liable for any special, consequential, or exemplary damages resulting, in whole or part, from the readers' use of, or reliance upon, this material.

Occupational Therapy Manual for Evaluation of Range of Motion and Muscle Strength

Table of Contents

Preface

As practicing Occupational Therapists and faculty members, we have desired for a long while to create our own manual for goniometry and manual muscle testing, incorporating our own philosophy and teaching styles. We firmly believe that the classroom should provide instruction in formal techniques as well as prepare the student for the practical aspects of the clinic. This teaching strategy should assist the student in the transition from the classroom to the affiliation site/clinic.

In the clinical environment today students need the traditional skills required for isolated manual muscle testing procedures; however, in addition, these students must have the capabilities to appropriately adapt to the often limited evaluation time provided. These clinical adaptations often require flexibility and higher clinical reasoning than the isolated manual muscle testing procedures, and these aspects must be incorporated into the educational process. In order to educate the students in a format which simulates the clinical environment, the range of motion and muscle testing are organized into categories. The range of motion assessment includes two categories called functional observation and goniometry evaluation. The strength assessment includes three categories called functional observation, gross manual muscle testing, and isolated manual muscle testing.

About the Authors

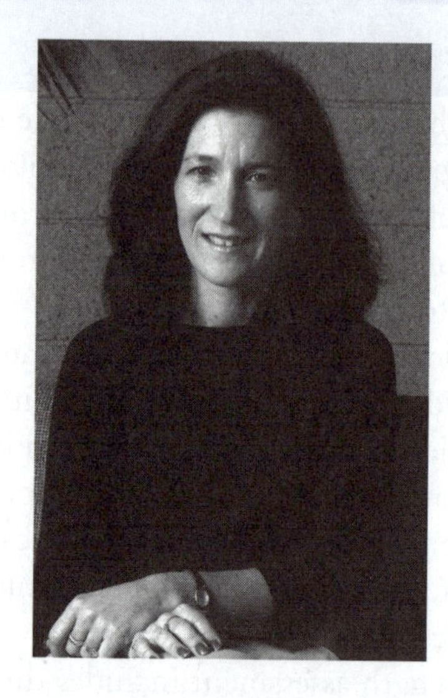

Donna Latella, MA, OTR/L is Assistant Clinical Coordinator and Assistant Professor in the Occupational Therapy Department of Quinnipiac University. Her clinical background is in acute care, outpatient rehab, and nursing homes. Donna, specifically, has expertise in areas such as orthopedics, geriatrics, dysphagia, and restorative dining programs. She teaches courses which include orthopedics, administration, and fieldwork. In addition, Donna is an Exercise Physiologist, and teaches human performance coursework. As a Clinical Coordinator, most recently, Donna has helped to create and supervise students in emerging practice areas, including an Adult Day Center in her hometown of Branford, Connecticut. At the same center, Donna and her golden retriever, Cody, also volunteer to provide animal-assisted therapy to the clients as a certified Pet Partner Team through the Delta Society. Her publications and presentations have been on topics such as leadership, teamwork, learning styles, educational malpractice, and dysphagia. Donna's most recent endeavor is focused on her doctoral dissertation toward the completion of her EdD in Educational Leadership at the University of Bridgeport in Connecticut. Donna enjoys jogging, boating, and spending time with her husband, two children, and two dogs.

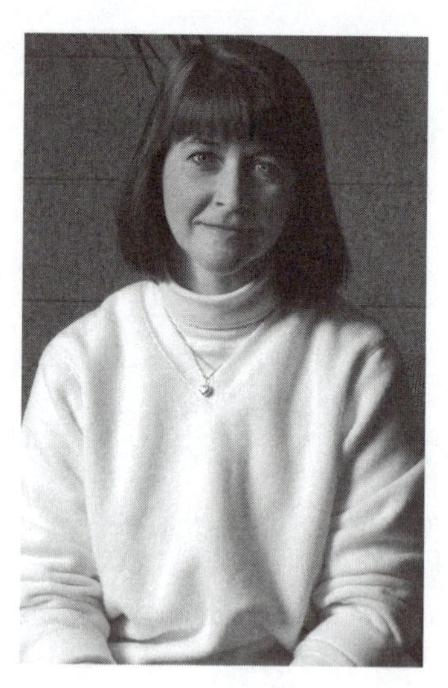

Catherine Meriano is a three-time graduate of Quinnipiac University with a BS degree in Occupational Therapy, an MHS degree in Education, and a JD from the School of Law. She is currently a tenured Associate Professor in the Department of Occupational Therapy and the University Director of Academic Integrity. Professor Meriano's primary area of practice and teaching has been in adult/geriatric physical disabilities. She has worked in a variety of settings, including acute care, home care, nursing homes, outpatient, and adult day centers. Professor Meriano lectures on the topics of "dysphagia" and "legal aspects of health care," and has recent or upcoming publications on these same topics.

Acknowledgments

We extend our thanks to Maria D'Angelico, developmental editor, as well as the team at Delmar Learning who assisted us in the creation of this manual. We wish to acknowledge the efforts of our professional peers who supported this endeavor. We appreciate the valuable feedback provided on early drafts by occupational therapists Gina Acampora and Signian McGeary. We wish to thank the following Quinnipiac University occupational therapy students for their specific assistance: Tara Tellefson, who created early artwork design, Thepdara Boriboun, the photography "client," and Jocelyn Costa, the photography "therapist." In addition, we wish to thank our families: Domenic, Kristy, and Dylan Latella, and John, Kathleen, and Jay Meriano. Your support throughout the writing of this manual was greatly appreciated.

Contributors

The following is a list of contributors to this manual:

Frank DeRubeis, OTR/L

Maria Cusson, JD, MS, RPT

Roberta Solimene, OTR/L, CHT

Introduction

The first category for both range of motion and strength assessments is **functional observation**. Once a student masters the anatomy, he/she can determine what joints and muscle groups are used for different functional tasks. Knowing this enables the student to observe the client completing a functional activity and to decide, based on that observation, whether a range of motion assessment, gross manual muscle testing, or isolated manual muscle testing is required. Examples of functional tasks are found in Table 1. Other factors, such as the facility requirements, the specific occupation or role of the client, and the client's own goals will also influence this decision; however, in this manual the concentration will center on range of motion and strength assessments.

TABLE 1 Functional Tasks

MOTION	EXAMPLE OF FUNCTIONAL ACTIVITY TO BE OBSERVED
Spinal flexion	Bending to pick up an object
Spinal extension	Sit-to-stand or lifting activities
Spinal lateral flexion	Getting in/out of a car
Spinal oblique rotation	Looking over the shoulder when driving
Neck flexion	Looking down to button a shirt or writing activities
Neck extension	During overhead activities or washing hair in the shower
Neck lateral flexion	Leaning head on hand or scratching head
Neck rotation	Looking over the shoulder when driving
Scapular elevation	While individuals rarely use the scapula in isolation during functional activities, observation of a client while he is shrugging his shoulders or carrying a backpack on one shoulder will indicate a functional weakness
Scapular depression	While individuals rarely use the scapula in isolation during functional activities, observation of a client while reaching into pants pockets may indicate a weakness of the scapular depressors.
Scapular adduction	While individuals rarely use the scapula in isolation during functional activities, observation of a client while posteriorly tucking in a shirt may indicate a weakness of the scapular adductors
Scapular abduction	While individuals rarely use the scapula in isolation during functional activities, observation of a client while reaching forward for an object may indicate a weakness of the scapular abductors
Humeral flexion	Brushing teeth and reaching into an overhead cabinet
Humeral extension	Bowling and donning a coat sleeve

(continues)

TABLE 1 Functional Tasks

MOTION	EXAMPLE OF FUNCTIONAL ACTIVITY TO BE OBSERVED
Humeral abduction	Scratching the back of neck and washing one's hair
Humeral adduction	Holding a book or paper under one's arm
Humeral external rotation	Brushing the back of one's head and pitching a ball
Humeral internal rotation	Hooking a bra or scratching one's back
Humeral horizontal abduction	Pulling open a door or swinging a tennis racquet
Humeral horizontal adduction	Giving a hug or applying earrings
Elbow flexion	Lifting a box or eating
Elbow extension	Pushing to stand or hammering
Forearm supination and pronation	Turning a doorknob, using a screwdriver, or playing cards
Wrist flexion	Pouring a cup of tea or zipping a jacket
Wrist extension	Shaving with a standard razor or swinging a tennis racquet
Wrist radial and ulnar deviation	Waving, washing a window, or wiping a table
Digit MCP flexion	Holding a book or cards, or puppetry
Digit PIP/DIP flexion	Handwriting or threading a needle
Digit MCP/DIP/PIP extension	Releasing a ball or typing
Hip flexion	Climbing stairs or attempting to don socks
Hip extension	Sit-to-stand activities including transferring from bed to chair and toilet
Hip abduction	Getting onto a bicycle or sidestepping in/out of the bath tub
Hip adduction	Sitting with ankles crossed or bracing an object between the legs
Hip external rotation	Sitting "pretzel" style or observing the bottom of the foot
Hip internal rotation	Getting into a kneeling position or performing a quadriceps stretch in standing
Knee flexion	Stand-to-sit movements or positioning to bathe feet
Knee extension	Kicking a ball or hiking pants
Ankle dorsiflexion	Pressing the gas pedal while driving or dancing
Ankle plantar flexion	Walking on the beach or donning shoes
Foot inversion/eversion	Activities which require foot stabilization such as walking on rough ground
Toe MTP flexion	Any functional mobility activity such as ambulating to the bathroom with an assistive device or climbing stairs
Toe IP flexion	Any functional activity which involves maintaining balance such as standing on a moving bus
Toe MTP abduction	May be observed with MTP flexors when walking on gravel, for example, as the MTP abductors are difficult to observe in isolation
Toe MTP and IP extension	Any functional mobility activity such as making a bed or climbing stairs. Weakness may also be noted when trimming toe nails

(continued)

When the student makes the decision regarding further assessment of the client, based on all the known factors and observations, this is called **clinical reasoning**. Clinical reasoning, simply stated, is thinking as a therapist. The therapist today is required to complete a client evaluation in a limited time and must use his/her clinical reasoning to determine what is the best use of that limited time. For example, if a therapist notes during an observation of a functional task that a client has limited range of motion, yet the client is functional in all activities of daily living (ADL), the therapist should not proceed with a goniometry or range of motion assessment at that time. The time is better spent addressing other areas that do affect the client's function.

The second category for the range of motion assessment is formal **goniometry**. This includes the use of the goniometer to measure the degrees of motion that are available at a particular joint. Goniometry is discussed in detail in chapter one of this manual.

The second category for strength assessment is **gross manual muscle testing**. This includes test grades of poor to normal (2–5), and includes testing of muscle groups as a whole rather than testing specific muscles. This again will save time for the therapist. Once skilled in gross muscle testing, the therapist can quickly evaluate a client for muscle group weakness. Depending on the needs of the client and the facility, this may be all that is necessary to formulate an appropriate intervention plan. If a therapist is working with a client who has had a head injury, it may not be necessary to determine which shoulder muscle is weak, but sufficient to know that the shoulder muscle group is weak and affecting function. On the other hand, if a client has a diagnosis of a recent rotator cuff repair, it is important that the therapist evaluate each muscle of the shoulder. The procedures for gross manual muscle testing are presented in chapter two of this manual.

This assessment of each specific muscle within a muscle group is the third category and is called **isolated manual muscle testing**. This includes tests for grades of trace to normal (1–5).

It is best to be proficient in all these methods to afford the efficiency that is demanded of therapists today without losing the accuracy due to all clients. Functional observation and gross muscle testing can quickly indicate or identify a problem group of muscles, which can then be tested individually using isolated manual muscle testing techniques. The procedures for isolated manual muscle testing are found in chapter three of this manual.

Refer to Figure 1 for a review of the decision tree necessary for appropriate clinical reasoning. In addition to clinical reasoning, occupational therapists also utilize frames of reference when providing evaluation and intervention to our clients. A **frame of reference** was clearly defined by Anne Mosey as "a set of interrelated internally consistent concepts, definitions, postulates, and principles that provide a systematic description of and prescription for a practitioner's interaction with his domain of concern." (1970, p5) The focus of a frame of reference is to act as a guide to the therapist for the evaluation and intervention process. In this manual, a small portion of that "practitioner's interaction" is discussed. That portion is the assessment of range of motion and muscle strength. Because of this, the most appropriate frame of reference for use during a range of motion or strength assessment is the **biomechanical frame of reference**. This frame of reference defines function and dysfunction in terms of an individual's range of motion, strength, and endurance. The biomechanical frame of reference is a building block on the way to other frames of reference because the components of range of motion, strength, and endurance are the building blocks to more functional activities.

The biomechanical frame of reference has four basic assumptions. The first is that purposeful activity will improve range of motion, strength, and endurance. It is important to note that this is purposeful activity, which has meaning to the client, not just activities created to provide a diversion for a client. The second assumption is that the improvement of range of motion, strength, and endurance will result in improved functional skills. This is why this frame of reference is considered a building block. Once the range of motion, strength, and endurance have improved, the functional skills will follow and the therapist can begin to utilize a frame of reference which can incorporate more functional skills and the client's

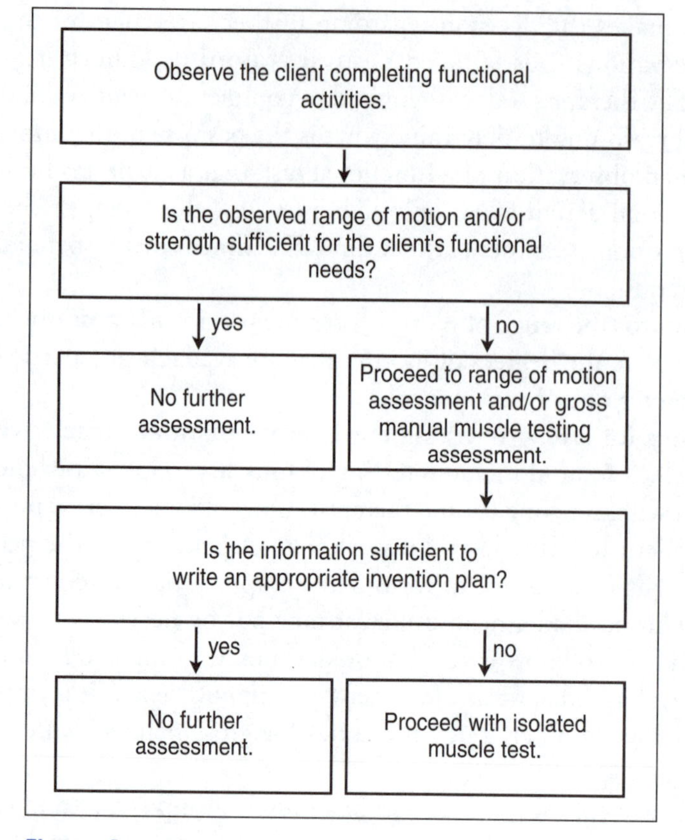

Figure 1 Decision Tree

occupation. The third assumption is called the "rest/stress principle." This principle dictates that while stress is necessary to avoid a loss of function, the body must also have time to rest and heal. This is especially important to consider in the health care environment of today. Many therapy referrals are occurring rapidly after the onset of a disease or injury. With shorter hospital stays, clients are pushed to progress earlier. As therapists, we must consider the needs of the body to heal while providing appropriate intervention to the client. The fourth and final assumption is that the client must have an intact central nervous system to utilize this frame of reference. This is because a client needs to demonstrate isolated and coordinated movement for the therapist to accurately measure an individual's range of motion, strength, and endurance. If the client has abnormal muscle tone or is unable to follow directions, this will influence the accuracy of all assessment areas.

Although this manual is for the assessment, and not the intervention, of deficits in the areas of range of motion and strength, the biomechanical frame of reference is appropriate because assessment is the first step in establishing a baseline on which to build an intervention plan. That intervention plan can then continue with the biomechanical frame of reference as well as other appropriate frames of reference.

Function and functional activities have been mentioned frequently in this introduction. Occupational therapists work toward the recovery of functional skills and occupations with individual clients. Because the focus of intervention is based on functional skills, there has been a deliberate attempt throughout this manual to position the clients against gravity for both goniometry and muscle testing. The majority of functional activities occur against gravity; therefore, it is most appropriate to test our clients in that position. There are times when this is not possible because of the client's comfort. In addition, the positioning in relationship to gravity is not as important when assessing the hands and feet because gravity does not have as large an effect on these smaller muscles. It is possible to find other reference materials that show different client and therapist positions for goniometry and muscle testing. These positions while not incorrect, are inappropriate for a manual such as this, which is concerned with the assessment of a client's *functional* range of motion and strength.

The following is a list of Key Terms used in this manual. Key Terms are defined in the glossary at the end of the book.

Key Terms

Active range of motion
Against gravity
Axis of the body
Biomechanical frame of reference
Clinical reasoning
Compensation
End feel
Frames of reference
Fulcrum
Functional observation
Goniometer
Goniometry
Gravity-eliminated
Gross manual muscle testing
Isolated manual muscle testing
Movable arm
Passive range of motion
Plane of the body
Resistance
Screening
Stabilization
Stationary arm

Finally, there are three icons that are used to designate features that appear intermittently throughout the text. They are: Note, Caution, and ASHT guidelines.

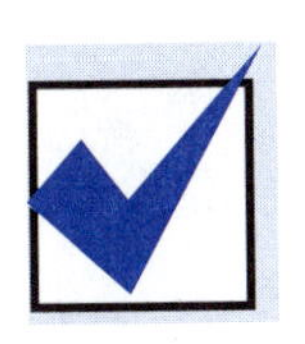

Note

Caution

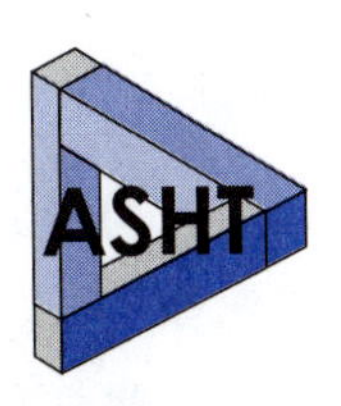

ASHT Guidelines

chapter 1

Goniometry

SECTION 1-1: Introduction to Goniometry

After completing this chapter the student should be able to accomplish the following:

- define the terms related to goniometry
- demonstrate the ability to observe a client during functional activities and estimate the areas of deficit
- demonstrate the ability to perform all steps of the goniometry process

Along with these specific skills, the student should begin practicing the use of terminology that clients can comprehend rather than medical terminology, as well as the skill of building client rapport.

DEFINITIONS

When evaluating a client's range of motion, a therapist should first observe the client during a functional activity. This functional observation may be referred to as a **screening** because it is not a formal assessment, but a method to allow the therapist to determine quickly which joints need further assessment. By demonstrating proficient observation skills a therapist will be able to save time in the fast-paced health care environment. If no deficits are noted during observation, the therapist can avoid spending excessive time on measuring the range of motion of each joint only to determine that all joints are functional or normal. In addition, this screening can be completed during another assessment such as activities of daily living (ADL).

Once a deficit joint or joints are noted, the therapist will need to complete a goniometry assessment. The purpose of **goniometry** is to measure the arc of motion of a joint. The word goniometry itself means the measurement of angles with gonia, meaning angle, and metron, meaning measure. In order to measure this arc of motion, the therapist utilizes bony landmarks on the human body to place the goniometer. The **goniometer** is the most commonly used instrument to measure joint motion. There are many sizes and shapes. Some goniometers are plastic while others are metal (see Figure 1-1-1). All goniometers have a body and two arms. The body is a full or semicircle with a center point called the axis or **fulcrum**. One arm is called the **stationary arm** and the other is the **movable arm**.

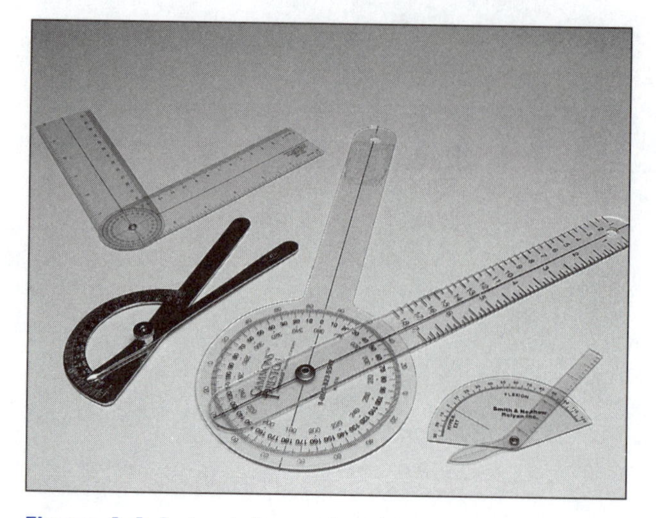

Figure 1-1-1 Sample finger and regular goniometer.

During the use of the goniometer, the axis or fulcrum is placed over the axis of motion being measured. The stationary arm stays fixed and aligned with the plane of motion proximal to the joint being measured. The movable arm is also aligned with the plane of motion, but is distal to the joint being measured and follows the arc of motion. For example, if shoulder flexion is measured, the axis is on the lateral aspect of the shoulder, the stable arm stays positioned with the trunk of the body, and the movable arm follows the humerus along the plane of motion.

Now that the goniometer placement has been determined, it is important to understand the planes and axis of joint motion. The **planes** are the surfaces along which movement occurs. They are imaginary sheets of glass that run through the body. There are different planes (of glass) running through the body in different directions because the body moves in different directions (Figure 1-1-2). The names and locations of these planes are listed in Table 1-1-1.

Movement of the body generally occurs in an arc or circular motion. The axis or fulcrum is the center of this motion. The **axis of the body** is a straight line running through the body like an arrow. This axis also runs through the plane (sheet of glass). Because the axis runs through the plane, it must be perpendicular to that plane. Each axis and plane that are perpendicular to each other create a partnership. The plane is the flat surface along which the movement occurs, and the axis is the location around which the movement occurs (Figure 1-1-3). Table 1-1-2 lists each axis, its location, and its partner plane.

Prior to the initiation of goniometry, the therapist must be knowledgeable about **passive range of motion** (PROM) and **active range of motion** (AROM). PROM is completed by the therapist alone. The therapist moves the extremity through the available arc of motion without the assistance of the client. AROM is the opposite of PROM. The client moves the extremity through the available arc of motion without the assistance of the therapist. In general, PROM is completed to assess the joint integrity/end feel, and to assess the tone or muscle tightness of the muscle groups. The **end feel** of a joint is, as the name describes, the feeling that is elicited when the joint is brought through the entire available range of motion. The end feel can be hard, firm, or soft. Table 1-1-3 lists the types of end feels along with a normal and abnormal example for each.

Some of the names for planes and axes are the same, which can create confusion; however, if you remember the frontal plane runs through the body dividing into front and back portions, then the frontal axis runs along the same area. Therefore, if these are parallel, they cannot be "partners."

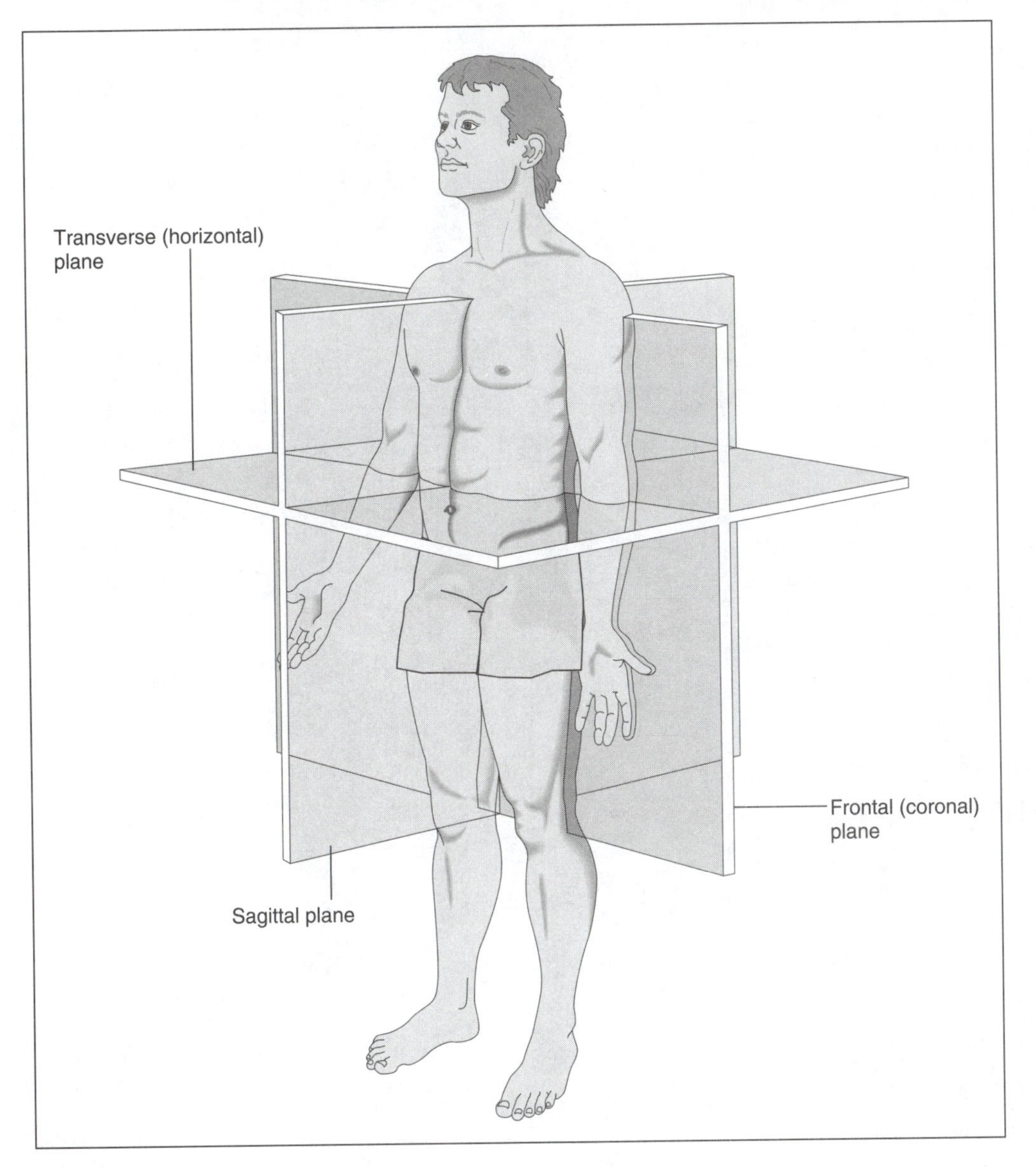

Figure 1-1-2 Planes of the body.

TABLE 1-1-1 Planes of the Body

PLANE NAME	LOCATION OF PLANE IN THE BODY
Sagittal (***Note***: a plane bisecting the body equally can be referred to as the median plane)	Dissects the body into right and left portions
Frontal or Coronal	Dissects the body into equal or unequal anterior and posterior portions
Transverse or Horizontal	Dissects the body into equal or unequal cranial and caudal portions

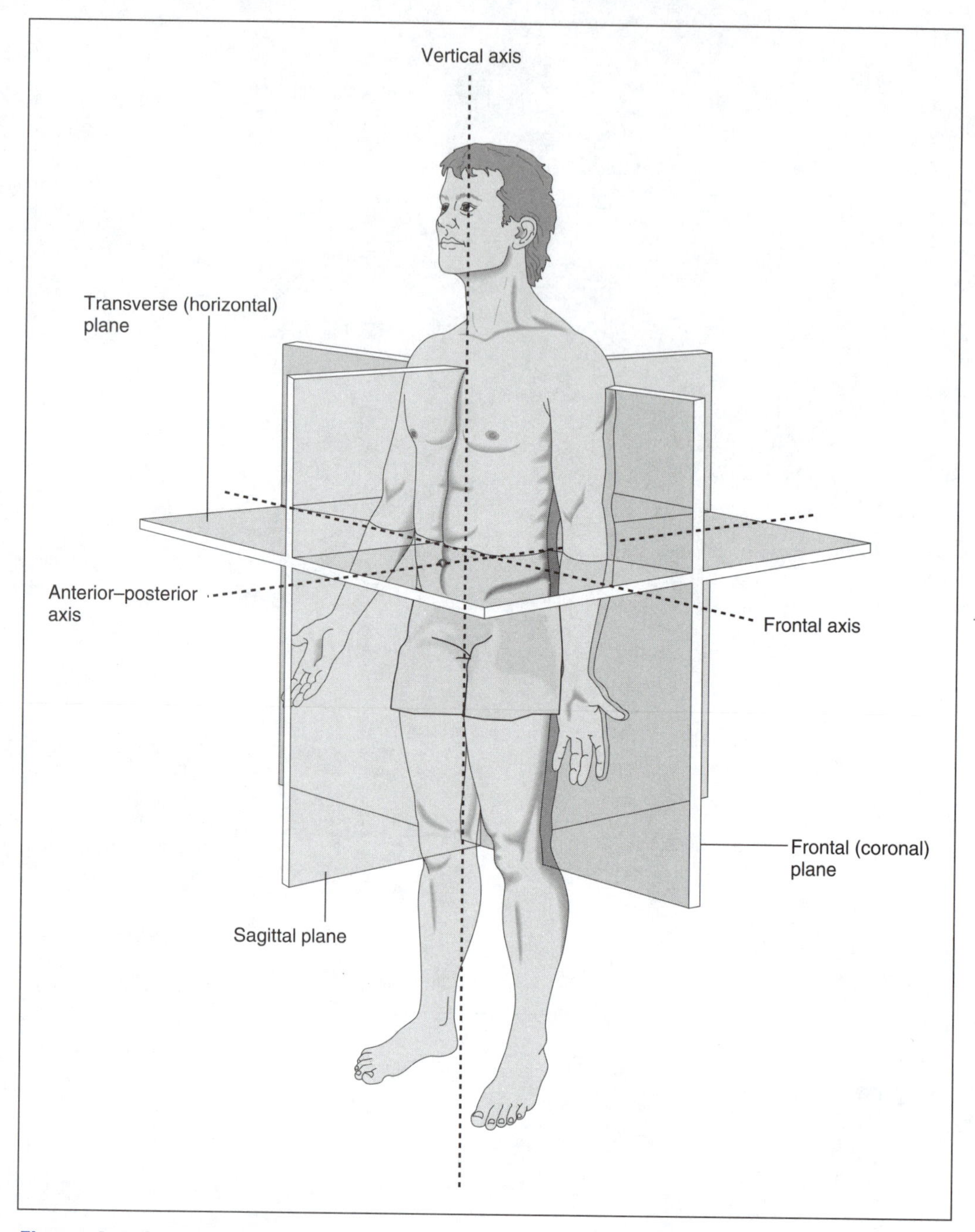

Figure 1-1-3 Planes and axes of the body.

TABLE 1-1-2 Axes of the Body

AXIS NAME	LOCATION OF AXIS	PARTNER PLANE
Frontal or Coronal	Runs side to side (right ↔ left)	Median and Sagittal planes
Anterior–Posterior	Runs front ↔ back	Frontal or Coronal plane
Vertical	Runs cranial ↔ caudal	Transverse or Horizontal plane

TABLE 1-1-3 Types of End Feels

Hard End Feel: when bone hits bone	*Normal Example*: elbow extension when the olecranon process enters the olecranon fossa to stop joint movement	*Abnormal Example*: bone hitting bone because of arthritis or a bone chip in a joint which causes joint movement to stop
Firm End Feel: a stretching or "springy" feeling	*Normal Example*: hip flexion when the hamstrings stretch to stop joint movement	*Abnormal Example*: elbow extension when bicep spasticity causes joint movement to stop
Soft End Feel: when soft tissue hits soft tissue	*Normal Example*: elbow or knee flexion when one muscle belly hits another to stop joint movement	*Abnormal Example*: hand edema causes joint movement to stop

PROCEDURE

As stated in the decision tree, observation is always the first step in the evaluative process. This observation occurs during a functional activity and is usually in combination with another assessment, such as ADL. During the observation, the therapist uses his/her clinical judgment to determine if the client has any functional limitations and if further formal assessment is appropriate. If the therapist determines that goniometric measurements are appropriate, the process begins with PROM of the extremity. As stated earlier, PROM is necessary to evaluate joint integrity/end feel, and muscle tone.

After the completion of PROM, the therapist asks the client to complete the same motion actively (AROM). This allows the therapist to determine if the client understands the proper motion, which is required for the assessment to take place. In addition, the therapist should observe the AROM for any compensation. **Compensation** is noted when the client uses alternative motions to achieve the AROM that has been requested by the therapist. For example, when a client is asked to flex the shoulder joint he/she may compensate by utilizing excessive scapular motion or trunk extension in an attempt to increase shoulder flexion. This is generally not a conscious act on the part of the client, and proper cueing by the therapist can usually eliminate the compensation. Once eliminated, a more accurate measurement can be achieved.

The next step in the goniometry process is the placement of the goniometer. The axis or fulcrum is placed over the axis of motion. The stationary arm and movable arms are placed along the plane of motion. The goniometer placement is specific to each joint motion being tested. The specifics are explained in the sections that follow. Once this process is completed, the contralateral side is evaluated and all results are recorded.

The format for recording is determined by individual facilities, but is always measured in degrees of motion. Because the motion is measured in degrees, the measurements are reported with a beginning and end measurement. The majority of motions begin at zero degrees. It is important for a therapist to be able to establish the zero point when initiating goniometry measurement. Different measurements require different placement of the goniometer arms. The goniometer arms may be closed with both arms together, open with both arms opposite each other, perpendicular to each other, or somewhere in-between. With each of these different placements of the goniometer arms, the zero point moves. Most goniometers have two sets of numbers labeled zero to 180 or 360 degrees (Figure 1-1-4). The two zero points are placed such that the zero starts with the goniometer arms either open or closed. Some goniometers will also have a zero point when the arms are perpendicular to each other. If a measurement begins away from a zero point, the therapist should document the exact beginning point in degrees.

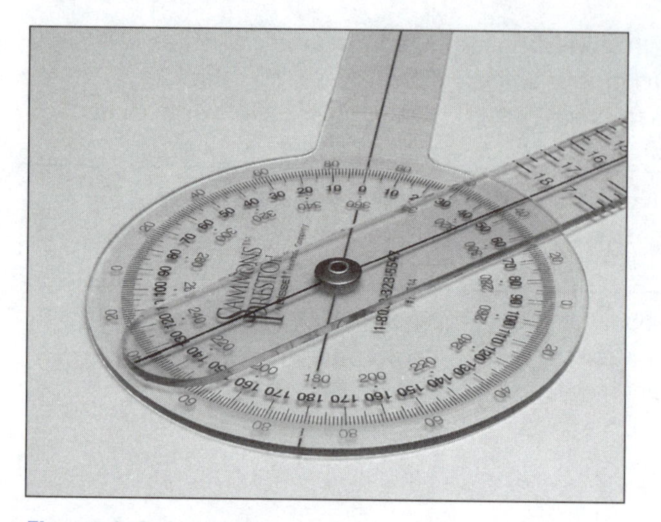

Figure 1-1-4 Goniometer numbers.

Typically AROM is measured; however, PROM can also be measured if limitations are noted. The measurements are completed in the same manner as the AROM evaluation.

Contraindications and Precautions

The following are contraindications to goniometry because the therapist can cause injury to the client if the assessment is attempted:

- dislocation of a joint
- diagnosis of myositis ossificans

The following are precautions to goniometry because injury to the client may occur:

- infection or inflammatory conditions
- surgical procedure has just been performed
- unhealed fracture
- marked osteoporosis
- carcinoma of the bone or any fragile bone condition
- significant hypermobility
- significant pain
- hemophilia
- hematoma
- acute muscular injuries

SECTION 1-2: Goniometric Measurements of the Trunk and Neck

Trunk: *spinal flexion*

Normal ROM: 0–80 degrees/4 inches

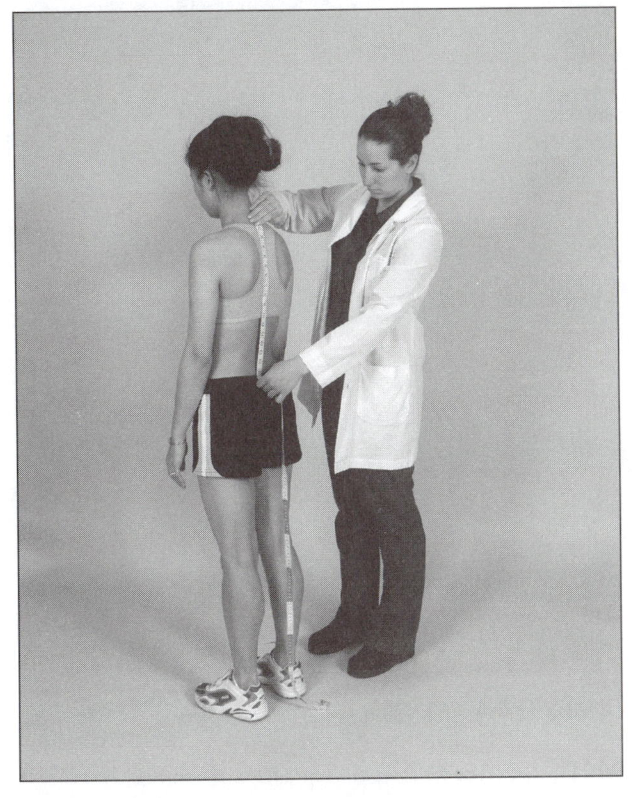

Figure 1-2-1 Start position for spinal flexion.

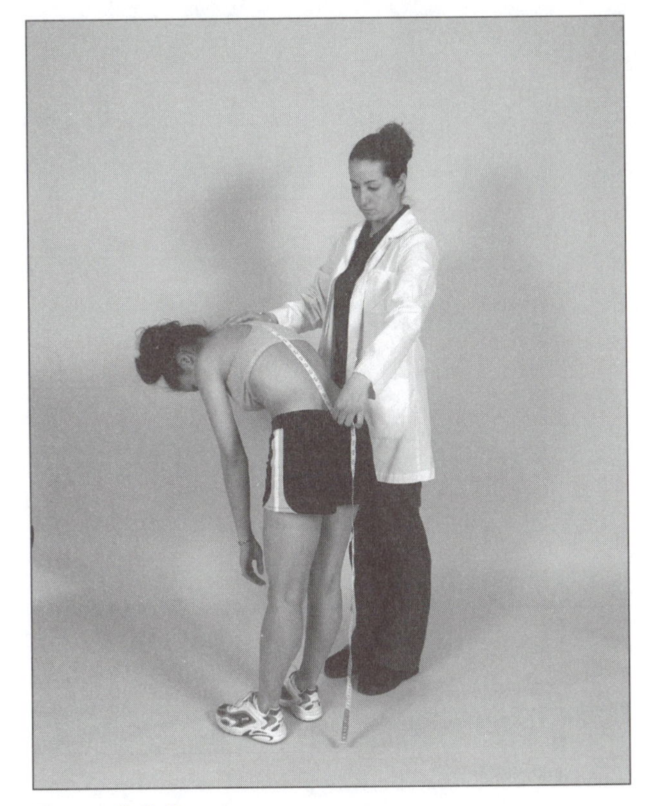

Figure 1-2-2 End position for spinal flexion.

Client Position: Client is standing with upper extremity resting at side. Cervical spine is in neutral. Feet are shoulder width apart.

Starting—spine is in neutral (Figure 1-2-1) .

Ending—client moves into maximum spinal flexion (Figure 1-2-2).

Therapist Position: Observe to prevent anterior tilt.

Measurement: A tape measure is placed between the spinous processes of C7 and S1. First the measurement is taken with the client in the upright position and a second one taken at maximal flexion. The difference between the two measurements is the amount of flexion present.

Trunk: *spinal extension*

Normal ROM: 0–25 degrees

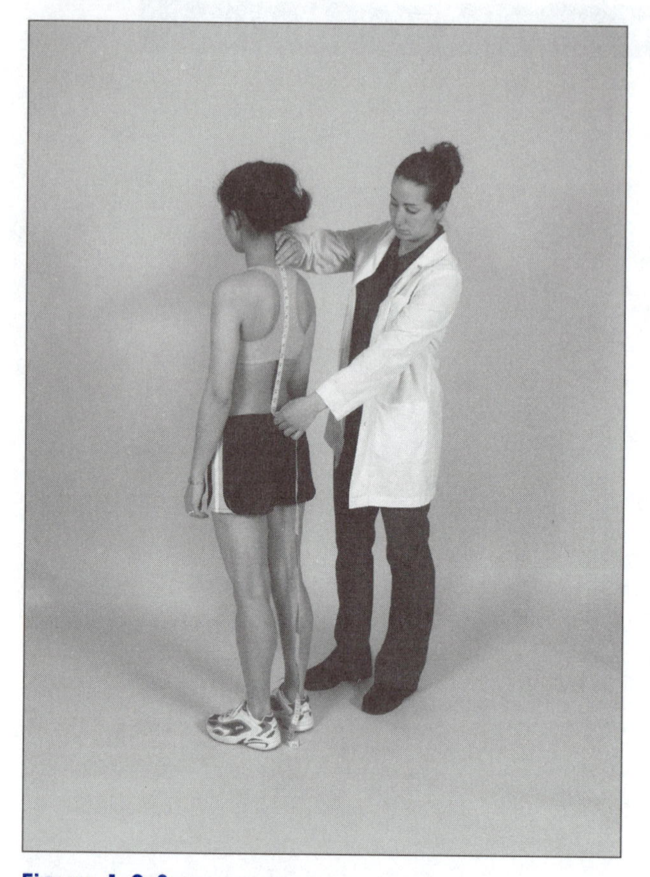

Figure 1-2-3 Start position for spinal extension.

Client Position: Client is standing with upper extremity resting at side. Cervical spine is in neutral. Feet are shoulder width apart.

Starting—spine is in neutral (Figure 1-2-3).

Ending—client moves into maximum spinal extension (Figure 1-2-4).

Therapist Position: Observe to prevent anterior tilt.

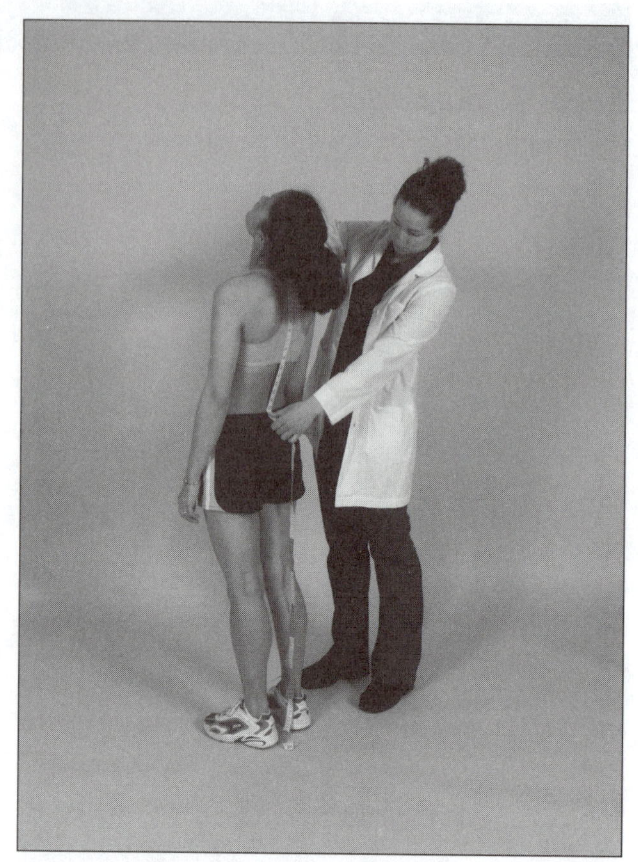

Figure 1-2-4 End position for spinal extension.

Measurement: A tape measure is placed between the spinous processes of C7 and S1. First the measurement is taken with the client in the upright position and a second one taken at maximal extension. The difference between the two measurements is the amount of extension present.

Trunk: *spinal lateral flexion*

Normal ROM: 0–35 degrees

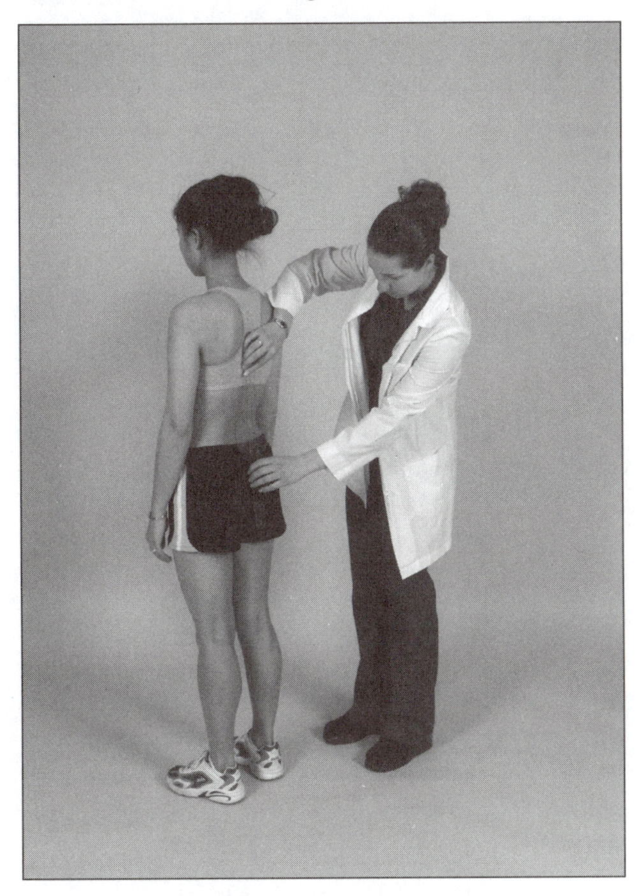

Figure 1-2-5 Start position for spinal lateral flexion.

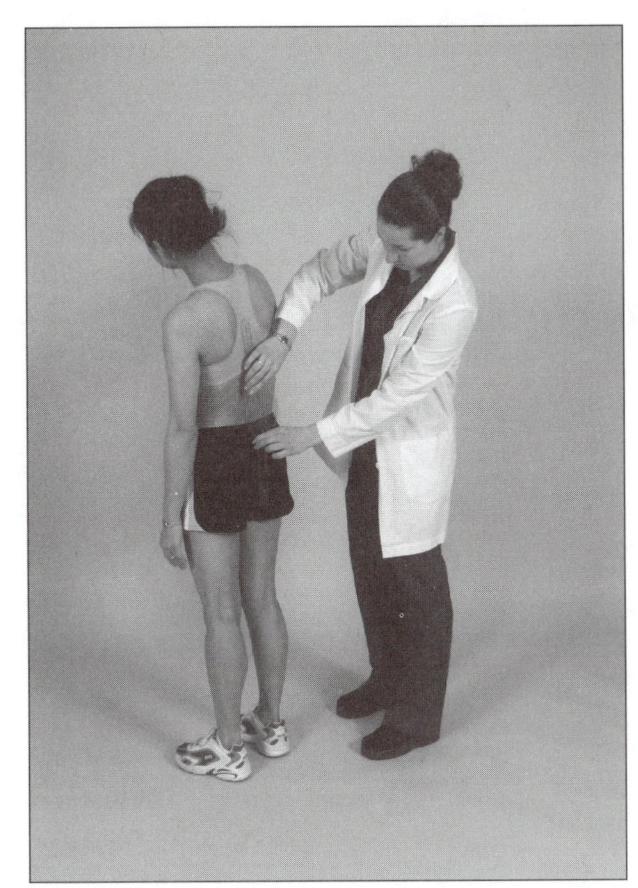

Figure 1-2-6 End position for spinal lateral flexion.

Client Position: Client is standing with upper extremity resting at side. Cervical spine is in neutral. Feet are shoulder width apart.

Starting—spine is in neutral (Figure 1-2-5).

Ending—client moves into maximum lateral flexion (Figure 1-2-6).

Therapist Position: Observe the pelvic region to prevent compensatory movements.

Goniometer Position:

FULCRUM: over the posterior aspect of the spinous process of S1

STABLE ARM: perpendicular to the floor

MOVABLE ARM: over the posterior aspect of the spinous process of C7

Alternate Test

A tape measure may be used to determine the distance from the tip of the middle finger and the floor as the client maintains maximum lateral flexion. The client's feet are flat on the ground and knees fully extended.

Trunk: *spinal rotation*
Normal ROM: 0–45 degrees

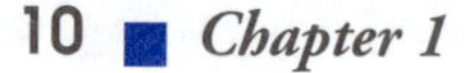

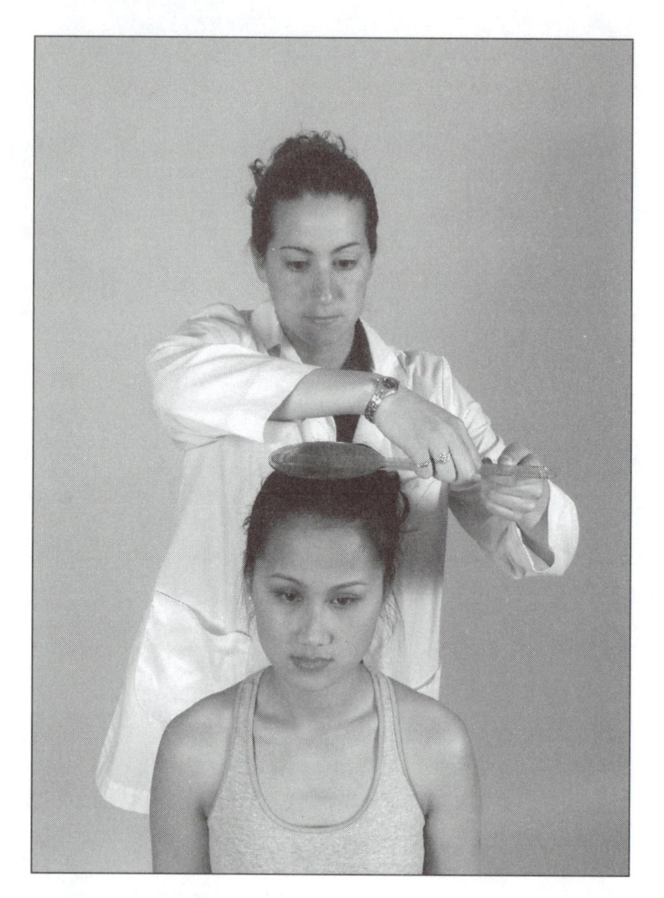

Figure 1-2-7 Start position for spinal rotation.

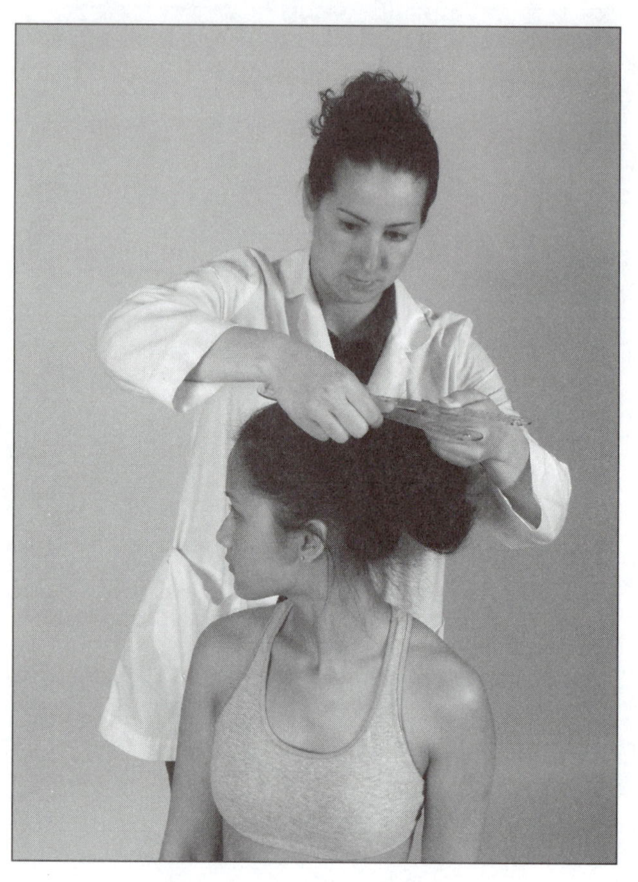

Figure 1-2-8 End position for spinal rotation.

Client Position: Client is sitting or standing with upper extremity resting at side. Cervical spine is in neutral. Feet are shoulder width apart.

Starting—Spine is in neutral (Figure 1-2-7).

Ending—client moves into maximum rotation (Figure 1-2-8).

Therapist Position: Observe the pelvic region to prevent compensatory movements.

Goniometer Position:

FULCRUM: over the center of the cranial aspect of the head

STABLE ARM: parallel to an imaginary line between the prominences of the iliac crests

MOVABLE ARM: along an imaginary line between the acromial processes

Neck: *cervical flexion*

Normal ROM: 0–45 degrees

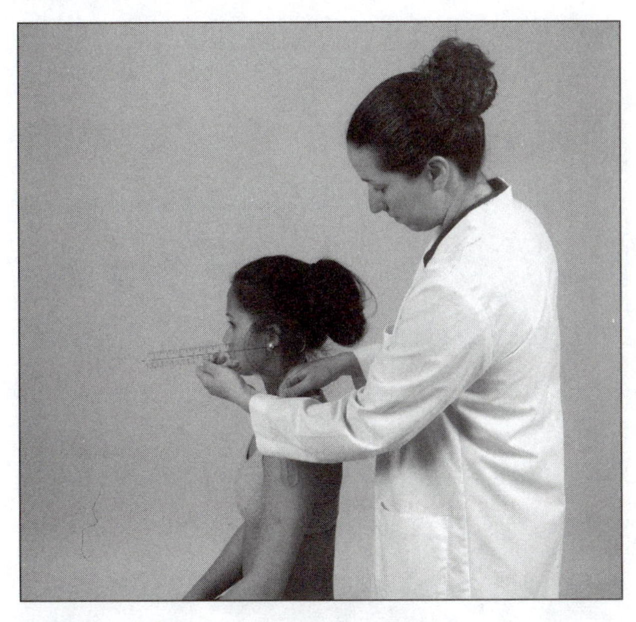

Figure 1-2-9 Start position for cervical flexion.

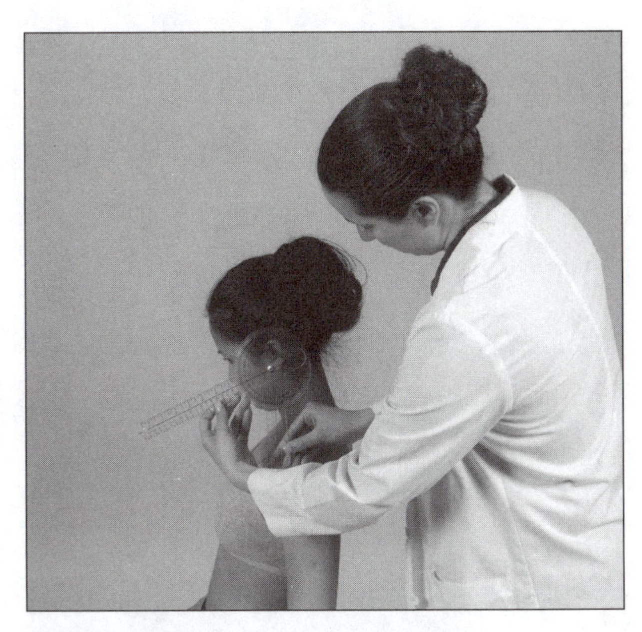

Figure 1-2-10 End position for cervical flexion.

Client Position: Client is sitting with upper extremity resting at side. Lumbar and thoracic spines are supported by the chair.

Starting—cervical spine is in neutral (Figure 1-2-9).

Ending—client moves into maximum cervical flexion (Figure 1-2-10).

Therapist Position: Observe the lumbar and thoracic regions to prevent compensatory movements.

Goniometer Position:

FULCRUM: over external auditory meatus

STABLE ARM: perpendicular or parallel to the floor

MOVABLE ARM: along the base of the nares

Alternate Test

A tape measure may be used to assess the distance between the tip of the chin and the sternal notch. Observe to ensure client's mouth is closed.

Neck: *cervical extension*

Normal ROM: 0–45 degrees

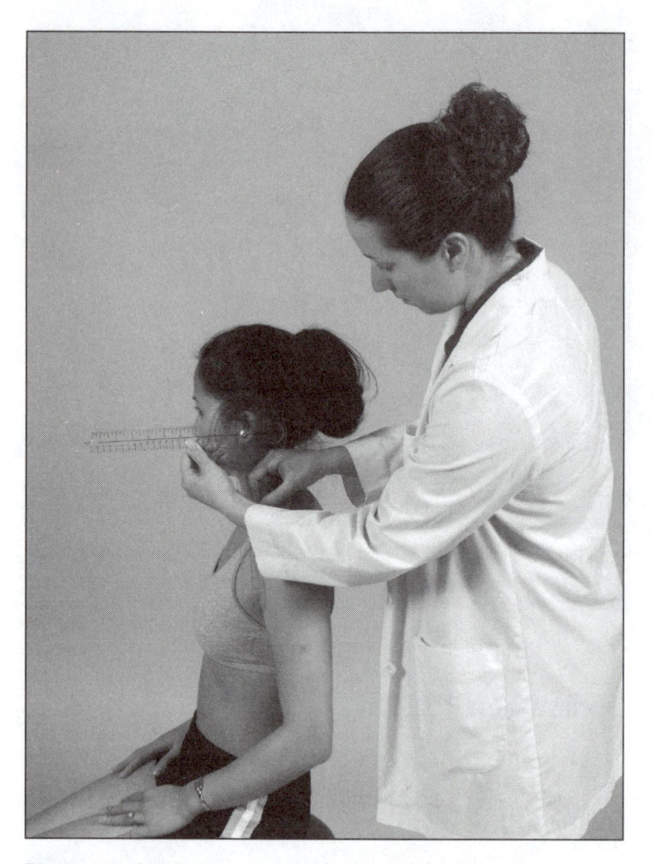

Figure 1-2-11 Start position for cervical extension.

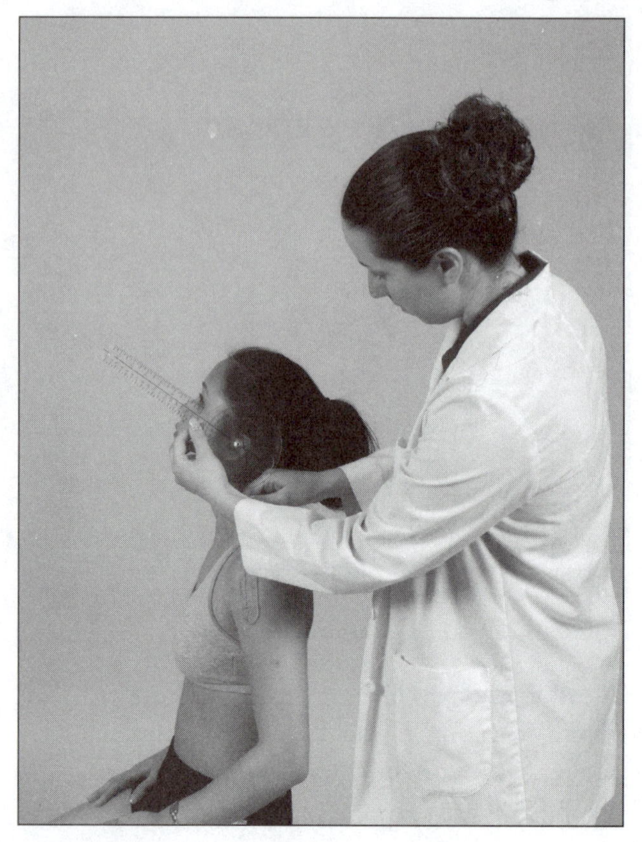

Figure 1-2-12 End position for cervical extension.

Client Position: Client is sitting with upper extremity resting at side. Lumbar and thoracic spines are supported by the chair.

Starting—cervical spine is in neutral (Figure 1-2-11).

Ending—client moves into maximum cervical extension (Figure 1-2-12).

Therapist Position: Observe the lumbar and thoracic regions to prevent compensatory movements.

Goniometer Position:

FULCRUM: over external auditory meatus

STABLE ARM: perpendicular or parallel to the floor

MOVABLE ARM: along the base of the nares

Alternate Test

A tape measure may be used to assess the distance between the tip of the chin and the sternal notch. Observe to ensure client's mouth is closed.

Neck: *cervical lateral flexion*

Normal ROM: 0–45 degrees

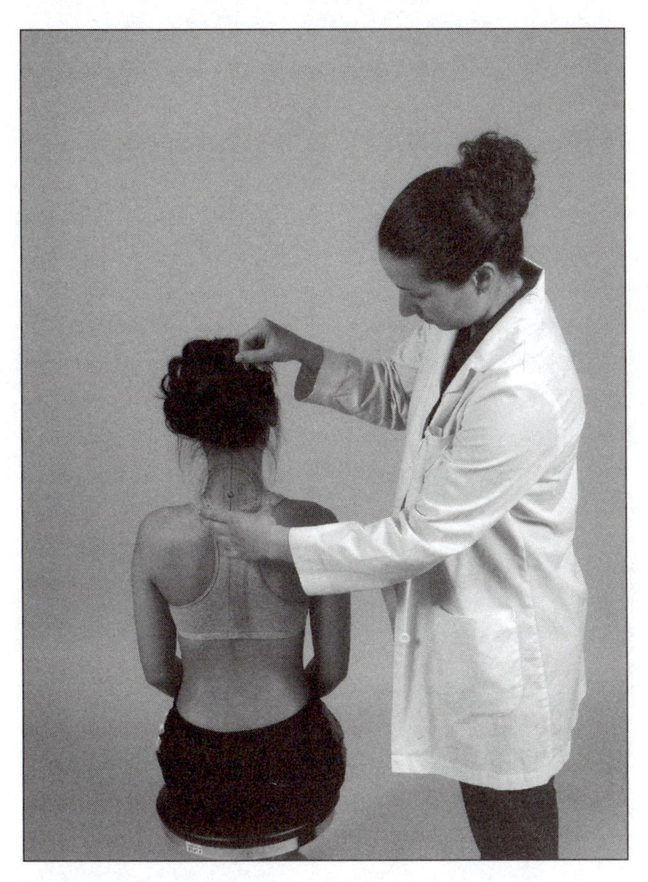

Figure 1-2-13 Start position for cervical lateral flexion.

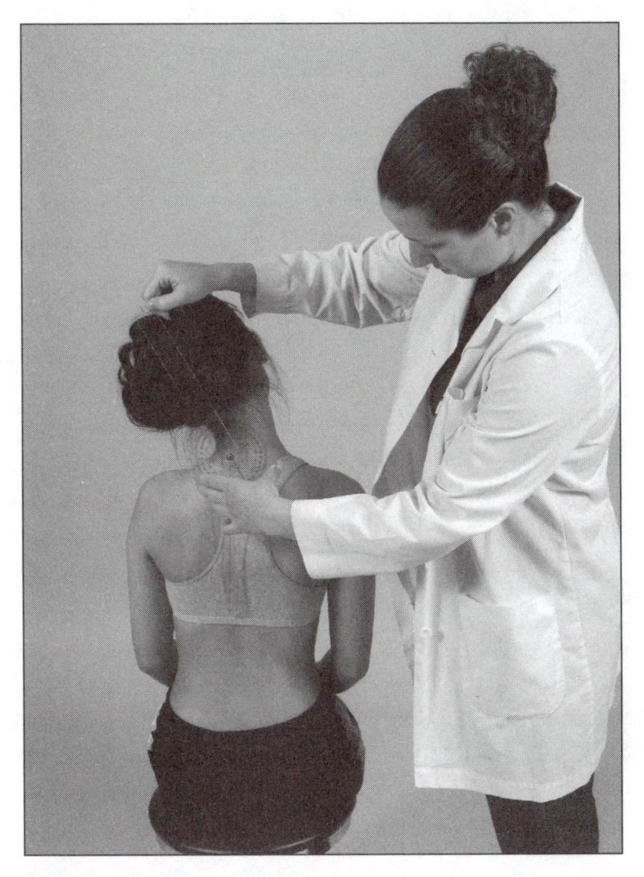

Figure 1-2-14 End position for cervical lateral flexion.

Client Position: Client is sitting with upper extremity resting at side. Lumbar and thoracic spines are supported by the chair.

Starting—cervical spine is in neutral (Figure 1-2-13).

Ending—client moves into maximum cervical lateral flexion (Figure 1-2-14).

Therapist Position: Observe the lumbar and thoracic regions to prevent compensatory movements.

Goniometer Position:

FULCRUM: over spinous process of C7 vertebrae

STABLE ARM: over spinous processes of the thoracic vertebrae with arm perpendicular to the floor

MOVABLE ARM: over dorsal midline of the head with the occipital protuberance as a guide

Alternate Test

A tape measure may be used to assess the distance between the mastoid process and the acromial process. Observe to ensure client's mouth is closed.

Neck: *cervical rotation*

Normal ROM: 0–60 degrees

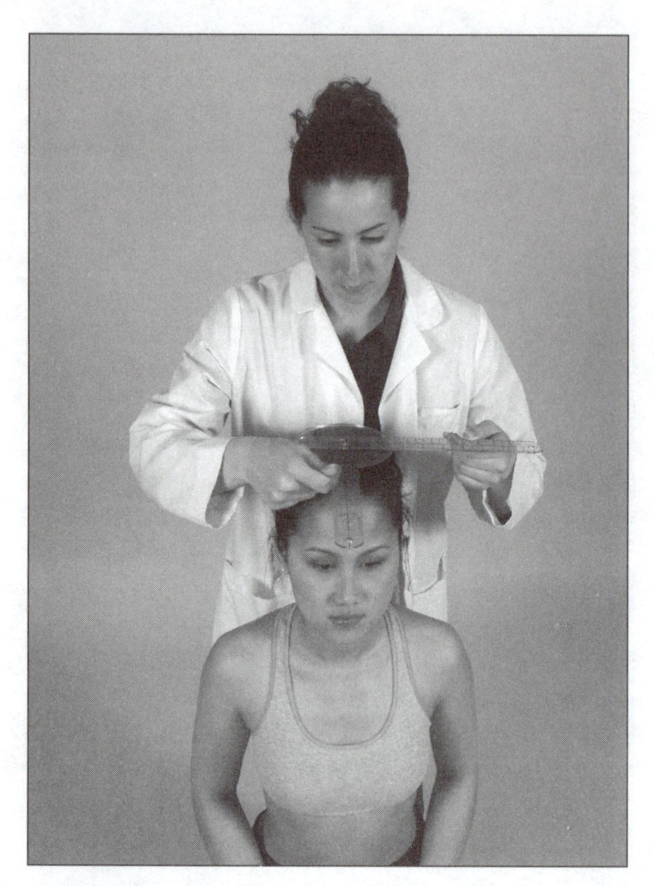

Figure 1-2-15 Start position for cervical rotation.

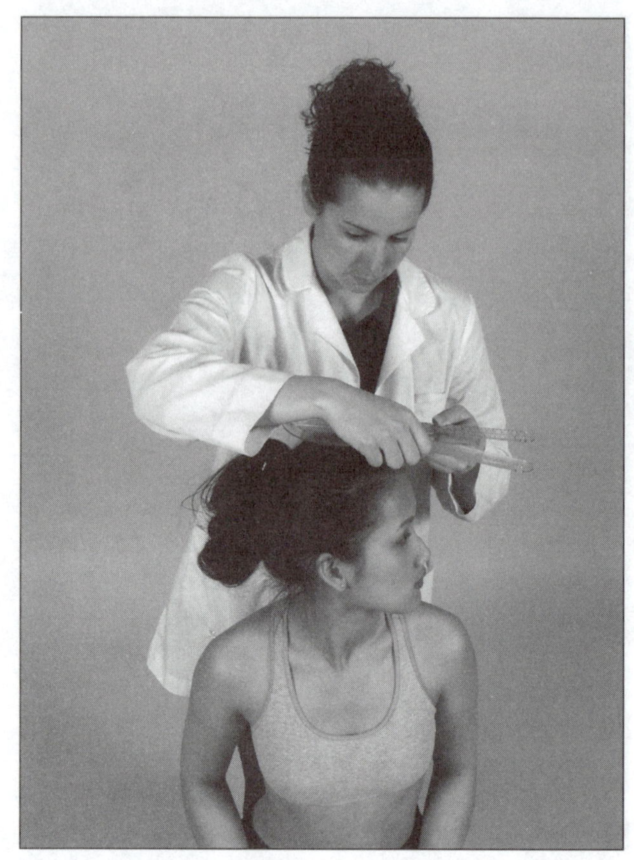

Figure 1-2-16 End position for cervical rotation.

Client Position: Client is sitting with upper extremity resting at side. Lumbar and thoracic spines are supported by the chair.

Starting—cervical spine is in neutral (Figure 1-2-15).

Ending—client moves into maximum cervical rotation (Figure 1-2-16).

Therapist Position: Observe the lumbar and thoracic regions to prevent compensatory movements.

Goniometer Position:

FULCRUM: centered over the middle of the cranial aspect of the head

STABLE ARM: parallel to an imaginary line between the acromial processes

MOVABLE ARM: in line with the tip of the nose

Alternate Test

A tape measure may be used to assess the distance between the tip of the chin and the acromial process. Observe to ensure client's mouth is closed.

SECTION 1-3: Goniometric Measurements of the Shoulder Complex

Shoulder: *humeral flexion*

End feel: firm

Normal ROM: 0–180 degrees

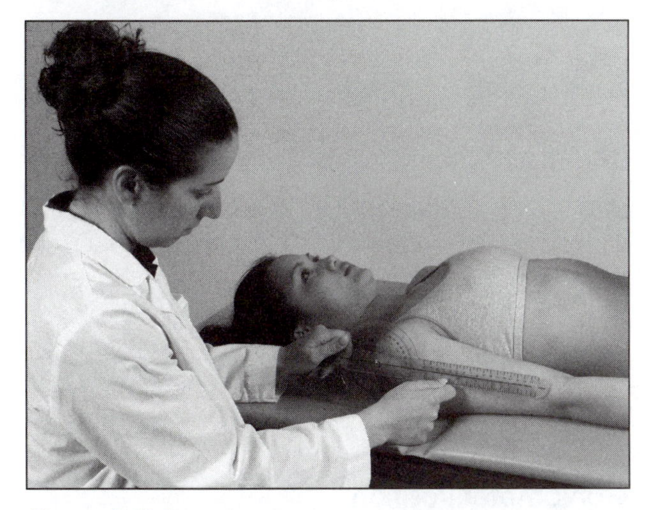

Figure 1-3-1 Start position for humeral flexion.

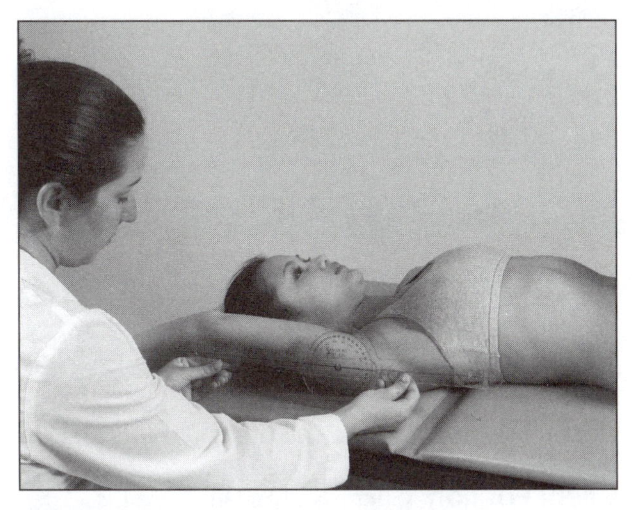

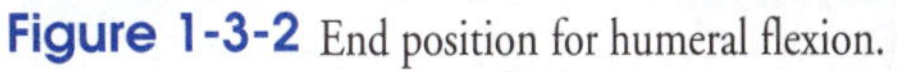

Figure 1-3-2 End position for humeral flexion.

Client Position: Client is supine with knees flexed or sitting.

Starting—testing extremity is at client's side, elbow extended and forearm in neutral (Figure 1-3-1).

Ending—client moves the testing extremity into maximum humeral flexion (Figure 1-3-2).

Therapist Position: Observe the scapula to prevent compensatory elevation, posterior tilt, and upward rotation.

Goniometer Position:

FULCRUM: lateral surface of the acromion process

STABLE ARM: mid axilla/thorax

MOVABLE ARM: lateral midline of the humerus

Shoulder: *humeral extension/hyperextension*

End feel: firm

Normal ROM: 0–60 degrees

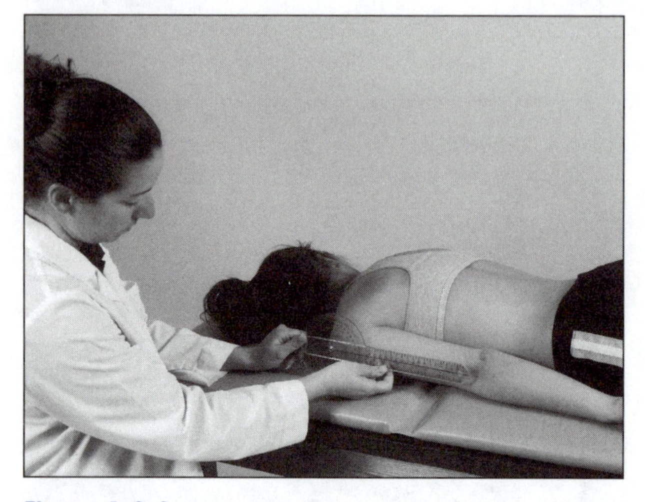

Figure 1-3-3 Start position for humeral extension/hyperextension.

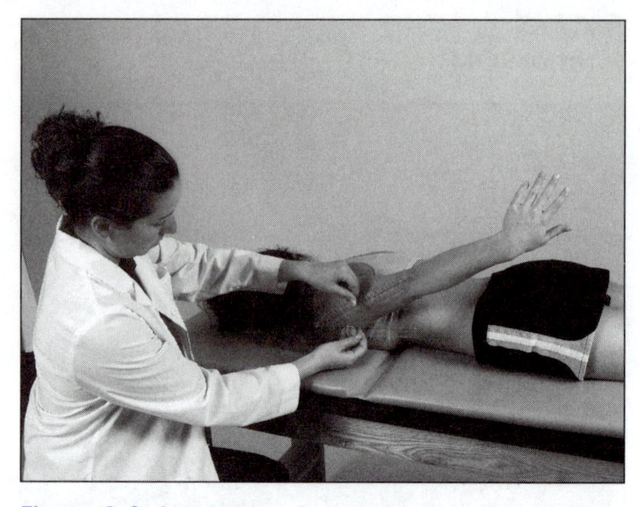

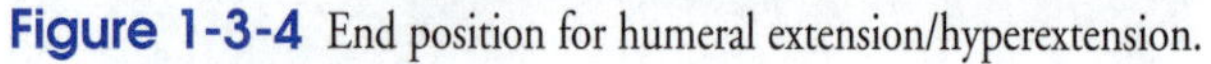

Figure 1-3-4 End position for humeral extension/hyperextension.

Client Position: Client is prone and head is turned away from testing side or sitting.

Starting—testing extremity is at client's side, elbow in slight flexion and forearm in neutral (Figure 1-3-3).

Ending—client moves the testing extremity into maximum humeral extension (Figure 1-3-4).

Therapist Position: Observe the scapula to prevent compensatory elevation and anterior tilt.

Goniometer Position:

FULCRUM: lateral surface of the acromion process

STABLE ARM: midline of axilla/thorax

MOVABLE ARM: lateral midline of the humerus

Shoulder: *humeral abduction*

End feel: firm

Normal ROM: 0–180 degrees

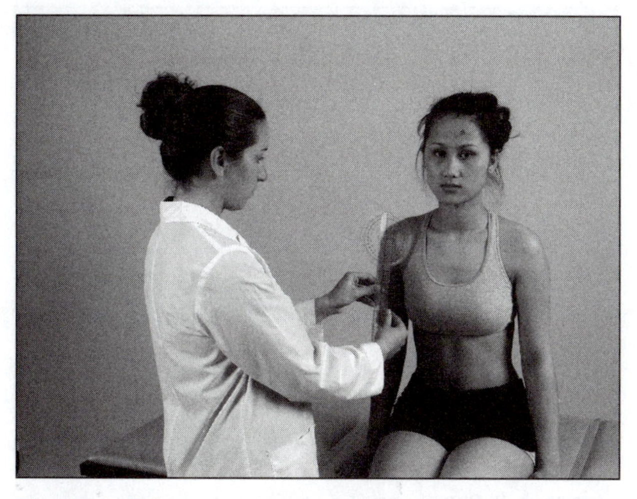

Figure 1-3-5 Start position for humeral abduction.

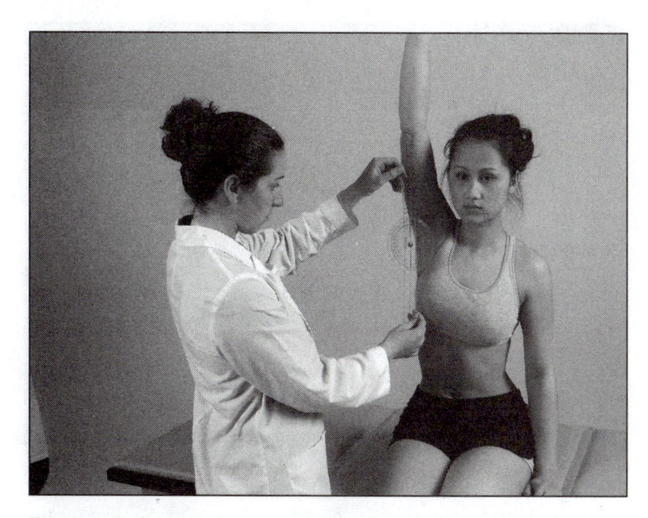

Figure 1-3-6 End position for humeral abduction.

Client Position: Client is sitting or standing.

Starting—testing extremity is at client's side, humerus is in full external rotation, elbow extension, and forearm in supination.

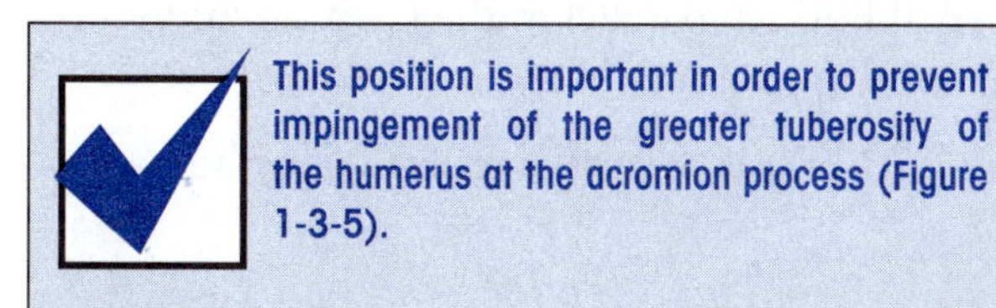

This position is important in order to prevent impingement of the greater tuberosity of the humerus at the acromion process (Figure 1-3-5).

Ending—client moves the testing extremity into maximum humeral abduction (Figure 1-3-6).

Therapist Position: Observe the scapula to prevent excessive compensatory upward rotation and elevation.

Goniometer Position:

FULCRUM: at anterior or posterior surface of the acromion process depending on the client's starting position

STABLE ARM: parallel to the sternum (anterior) or spine (posterior)

MOVABLE ARM: medial aspect of the humerus

Shoulder: *humeral adduction*

End feel: soft

Normal ROM: 180–0 degrees

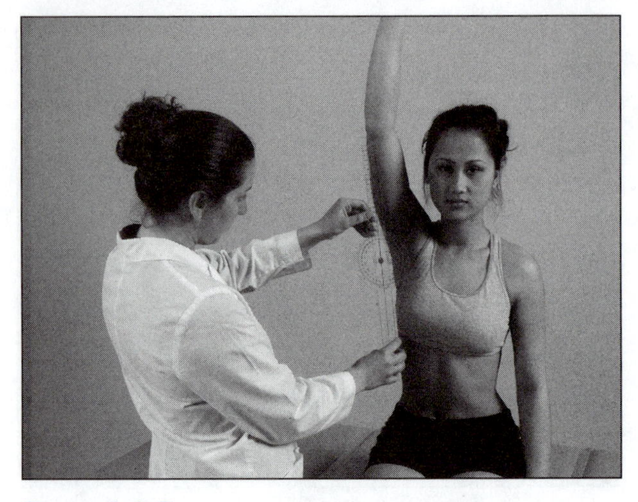

Figure 1-3-7 Start position for humeral adduction.

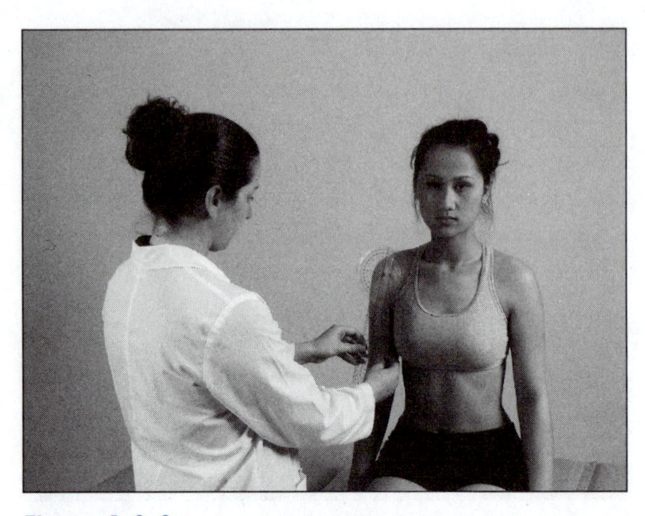

Figure 1-3-8 End position for humeral adduction.

Client Position: Client is sitting or standing.

Starting—testing extremity is in maximal humeral abduction and external rotation, elbow extension and forearm in supination (Figure 1-3-7).

Ending—client moves the testing extremity into maximum humeral adduction (Figure 1-3-8).

Therapist Position: Observe the scapula to prevent excessive compensatory downward rotation and depression.

Goniometer Position:

FULCRUM: at the anterior or posterior surface of the acromion process depending on the client's starting position

STABLE ARM: parallel to the sternum (anterior) or spine (posterior)

MOVABLE ARM: medial aspect of the humerus

Shoulder: *humeral external rotation*

End feel: firm

Normal: 0–90 degrees

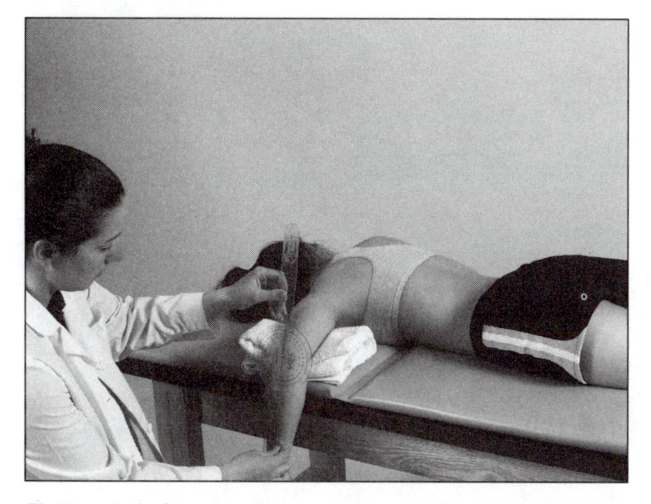

Figure 1-3-9 Start position for humeral external rotation.

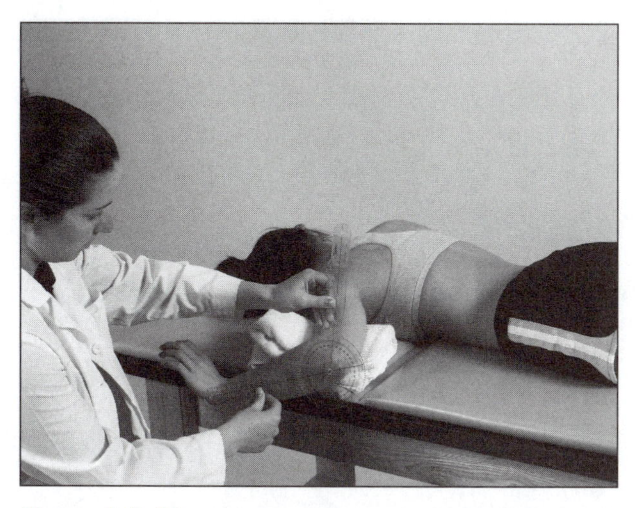

Figure 1-3-10 End position for humeral external rotation.

Client Position: Client is prone.

Starting—testing extremity is in 90 degrees of humeral abduction, elbow flexed to 90 degrees, forearm perpendicular to the plinth. A pad is placed under the humerus (Figure 1-3-9).

Ending—client moves the testing extremity into maximum humeral external rotation (Figure 1-3-10).

Therapist Position: Observe the distal end of humerus to maintain 90 degrees of abduction and to prevent compensation of excessive scapular depression.

Goniometer Position:

FULCRUM: midline of the olecranon process

STABLE ARM: perpendicular to the floor

MOVABLE ARM: midline of the lateral ulna

Alternate Position

Some references start the procedure in sitting or standing position and the forearm is parallel to the floor.

FULCRUM: midline of the olecranon process

STABLE ARM: parallel to the floor

MOVABLE ARM: midline of the lateral ulna

Shoulder: *humeral internal rotation*

End feel: firm

Normal ROM: 0–70 degrees

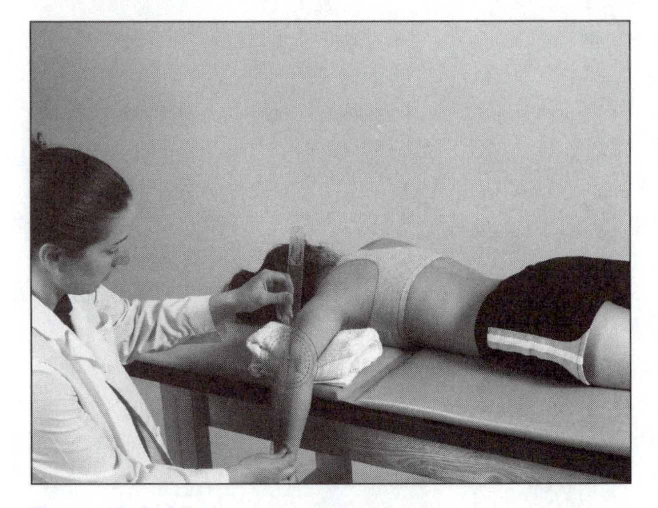

Figure 1-3-11 Start position for humeral internal rotation.

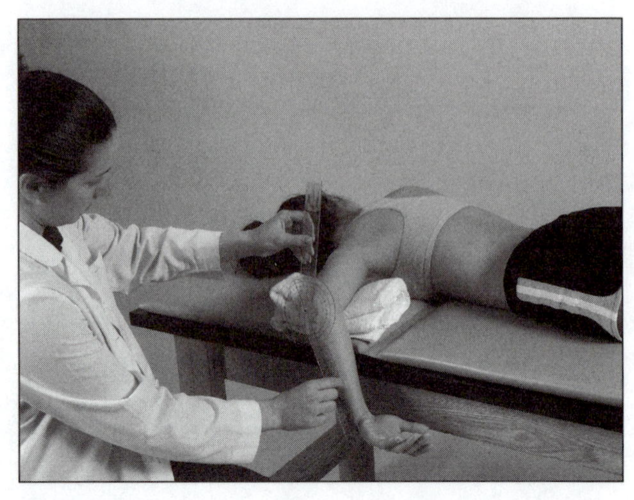

Figure 1-3-12 End position for humeral internal rotation.

Client Position: Client is prone.

Starting—testing extremity is in 90 degrees of humeral abduction, elbow flexed to 90 degrees, forearm is perpendicular to the plinth (Figure 1-3-11).

Ending—client moves the testing extremity into maximum humeral internal rotation (Figure 1-3-12).

Therapist Position: Observe the distal end of the humerus to maintain 90 degrees of shoulder abduction and to prevent scapular compensation.

Goniometer Position:

FULCRUM: midline of the olecranon process

STABLE ARM: perpendicular to the floor

MOVABLE ARM: midline of the lateral ulna

Alternate Position

Some references start the procedure in sitting or standing position and the forearm is parallel to the floor.

FULCRUM: midline of the olecranon process

STABLE ARM: parallel to the floor

MOVABLE ARM: midline of the lateral ulna

Shoulder: *humeral horizontal abduction*

End feel: firm

Normal ROM: 0–45 degrees

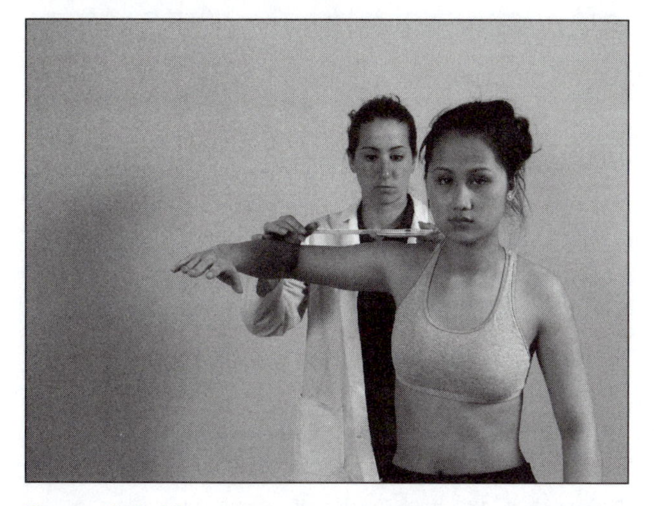

Figure 1-3-13 Start position for humeral horizontal abduction.

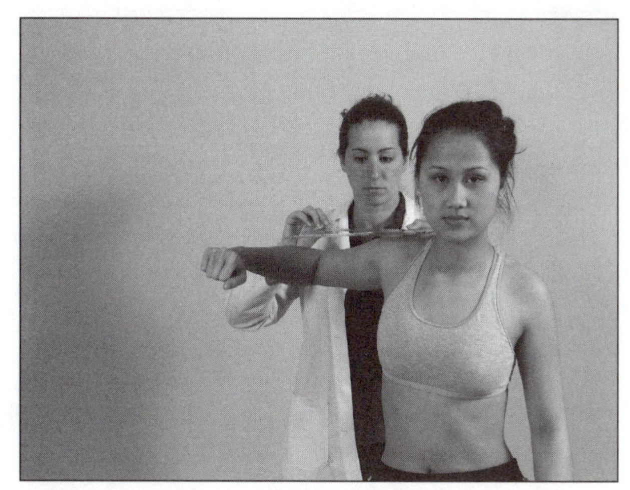

Figure 1-3-14 End position for humeral horizontal abduction.

Client Position: Client is sitting.

Starting—testing extremity is in 90 degrees of humeral abduction and neutral rotation, elbow flexed to 90 degrees, forearm pronated (Figure 1-3-13).

Ending—client moves the testing extremity into maximum humeral horizontal abduction (Figure 1-3-14).

Therapist Position: Support the testing extremity in 90 degrees of abduction to prevent compensation.

Goniometer Position:

FULCRUM: superior aspect of the acromion process

STABLE ARM: parallel to humerus

MOVABLE ARM: parallel to the humerus (goniometer arms start parallel to the humerus, once the extremity moves, the stable arm remains in the initial position)

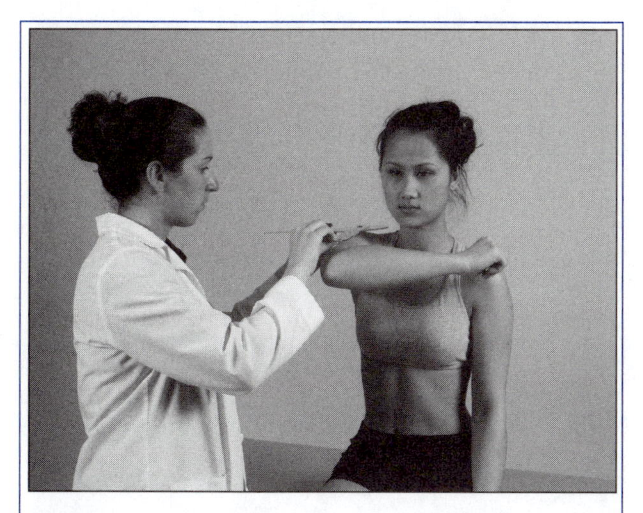

Figure 1-3-13a ASHT start position for humeral horizontal abduction.

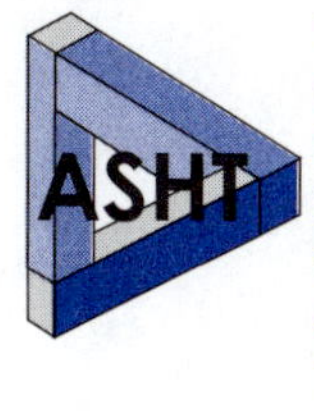

The American Society of Hand Therapy (ASHT) guidelines recommend starting horizontal abduction in full horizontal adduction (Figure 1-3-13a). This starting position will modify the norm as listed above. (The American Society of Hand Therapists, 1992).

Shoulder: *humeral horizontal adduction*

End feel: firm/soft

Normal ROM: 0–135 degrees

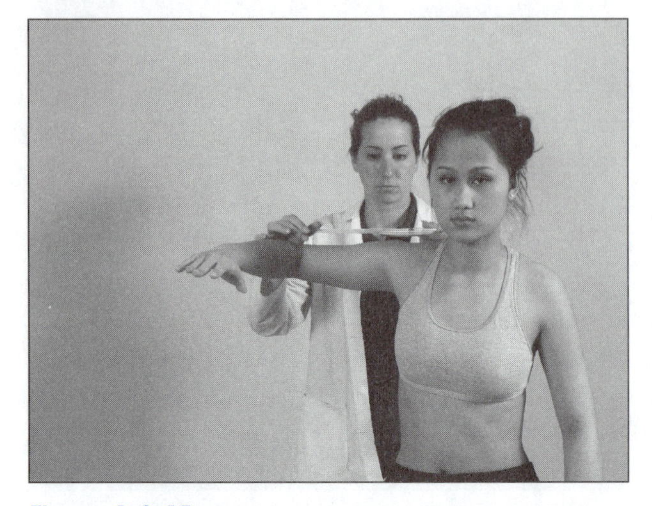

Figure 1-3-15 Start position for humeral horizontal adduction.

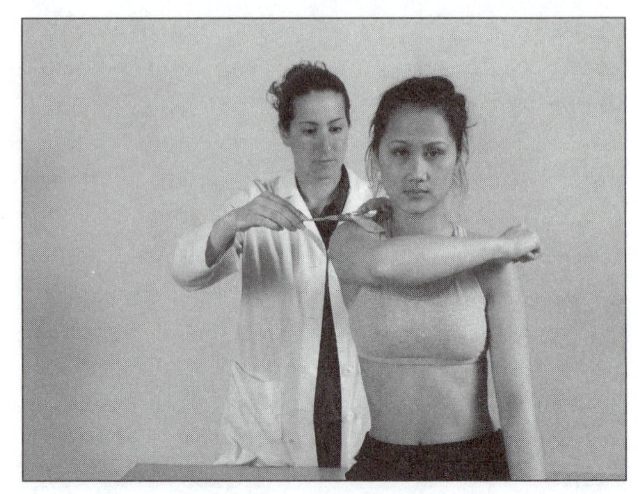

Figure 1-3-16 End position for humeral horizontal adduction.

Client Position: Client is sitting.

Starting—testing extremity is in 90 degrees of humeral abduction and neutral rotation, the elbow flexed, forearm pronated (Figure 1-3-15).

Ending—client moves the testing extremity into maximum humeral horizontal adduction (Figure 1-3-16).

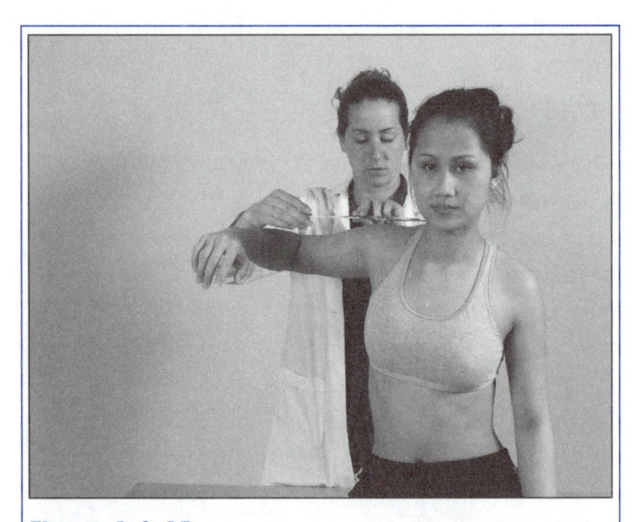

Figure 1-3-15a ASHT start position for humeral horizontal adduction.

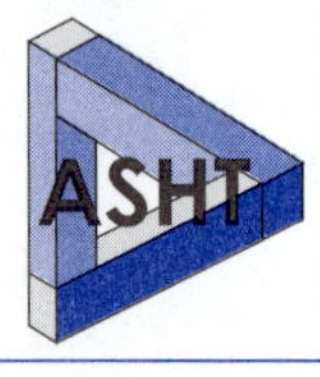

The ASHT guidelines recommend starting horizontal adduction in full horizontal abduction (Figure 1-3-15a). This starting position will modify the norm as listed above. (The American Society of Hand Therapists, 1992).

Therapist Position: Support the testing extremity in 90 degrees of abduction to prevent compensation.

Goniometer Position:

FULCRUM: superior aspect of the acromion process

STABLE ARM: parallel to humerus

MOVABLE ARM: parallel to the humerus (goniometer arms start parallel to the humerus, once the extremity moves, the stable arm remains in the initial position)

SECTION 1-4: Goniometric Measurements of the Elbow and Forearm

Elbow: *flexion*

End feel: Soft

Normal ROM: 0–135 degrees

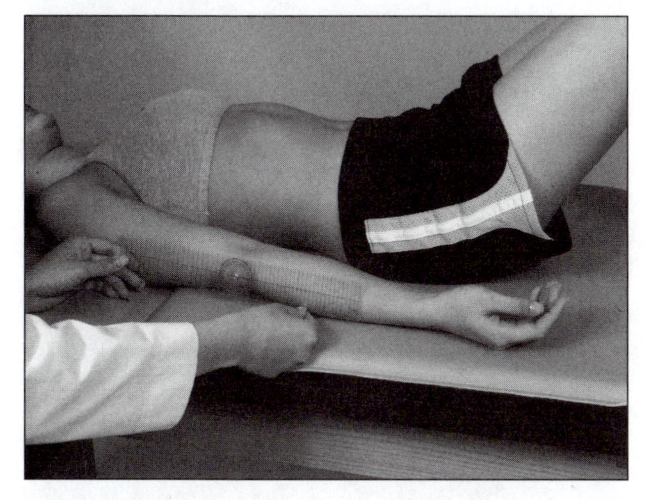

Figure 1-4-1 Start position for elbow flexion.

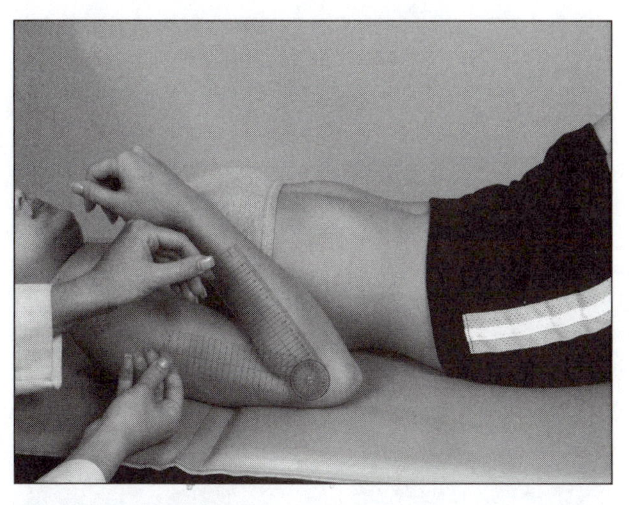

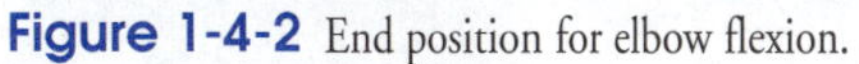

Figure 1-4-2 End position for elbow flexion.

Client Position: Client is supine with knees flexed or sitting.

Starting—testing extremity is fully extended at client's side and forearm is in neutral (Figure 1-4-1).

Ending—client moves the testing extremity into maximum elbow flexion (Figure 1-4-2).

Therapist Position: Observe at the humerus and shoulder to prevent compensation.

Goniometer Position:

FULCRUM: lateral epicondyle of the humerus

STABLE ARM: midline of lateral surface of the humerus

MOVABLE ARM: midline of lateral surface of the radius

Elbow: *extension*

End feel: firm

Normal ROM: 135–0 degrees

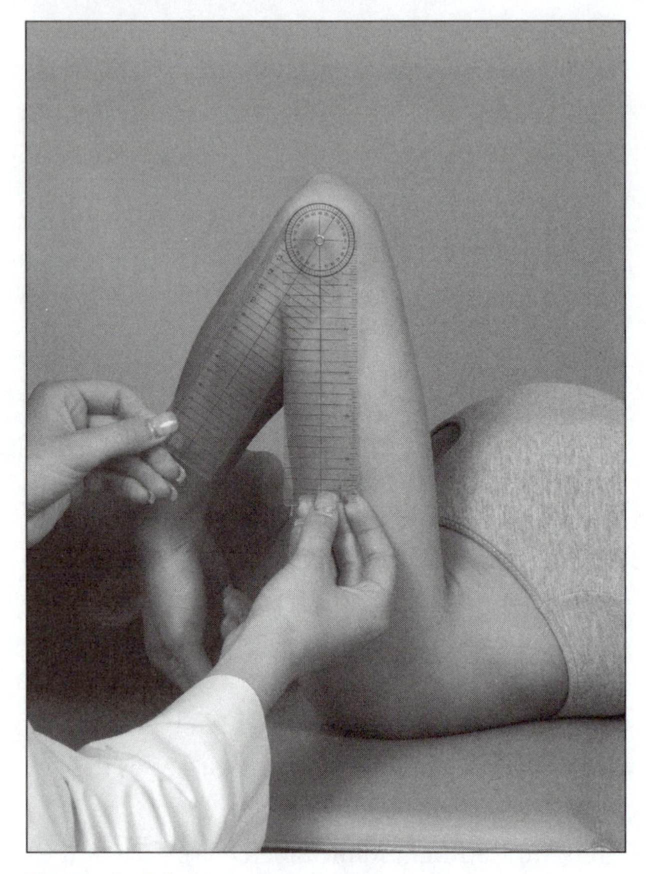

Figure 1-4-3 Start position for elbow extension.

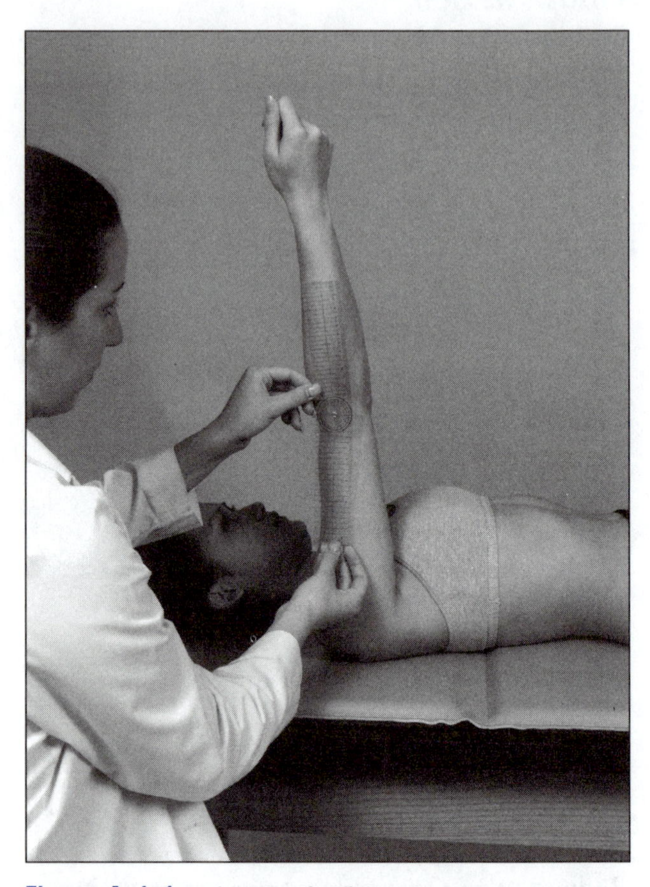

Figure 1-4-4 End position for elbow extension.

Client Position: Client is supine with knees flexed.

Starting—testing extremity is in 90 degrees of humeral flexion, elbow fully flexed, forearm supinated (Figure 1-4-3).

Ending—client moves the testing extremity into maximum elbow extension (Figure 1-4-4).

Therapist Position: Observe at the humerus and shoulder to prevent compensation.

Goniometer Position:

FULCRUM: lateral epicondyle of the humerus

STABLE ARM: midline of lateral surface of the humerus

MOVABLE ARM: midline of lateral surface of the radius

Forearm: *supination*

End feel: firm

Normal ROM: 0–90 degrees

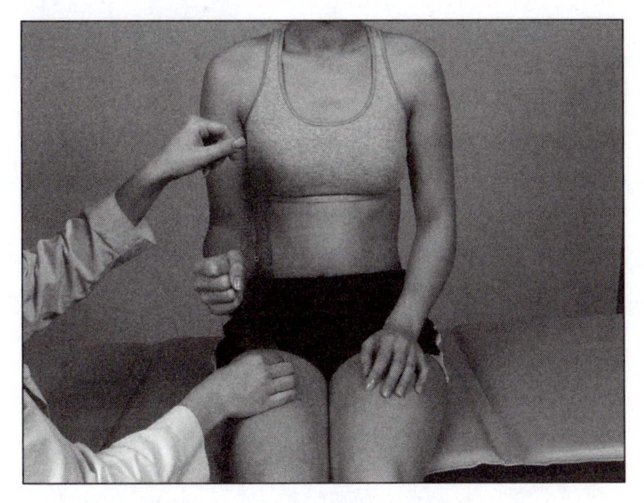

Figure 1-4-5 Start position for forearm supination.

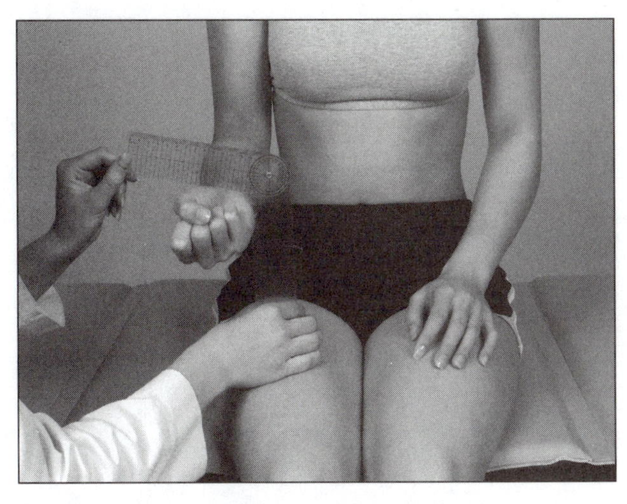

Figure 1-4-6 End position for forearm supination.

Client Position: Client is sitting with feet on the floor.

Starting—testing extremity is at client's side, humerus adducted, elbow flexed to 90 degrees, forearm in neutral (Figure 1-4-5).

Ending—client moves the testing extremity into maximum forearm supination (Figure 1-4-6).

Therapist Position: Observe at the humerus and elbow to prevent compensation of humerus moving away from the trunk.

Goniometer Position:

FULCRUM: volar surface of distal forearm one centimeter proximal to the pisiform

STABLE ARM: perpendicular to the floor

MOVABLE ARM: across the volar aspect of the distal forearm

Alternate Test

Client holds a pencil tightly in a closed fist of the testing extremity (Figures 1-4-5a and 1-4-6a).

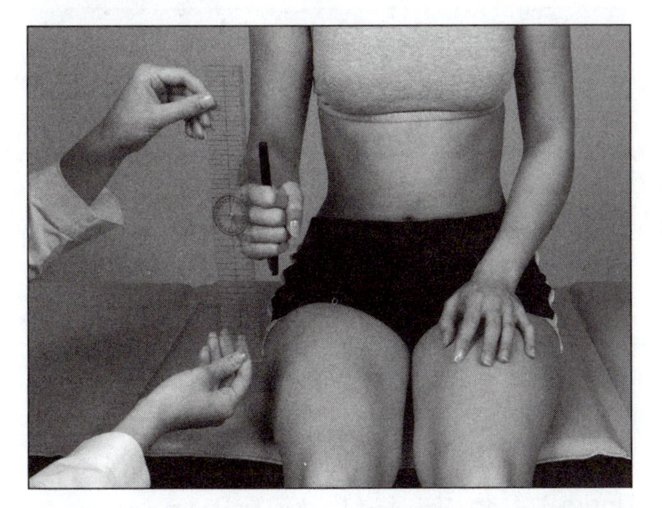

Figure 1-4-5a Alternate start position for forearm supination.

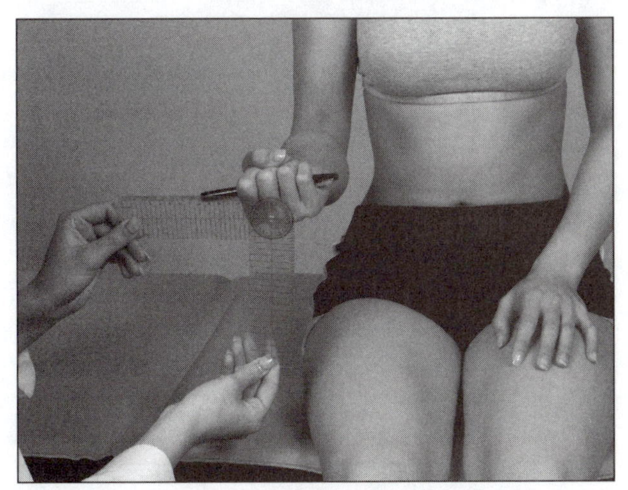

Figure 1-4-6a Alternate end position for forearm supination.

FULCRUM: over the head of the third metacarpal

STABLE ARM: perpendicular to the floor

MOVABLE ARM: parallel to the pencil

Forearm: *pronation*

End feel: hard

Normal ROM: 0–90 degrees

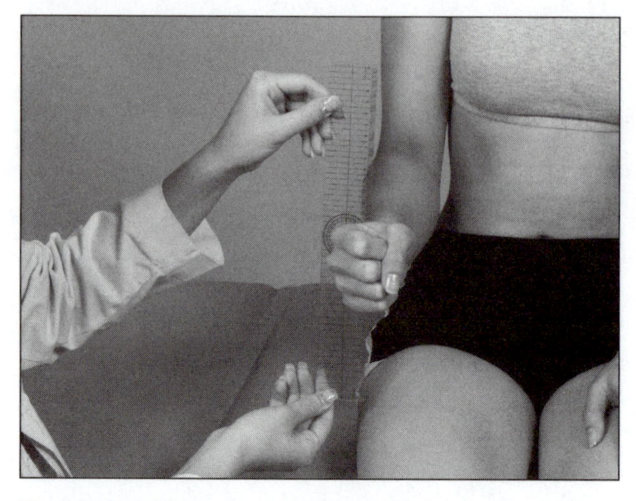

Figure 1-4-7 Start position for forearm pronation.

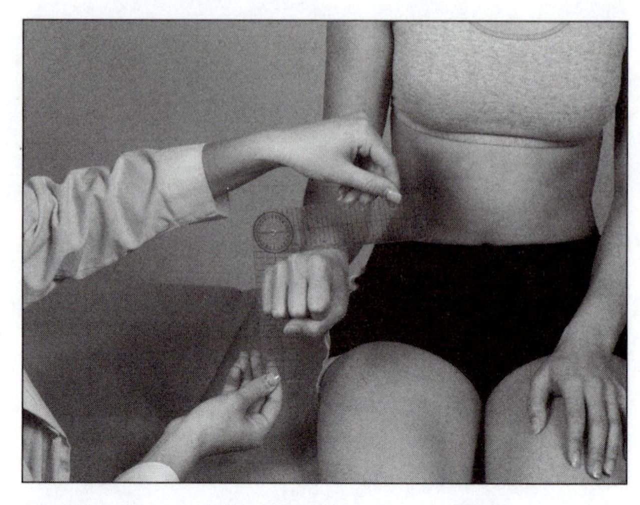

Figure 1-4-8 End position for forearm pronation.

Client Position: Client is sitting with feet on the floor.

Starting—testing extremity is at client's side, humerus adducted, elbow flexed to 90 degrees, forearm in neutral (Figure 1-4-7).

Ending—client moves the testing extremity into maximum forearm pronation (Figure 1-4-8).

Therapist Position: Observe at the humerus and elbow to prevent compensation of humerus moving away from the trunk.

Goniometer Position:

FULCRUM: ulnar styloid process

STABLE ARM: perpendicular to the floor

MOVABLE ARM: across dorsal surface of the distal forearm

Alternate Test

Client holds a pencil tightly in a closed fist of the testing extremity (Figures 1-4-7a and 1-4-8a).

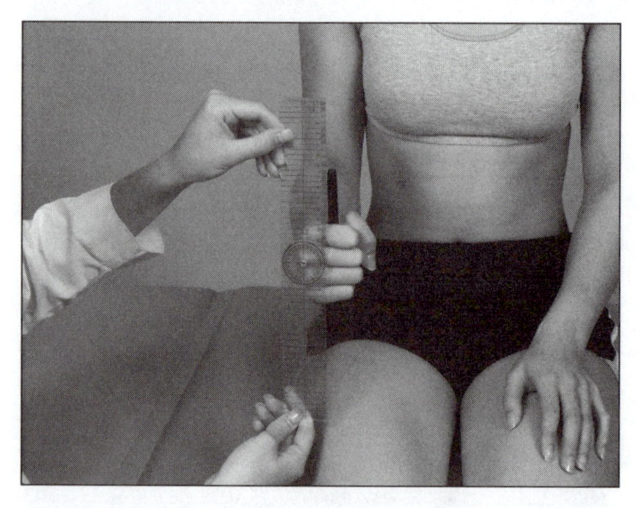

Figure 1-4-7a Alternate start position for forearm pronation.

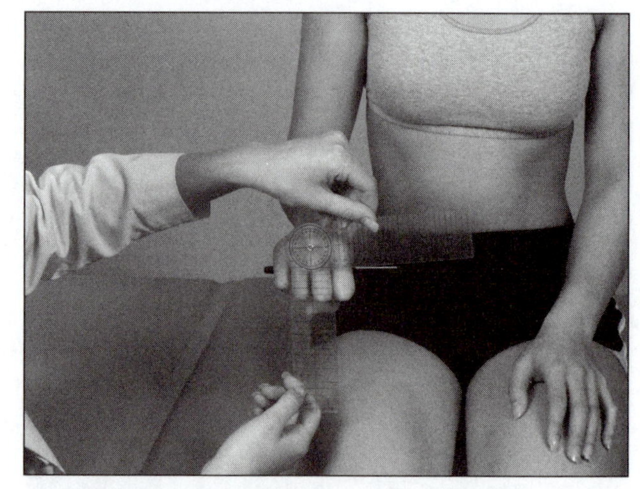

Figure 1-4-8a Alternate end position for forearm pronation.

FULCRUM: over the head of the third metacarpal

STABLE ARM: perpendicular to the floor

MOVABLE ARM: parallel to the pencil

SECTION 1-5: Goniometric Measurements of the Wrist and Hand

Wrist: *flexion/extension*

End feel: both are firm

Normal ROM: Flexion 0–80 degrees
Extension 0–70 degrees

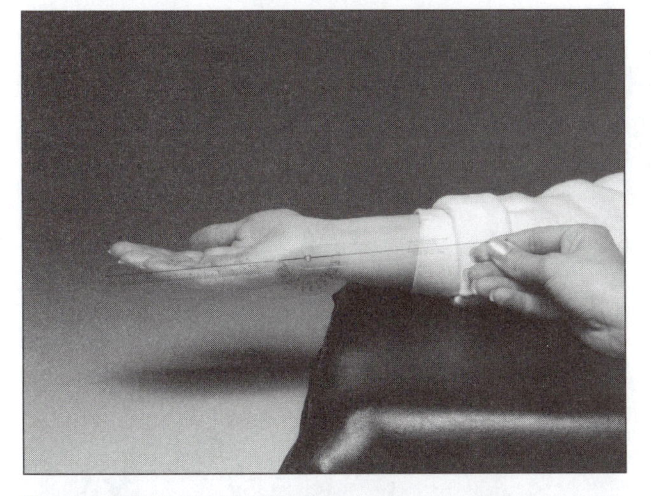

Figure 1-5-1 Start position for wrist flexion.

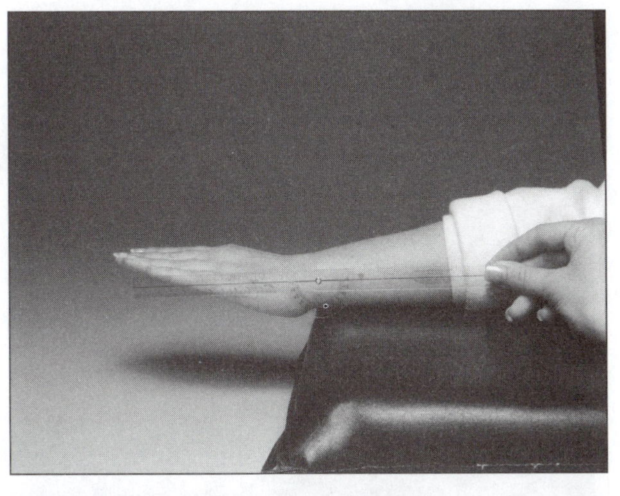

Figure 1-5-2 Start position for wrist extension.

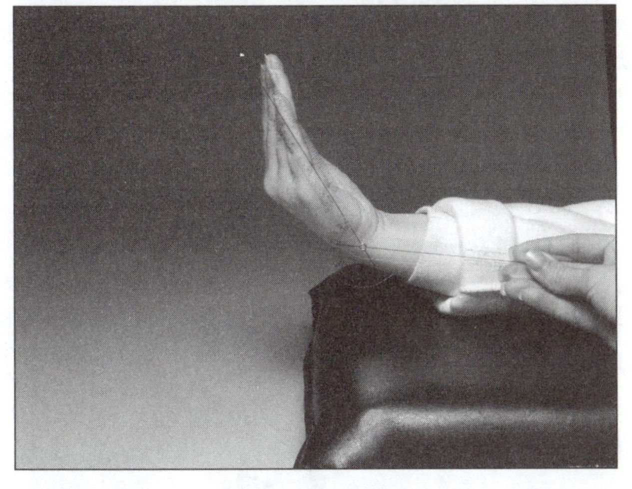

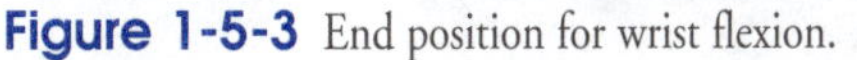

Figure 1-5-3 End position for wrist flexion.

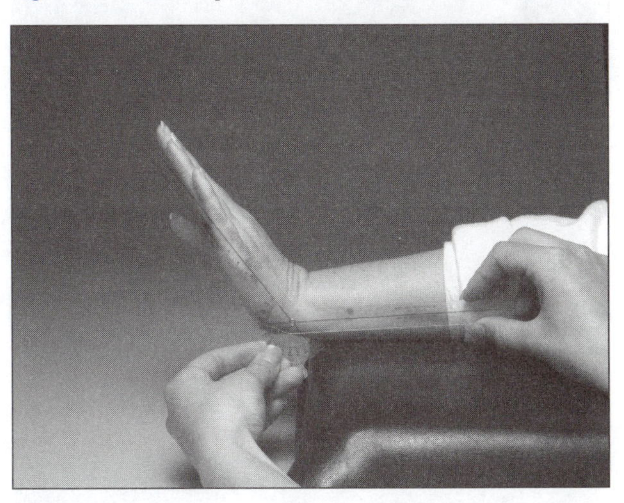

Figure 1-5-4 End position for wrist extension.

Client Position: Client is sitting with feet on the floor.

Starting—testing extremity is resting on table with the humerus abducted, elbow flexed, forearm supinated for wrist flexion (Figure 1-5-1)/ pronated for wrist extension (Figure 1-5-2). The distal forearm is placed on the end of a table so that the wrist is free to move through the full range.

Ending—client moves the testing extremity through maximum wrist flexion (Figure 1-5-3) or extension (Figure 1-5-4).

Therapist Position: Observe at the forearm to prevent compensation.

Goniometer Position:

FULCRUM: medial aspect of ulnar styloid process

STABLE ARM: midline of ulna

MOVABLE ARM: midline of fifth metacarpal

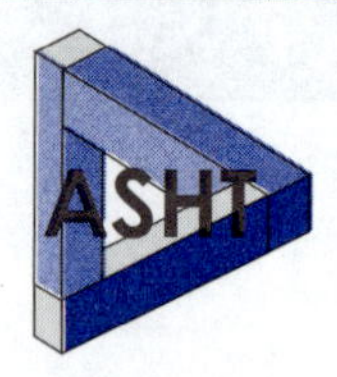

ASHT guideline recommendation for the measurement of wrist flexion places the goniometer on the dorsal surface of the wrist with the stable arm parallel to the radius and the movable arm parallel to the third metacarpal (Figures 1-5-1a and 1-5-3a). The guideline recommendation for the measurement of wrist extension places the goniometer on the volar surface of the wrist with the stable arm parallel to the radius and the movable arm parallel to the third metacarpal (Figures 1-5-2a and 1-5-4a). (The American Society of Hand Therapists, 1992).

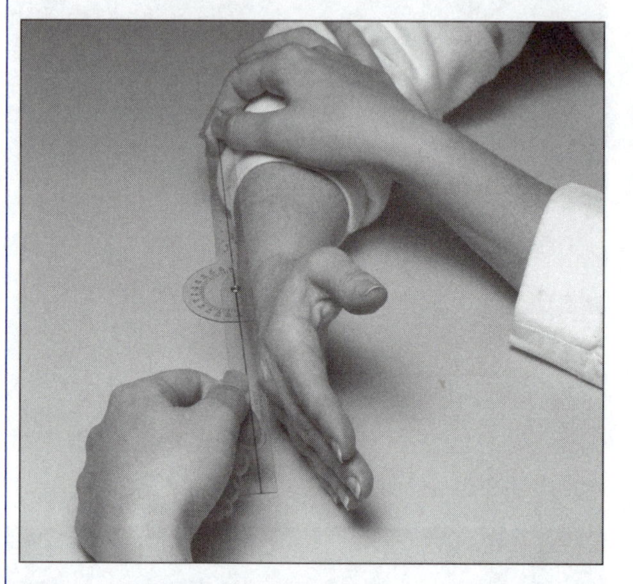

Figure 1-5-1a ASHT start position for wrist flexion.

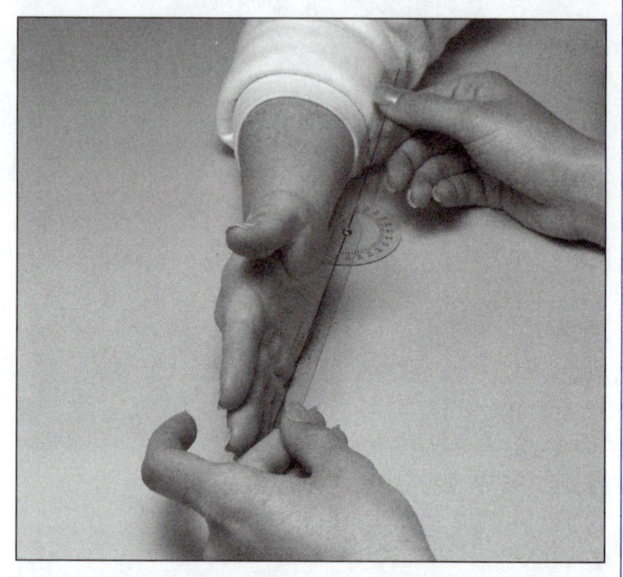

Figure 1-5-2a ASHT start position for wrist extension.

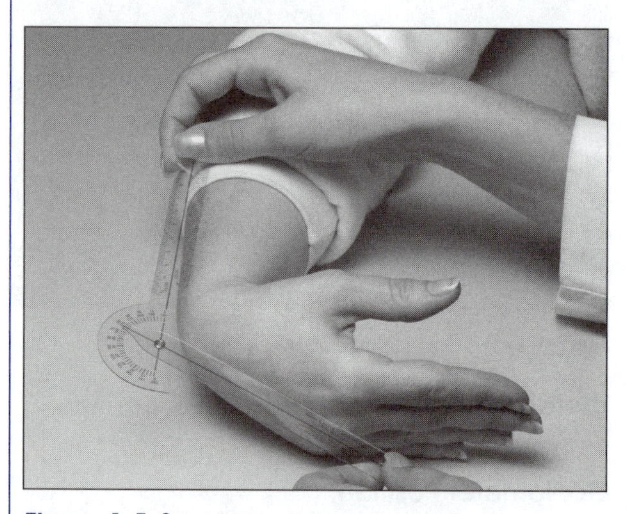

Figure 1-5-3a ASHT end position for wrist flexion.

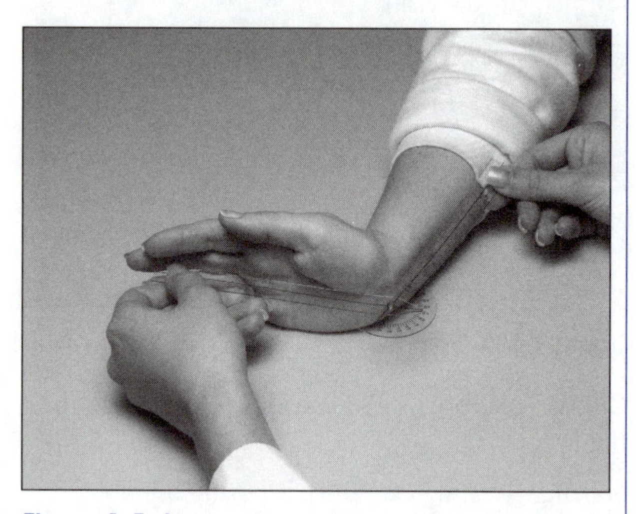

Figure 1-5-4a ASHT end position for wrist extension.

Wrist: *radial/ulnar deviation*

End feel: Radial—hard
Ulnar—firm

Normal ROM: Radial 0–20 degrees
Ulnar 0–30 degrees

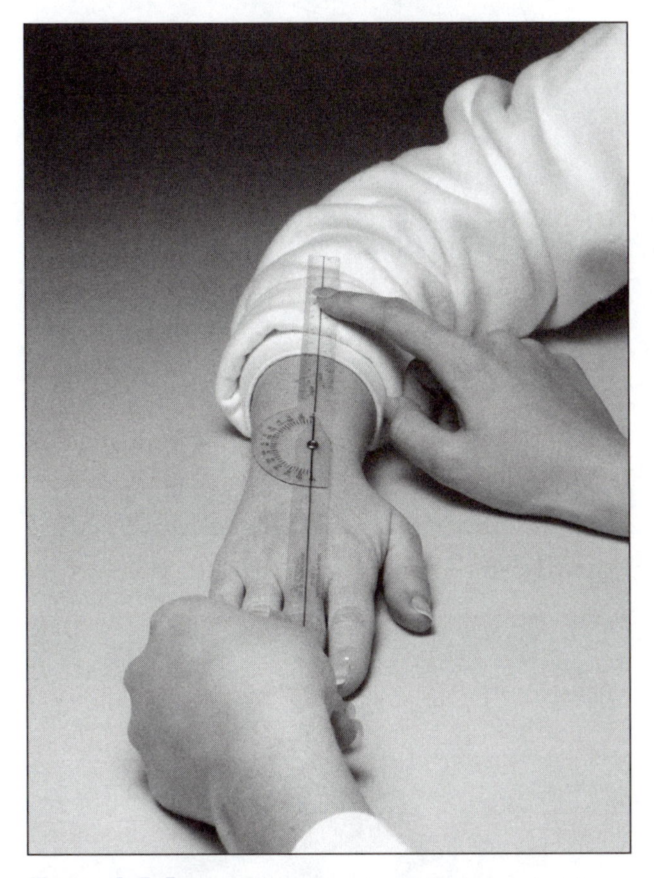

Figure 1-5-5 Start position for wrist radial and ulnar deviation.

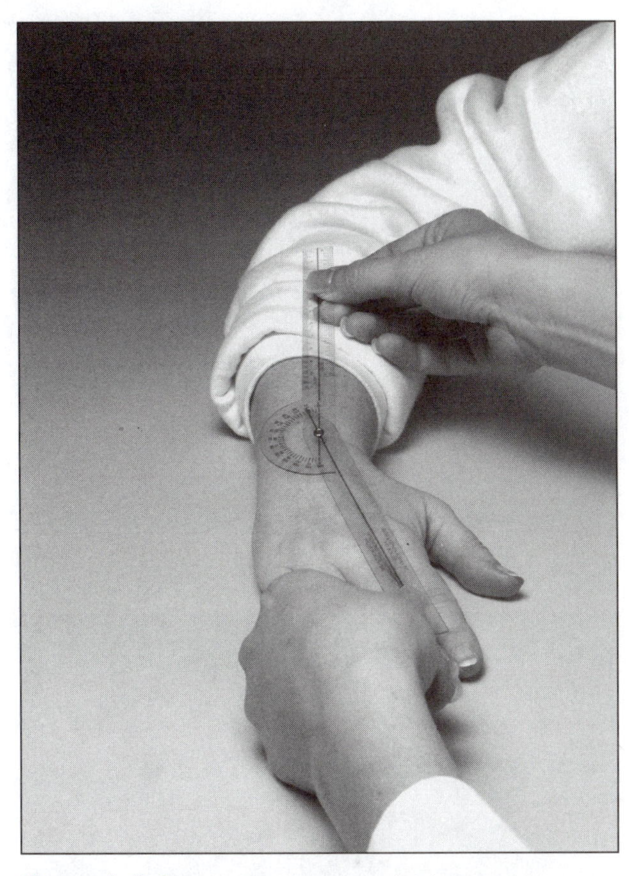

Figure 1-5-6 End position for wrist radial deviation (ulnar not shown).

Client Position: Client is sitting with feet on the floor.

Starting—testing extremity is resting on the table with the humerus abducted, elbow flexed, forearm pronated. Forearm is placed on the table with the palm flat. Wrist is in neutral (Figure 1-5-5).

Ending—client moves the testing extremity through maximum wrist ulnar or radial deviation (Figure 1-5-6).

Therapist Position: Observe at the distal forearm to prevent compensation.

Goniometer Position:

FULCRUM: base of the third metacarpal, over the capitate bone

STABLE ARM: midline of the forearm

MOVABLE ARM: midline of the third metacarpal

Digit and thumb: *MCP (metacarpal) flexion/extension*

End feel: Flexion—hard
Extension—firm

Normal ROM: Flexion 0–90 degrees,
Extension 90–0 degrees

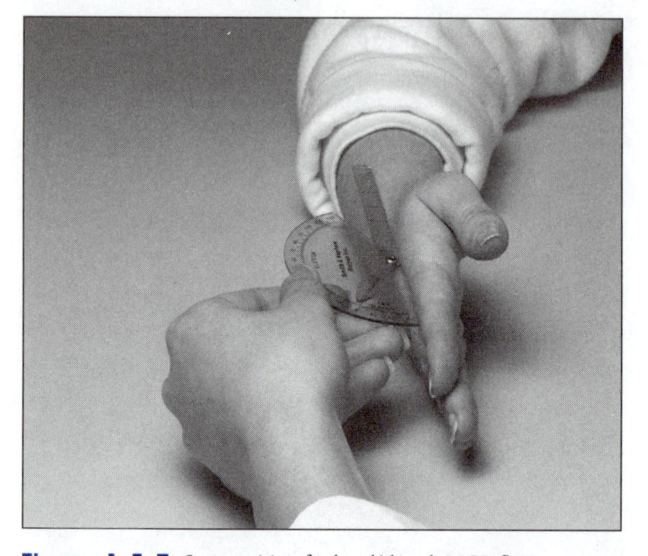

Figure 1-5-7 Start position for hand/thumb MCP flexion.

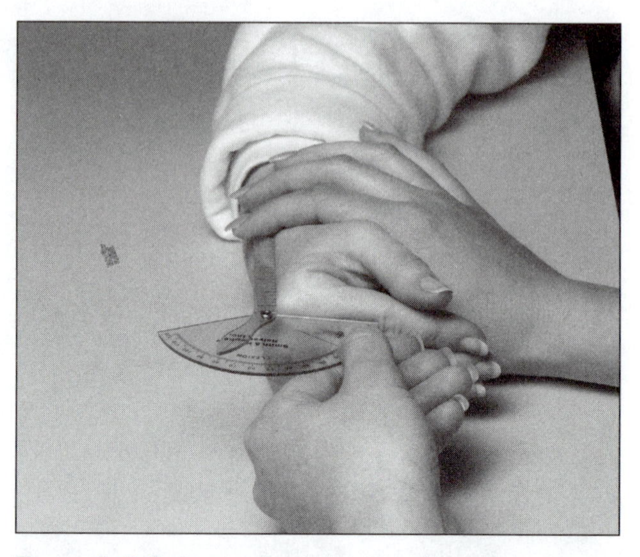

Figure 1-5-8 Start position for hand/thumb MCP extension.

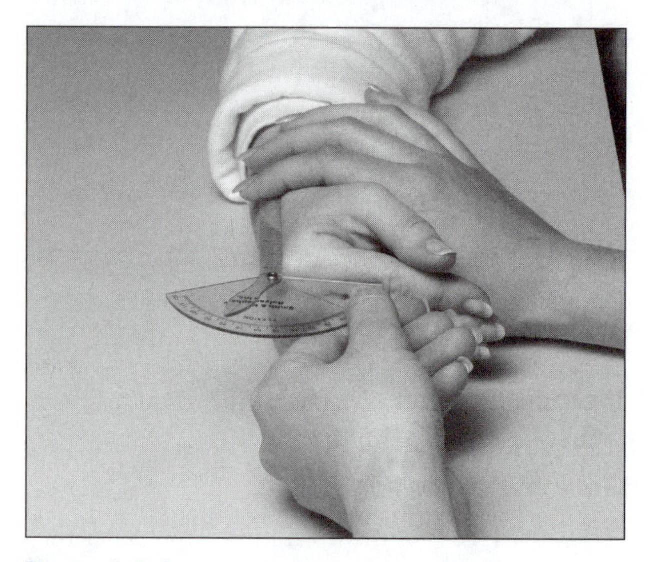

Figure 1-5-9 End position for hand/thumb MCP flexion.

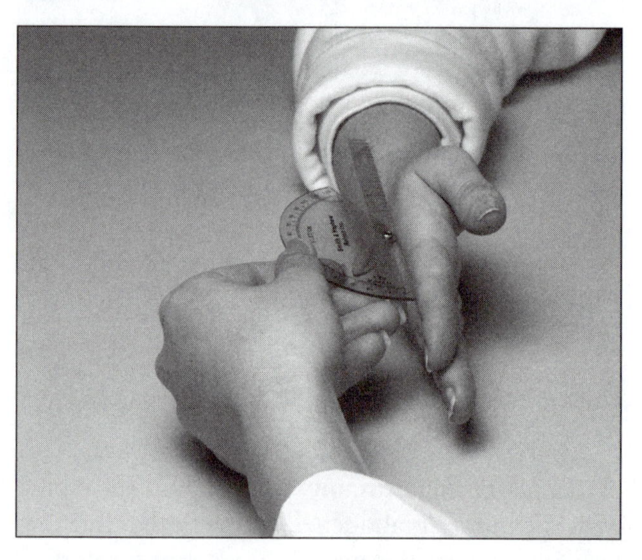

Figure 1-5-10 End position for hand/thumb MCP extension.

Client Position: Client is sitting with feet on the floor.

Starting—elbow of testing extremity is resting on table with the humerus slightly flexed and forearm in neutral. MCPs are in neutral when measuring MCP flexion (Figure 1-5-7), or in flexion when measuring MCP extension (Figure 1-5-8).

Ending—client moves the testing extremity through maximal MCP flexion (Figure 1-5-9) or extension (Figure 1-5-10).

Therapist Position: Observe at the metacarpals and the wrist to prevent compensation.

Goniometer Position:

FULCRUM: dorsal surface of the MCP joint that is being measured

STABLE ARM: midline and dorsal surface of the metacarpal of the digit being measured

MOVABLE ARM: midline and dorsal surface of the proximal phalanx of the digit being measured

Digit and thumb: *MCP hyperextension*

End feel: firm

Normal ROM: 0–30 degrees

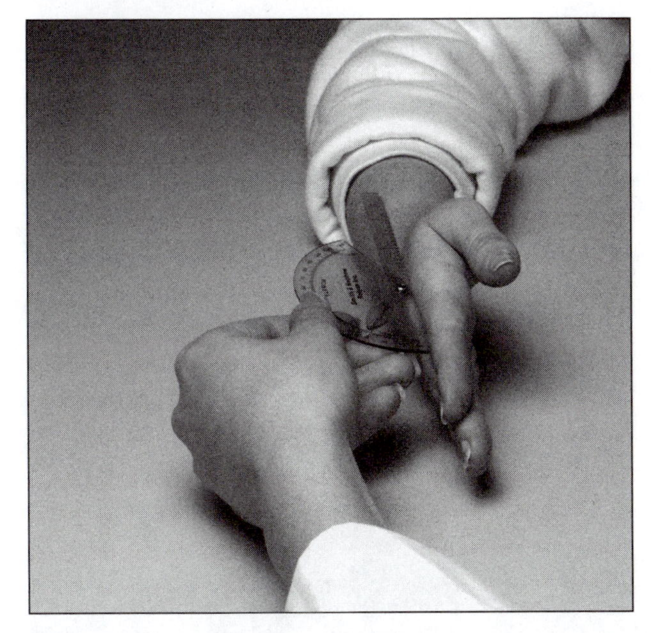

Figure 1-5-11 Start position for hand/thumb MCP hyperextension.

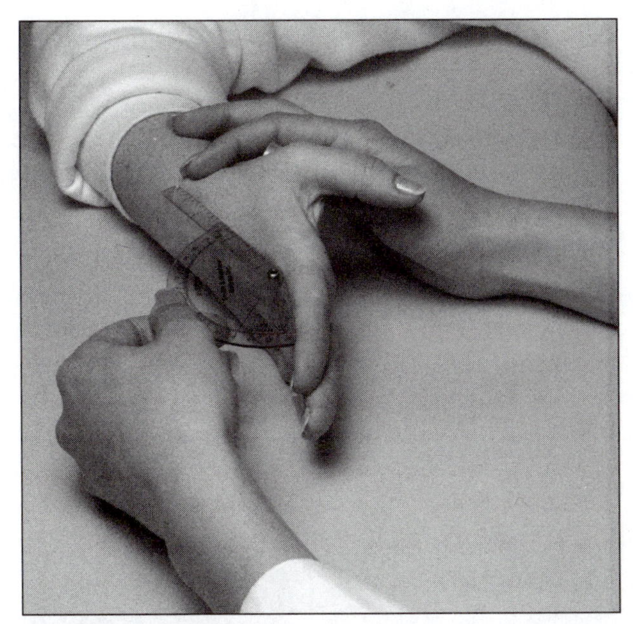

Figure 1-5-12 End position for hand/thumb MCP hyperextension.

Client Position: Client is sitting with feet on the floor.

Starting—elbow of the testing extremity is resting on the table with the humerus slightly flexed and forearm in neutral. MCPs are in extension/neutral (Figure 1-5-11).

Ending—client moves the testing extremity through maximum MCP hyperextension (Figure 1-5-12).

Therapist Position: Observe at the metacarpals and wrist to prevent compensation.

Goniometer Position:

FULCRUM: dorsal surface of the MCP joint that is being measured

STABLE ARM: midline and dorsal surface of the metacarpal of the digit being measured

MOVABLE ARM: midline and dorsal surface of the proximal phalanx of the digit being measured

Digit: *proximal interphalangeal (PIP) flexion*

End feel: hard

Normal ROM: 0–100 degrees

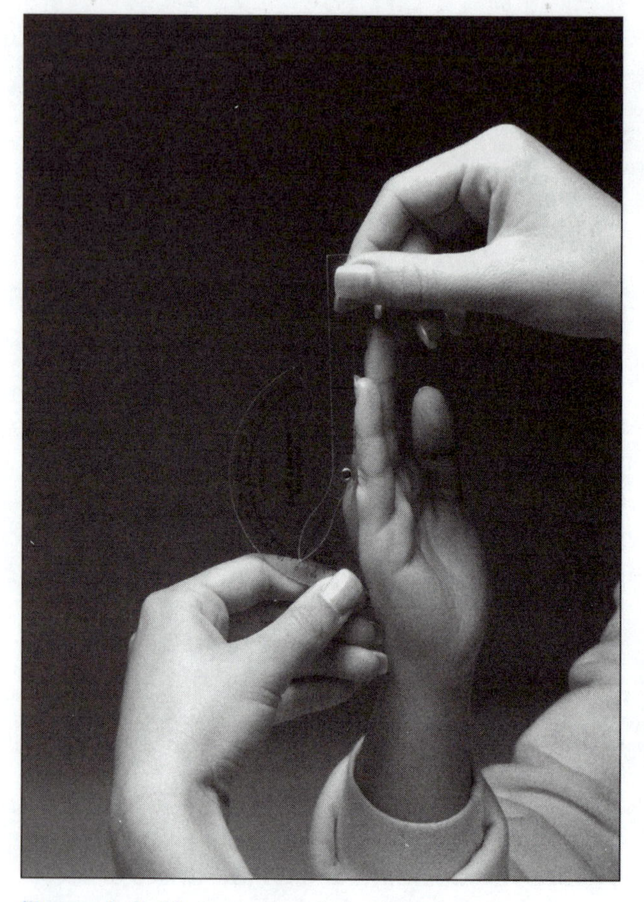

Figure 1-5-13 Start position for hand PIP flexion.

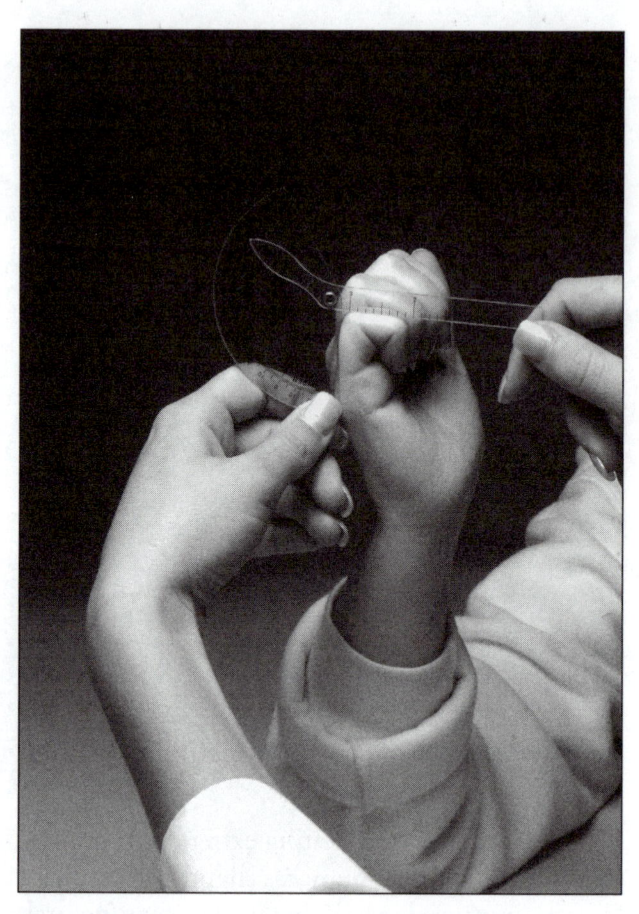

Figure 1-5-14 End position for hand PIP flexion.

Client Position: Client is sitting with feet on the floor.

Starting—elbow of the testing extremity is resting on the table with the humerus slightly flexed and forearm in neutral. The PIPs are in neutral or extension (Figure 1-5-13).

Ending—client moves the testing extremity through maximum PIP flexion (Figure 1-5-14).

Therapist Position: Observe and possibly stabilize at the MCPs to prevent compensation.

Goniometer Position:

FULCRUM: dorsal surface of the PIP joint that is being measured

STABLE ARM: dorsal and the midline of the proximal phalanx of the digit being measured

MOVABLE ARM: dorsal and the midline of the middle phalanx of the digit being measured

Digit: *PIP extension*

End feel: firm
Normal ROM: 90–0 degrees

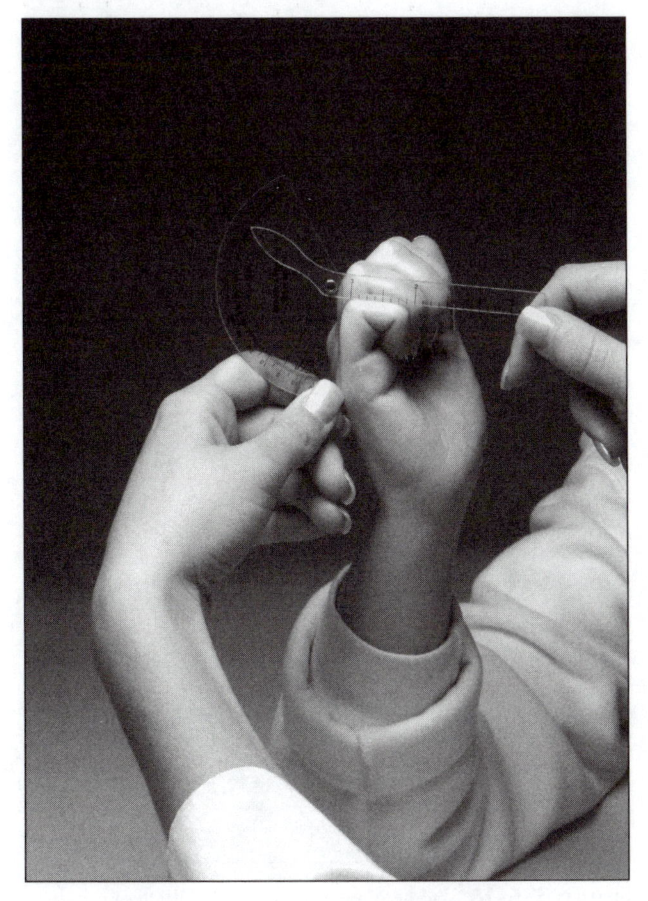

Figure 1-5-15 Start position for hand PIP extension.

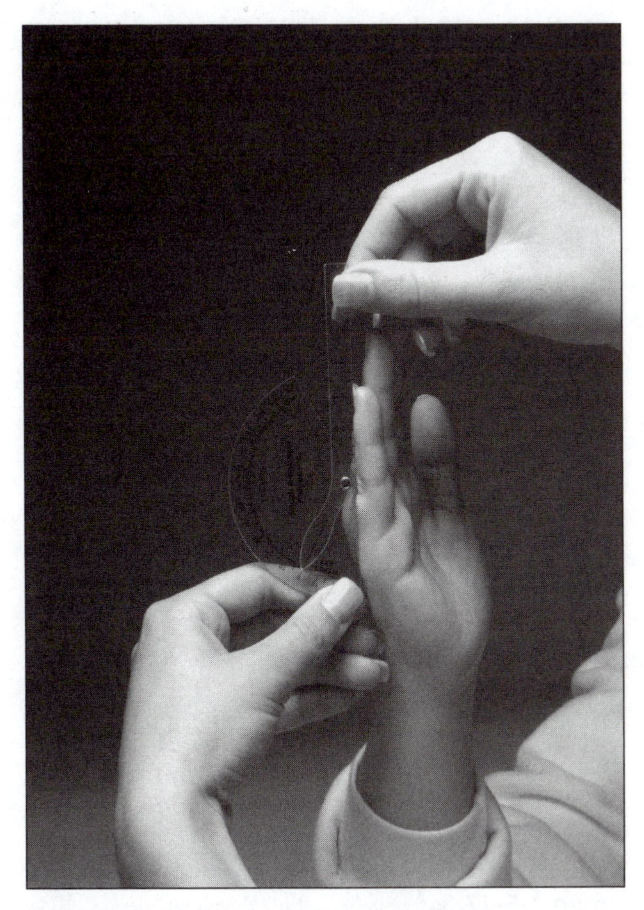

Figure 1-5-16 End position for hand PIP extension.

Client Position: Client is sitting with feet on the floor.

Starting—elbow of the testing extremity is resting on the table with the humerus slightly flexed and forearm in neutral. The PIPs are in flexion (Figure 1-5-15).

Ending—client moves the testing extremity through maximum PIP extension, but not into PIP hyperextension (Figure 1-5-16).

Therapist Position: Observe and possibly stabilize the MCPs in extension to prevent compensation.

Goniometer Position: Placed as above for PIP flexion.

Digit: *distal interphalangeal (DIP) flexion/Thumb: IP flexion*

End feel: firm

Normal ROM: 0–90 degrees

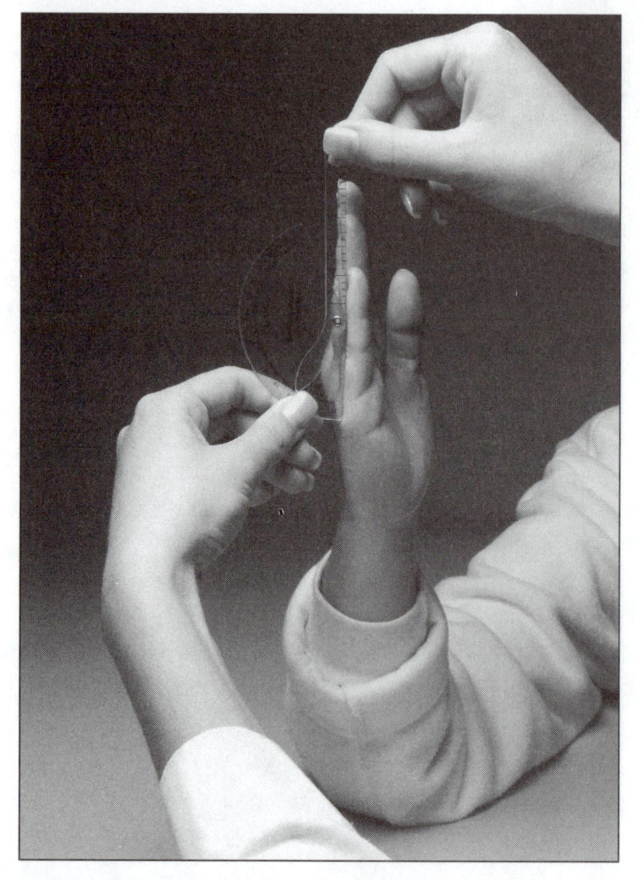

Figure 1-5-17 Start position for hand/thumb DIP flexion.

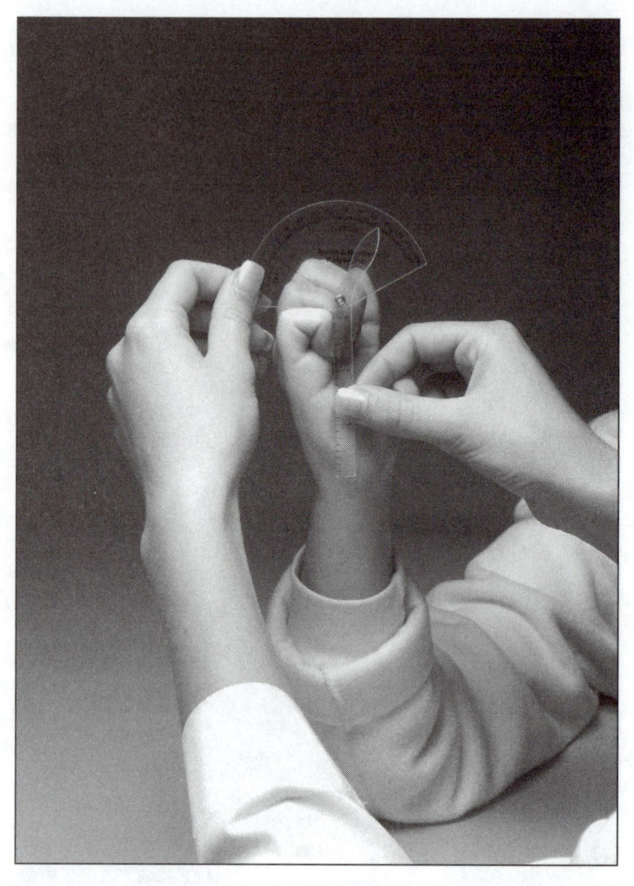

Figure 1-5-18 End position for hand/thumb DIP flexion.

Client Position: Client is sitting with feet on the floor.

Starting—elbow of the testing extremity is resting on the table with the humerus slightly flexed and forearm in neutral. The DIPs are in neutral or extension (Figure 1-5-17).

Ending—client moves the testing extremity through maximum DIP flexion (Figure 1-5-18).

Therapist Position: Stabilize at the PIP joint as necessary.

Goniometer Position:

FULCRUM: dorsal DIP joint that is being measured

STABLE ARM: dorsal and the midline of middle phalanx of joint being measured

MOVABLE ARM: dorsal and the midline of distal phalanx of joint being measured

Some clients may not achieve full DIP motion unless PIP joint is stabilized in extension or client is allowed to flex both the PIP joint and DIP joint while MCP joint is in extension.

Hand: *DIP extension/Thumb: IP extension*

End feel: firm

Normal ROM: 90–0 degrees

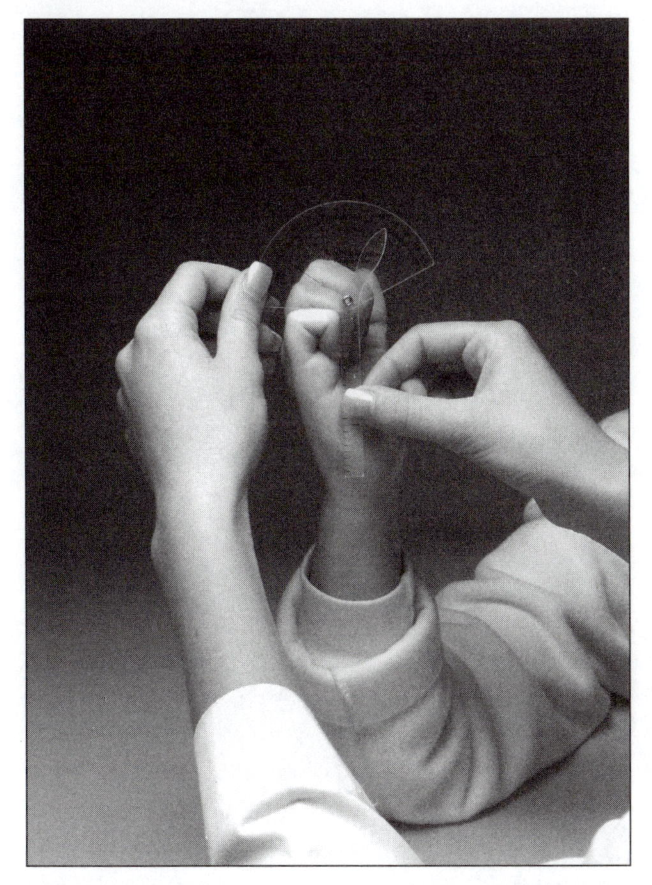

Figure 1-5-19 Start position for hand/thumb DIP extension.

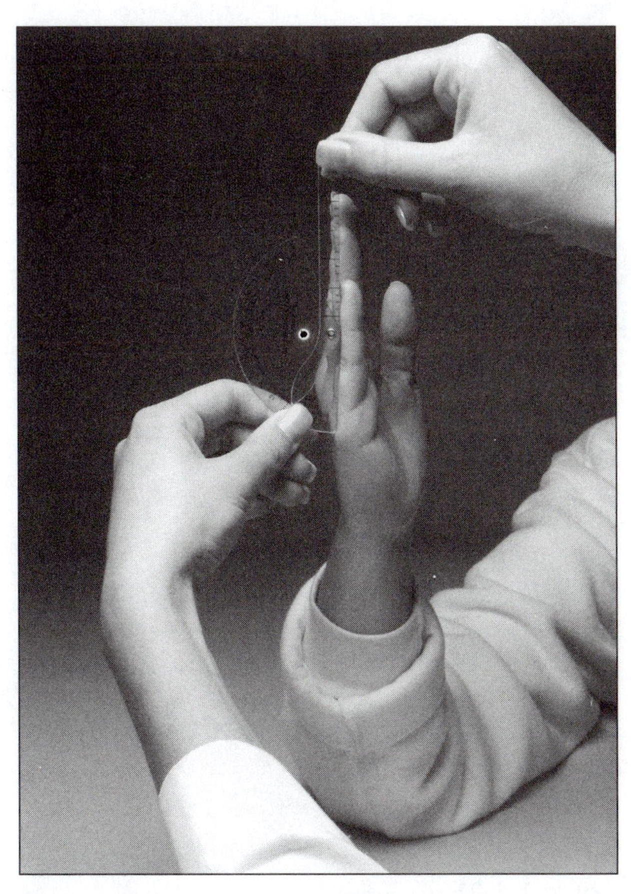

Figure 1-5-20 End position for hand/thumb DIP extension.

Client Position: Client is sitting with feet on the floor.

Starting—elbow of the testing extremity is resting on the table with the humerus slightly flexed and forearm in neutral. The DIPs are in flexion (Figure 1-5-19).

Ending—client moves the testing extremity through maximum DIP extension, but not into DIP hyperextension (Figure 1-5-20).

Therapist Position: Observe at the PIPs to prevent compensation.

Goniometer Position: Placed as above for DIP flexion

Digit: *MCP adduction*

End feel: firm

Normal ROM: As compared to the unaffected extremity.

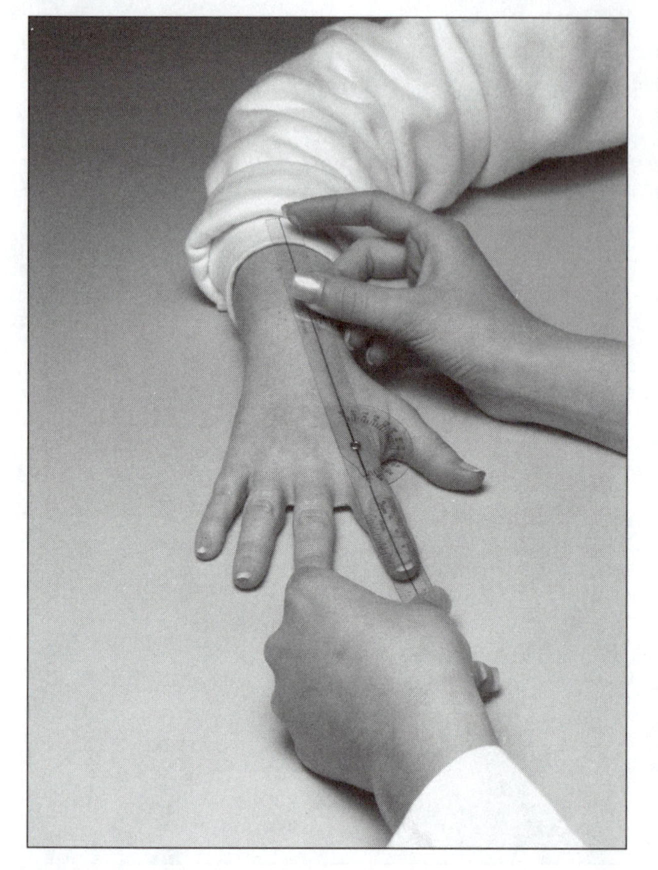

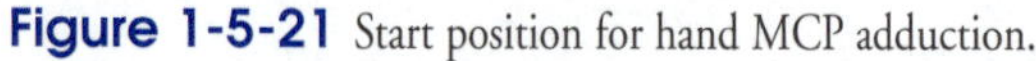

Figure 1-5-21 Start position for hand MCP adduction.

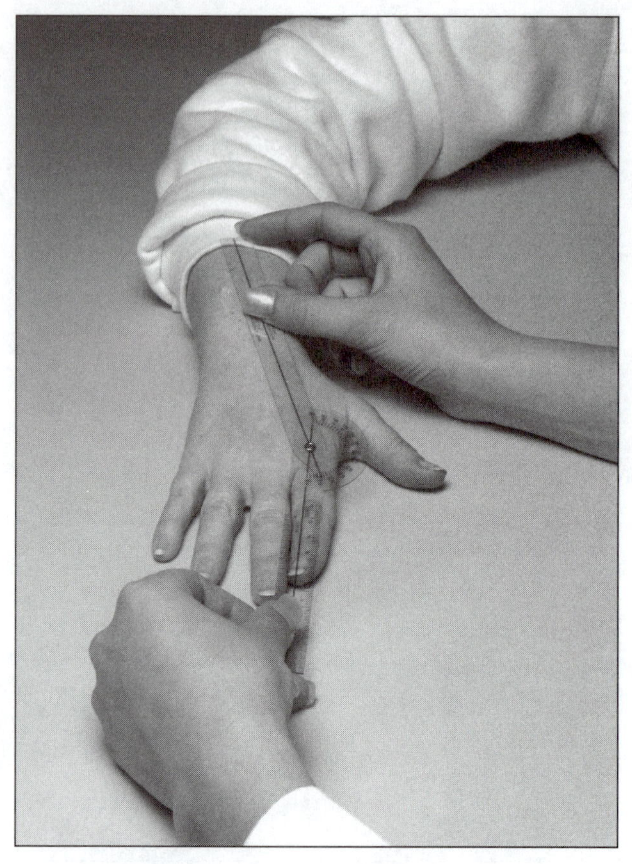

Figure 1-5-22 End position for hand MCP adduction.

Client Position: Client is sitting with feet on the floor.

Starting—testing extremity is resting on the table with the humerus abducted, elbow flexed, and forearm pronated. Digits are in abduction (Figure 1-5-21).

Ending—client moves the testing extremity digits into maximum MCP adduction (Figure 1-5-22). Note that the third digit does not adduct.

Therapist Position: Observe at the metacarpal to avoid compensation.

Goniometer Position:

FULCRUM: dorsal to the MCP joint

STABLE ARM: dorsal and parallel to the metacarpal

MOVABLE ARM: dorsal and parallel to the proximal phalanx

Digit: *MCP abduction*

End feel: soft

Normal ROM: As compared to the unaffected extremity.

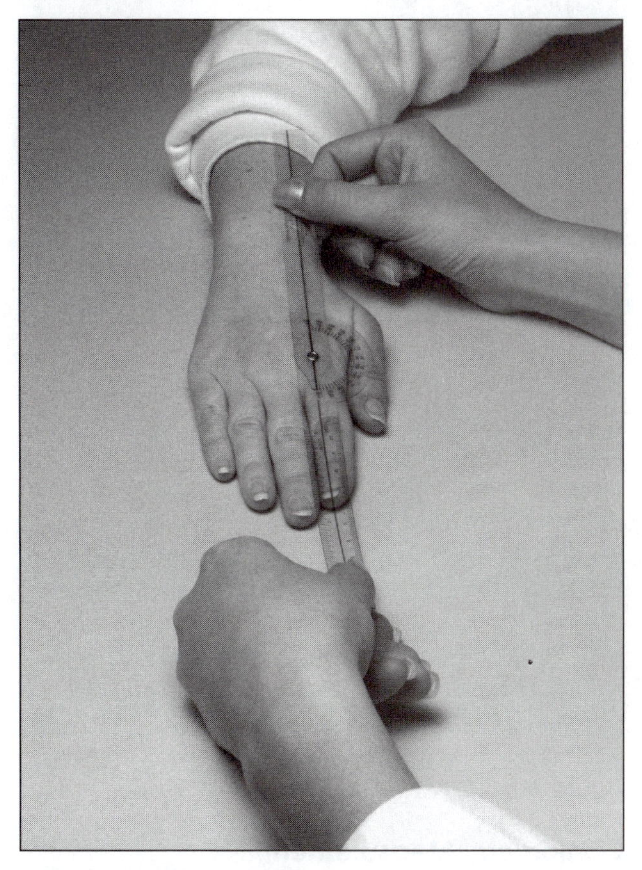

Figure 1-5-23 Start position for hand MCP abduction.

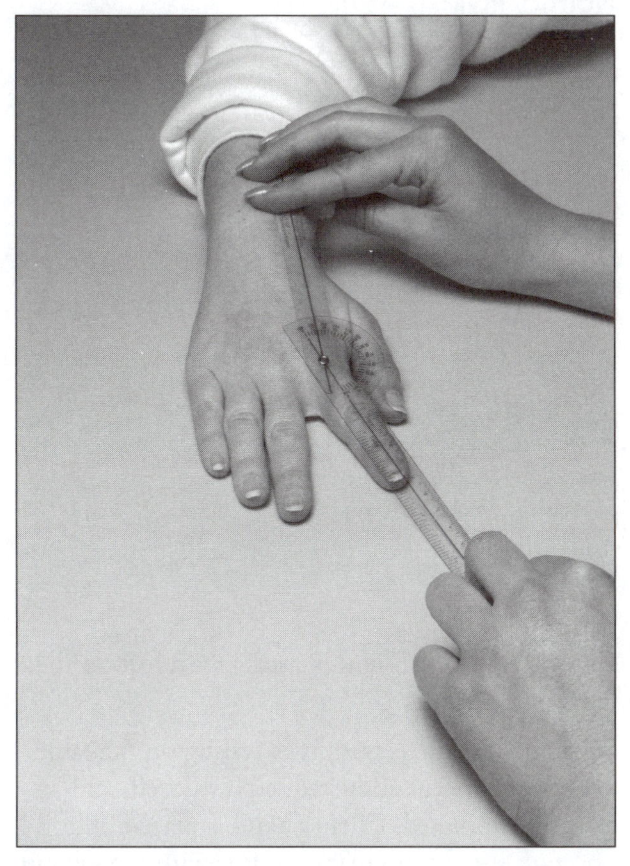

Figure 1-5-24 End position for hand MCP abduction.

Client Position: Client is sitting with feet on the floor.

Starting—testing extremity is resting on the table with the humerus abducted, elbow flexed, and forearm pronated. Digits are in MCP adduction (Figure 1-5-23).

Ending—client moves the testing extremity digits into maximum MCP abduction (Figure 1-5-24). Note that the third digit adducts in both the radial and ulnar directions.

Therapist Position: Observe at the metacarpal to avoid compensation.

Goniometer Position:

FULCRUM: dorsal to the MCP joint

STABLE ARM: dorsal and parallel to the metacarpal

MOVABLE ARM: dorsal and parallel to the proximal phalanx

Thumb: *CMC (carpometacarpal) flexion (ASHT guideline does not include this motion)*

End feel: soft

Normal ROM: 0–45 degrees

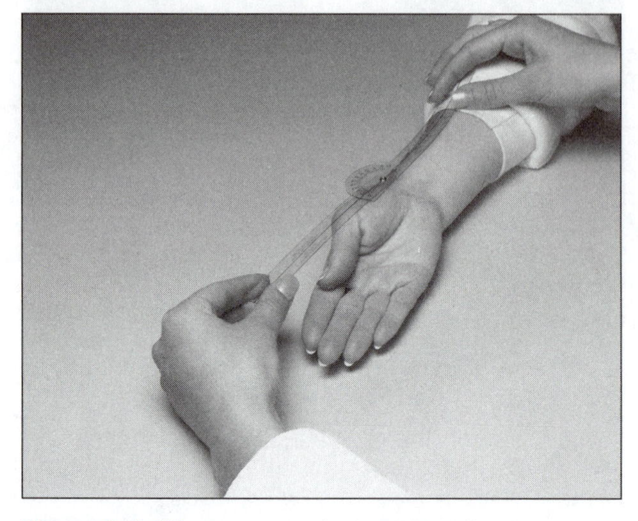

Figure 1-5-25 Start position for thumb CMC flexion.

Client Position: Client is sitting with feet on the floor.

Starting—testing extremity is resting on the table with the humerus abducted, elbow flexed, and forearm supinated. Client's hand is placed "palm up" with the thumb placed in line with the second digit (Figure 1-5-25).

Ending—client moves the testing extremity thumb across the palm into maximum CMC flexion (Figure 1-5-26).

Therapist Position: Observe at the forearm/wrist to prevent compensation.

Goniometer Position:

FULCRUM: base of the CMC joint

STABLE ARM: midline of radius

MOVABLE ARM: midline of first metacarpal

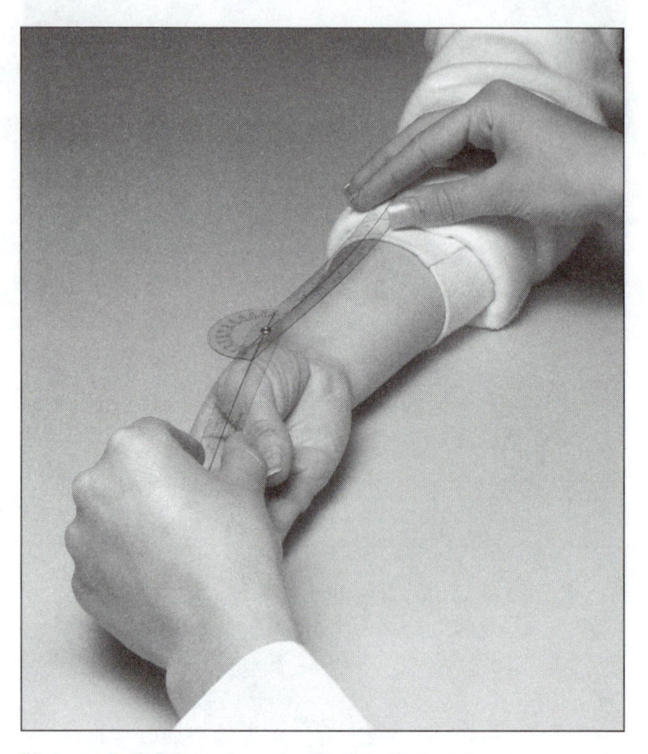

Figure 1-5-26 End position for thumb CMC flexion.

Goniometry Measurement:

This measurement is unusual because it does not start at zero, but starts in a negative position. The measurement starts to the right of the zero (negative), crosses the zero mark, and ends left of the zero (positive). The negative beginning point and the positive ending point should both be recorded.

It is important to stay in line with the metacarpal and *not* the thumb phalanges.

Thumb: *CMC extension (also referred to by ASHT guideline as radial abduction)*

End feel: firm

Normal ROM: 0–20 degrees

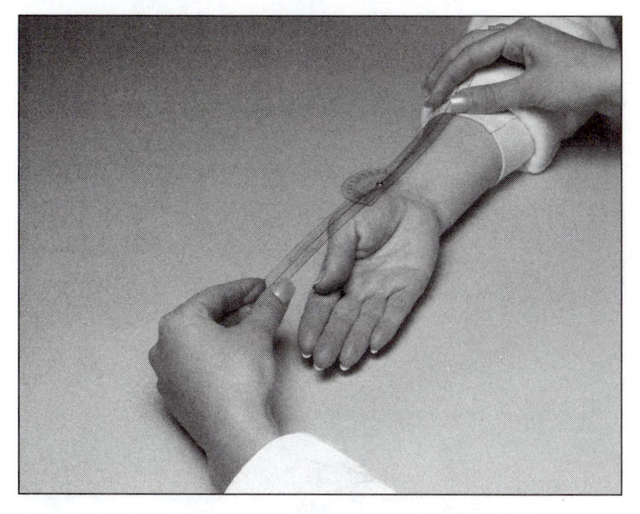

Figure 1-5-27 Start position for thumb CMC extension.

Client Position: Client is sitting with feet on the floor.

Starting—testing extremity is resting on the table with the humerus abducted, elbow flexed, and forearm supinated. Client's hand is placed "palm up" with the thumb placed in line with the second digit (Figure 1-5-27).

Ending—client moves the testing extremity thumb into maximum CMC extension (Figure 1-5-28).

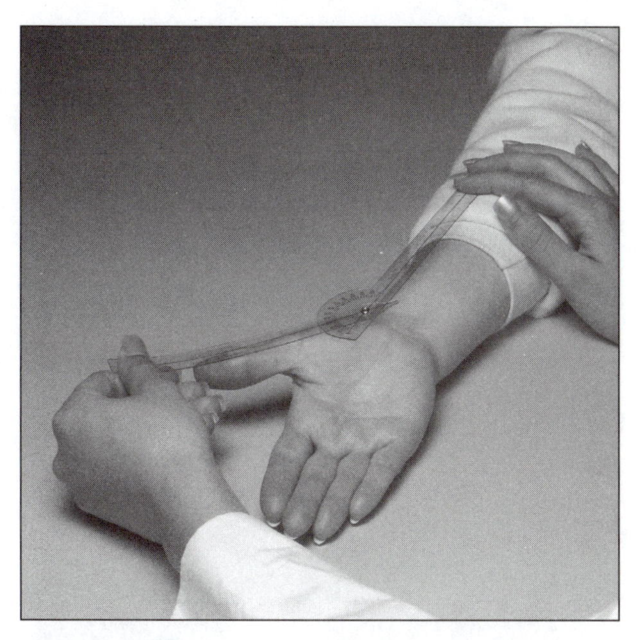

Figure 1-5-28 End position for thumb CMC extension.

Therapist Position: Observe at the forearm/wrist to prevent compensation.

Goniometer Position: Same position as thumb CMC flexion above. The goniometer readings for thumb CMC extension should be positive, but do not necessarily start at zero.

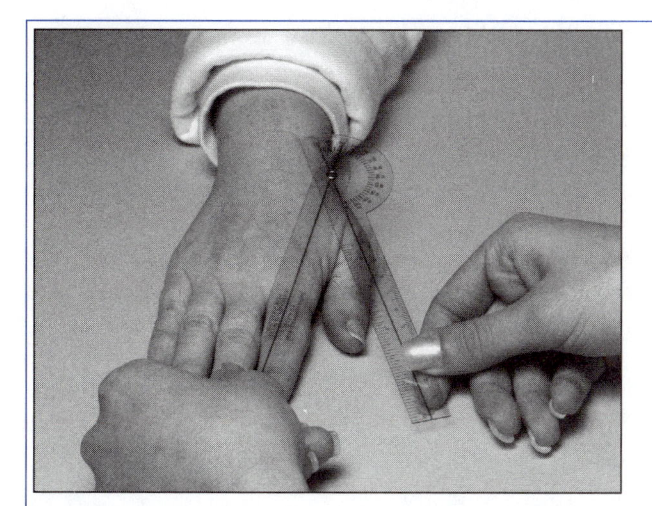

Figure 1-5-27a ASHT start position for thumb CMC extension or radial abduction.

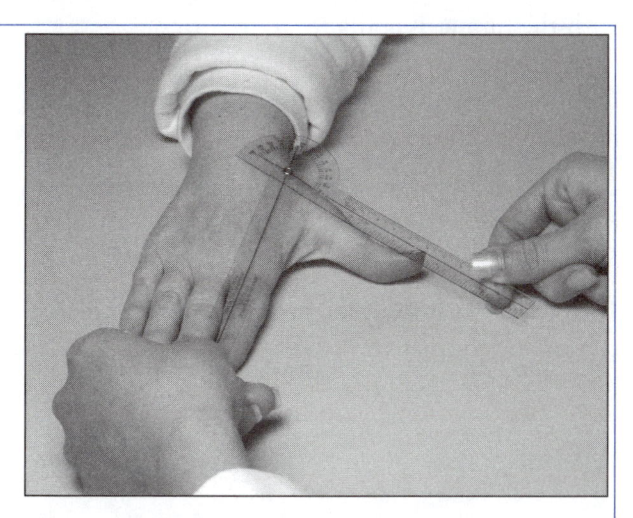

Figure 1-5-28a ASHT end position for thumb CMC extension or radial abduction.

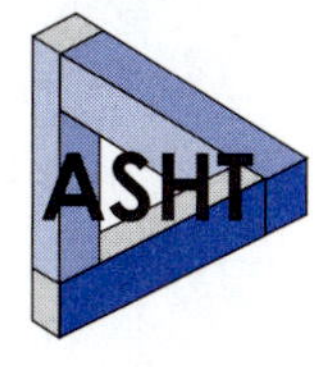

ASHT guideline recommendation for the measurement of thumb CMC extension or radial abduction places the goniometer on the dorsal surface of the CMC joint with the stable arm parallel to the second metacarpal and the movable arm parallel to the first metacarpal (Figures 1-5-27a and 1-5-28a). (The American Society of Hand Therapists, 1992).

Thumb: *CMC abduction (also referred to by ASHT guideline as palmar abduction)*

End feel: firm

Normal ROM: 0–70 degrees

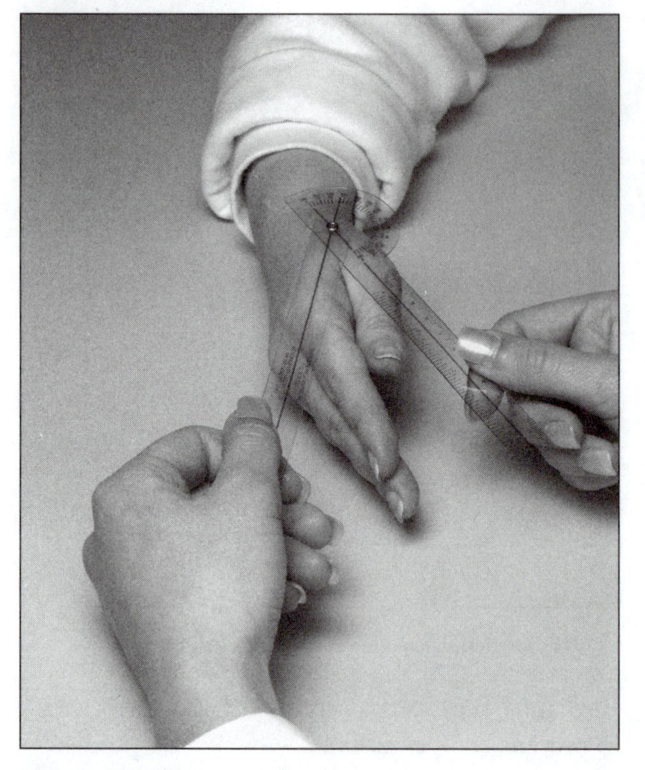

Figure 1-5-29 Start position for thumb CMC abduction.

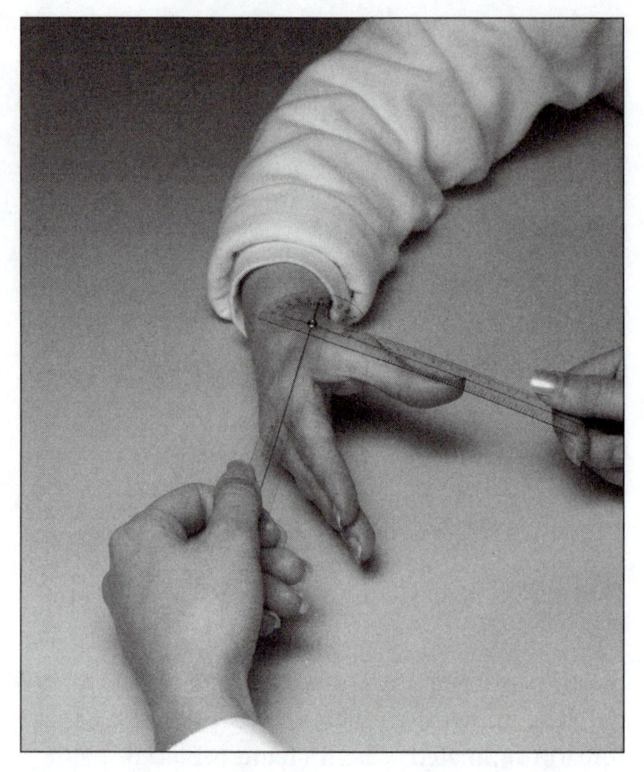

Figure 1-5-30 End position for thumb CMC abduction.

Client Position: Client is sitting with feet on the floor.

Starting—testing extremity is resting on the table with the humerus abducted, elbow flexed, and forearm supinated. Client's hand is placed with the ulnar aspect on the table. The thumb is placed in line with the second digit (Figure 1-5-29).

Ending—client moves the testing extremity thumb into maximum CMC abduction (Figure 1-5-30).

Therapist Position: Observe at the wrist/forearm to prevent compensation.

Goniometer Position:

FULCRUM: Base of the first and second metacarpals

STABLE ARM: midline of the second metacarpal, along the radial border

MOVABLE ARM: midline of the first metacarpal, along the radial border

Thumb: *CMC adduction (ASHT guideline does not include this motion)*

End feel: Soft

Normal ROM: As compared to unaffected side. There is no normal because this ROM is often not tested; however, it has been included for completeness.

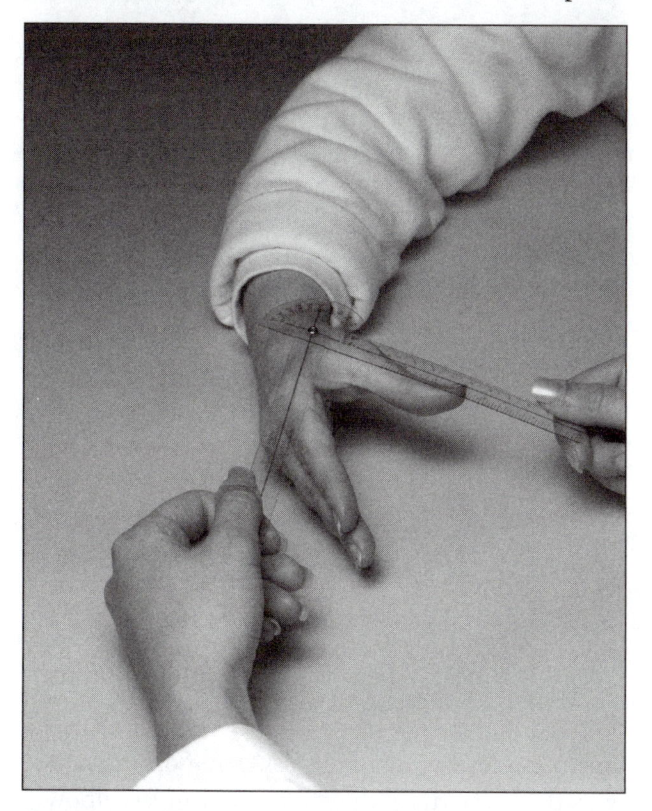

Figure 1-5-31 Start position for thumb CMC adduction.

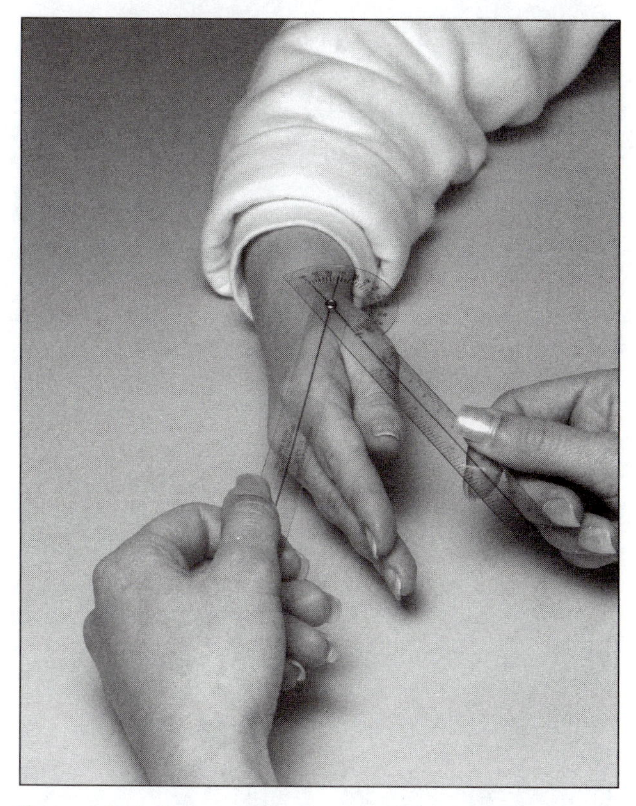

Figure 1-5-32 End position for thumb CMC adduction.

Client Position: Client is sitting with feet on the floor.

Starting—testing extremity is resting on the table with the humerus abducted to 90 degrees, elbow flexed, and forearm supinated. Client's hand is placed with the medial aspect on the table. The thumb is placed in full abduction (Figure 1-5-31).

Ending—client moves the testing extremity thumb into maximum CMC adduction (ending with thumb parallel with the second metacarpal) (Figure 1-5-32).

Therapist Position: Observe at the wrist/forearm to prevent compensation.

Goniometer Position: Same position as thumb CMC abduction above.

Hand: *opposition of first and fifth digits*

End feel: soft

Normal ROM: zero centimeters

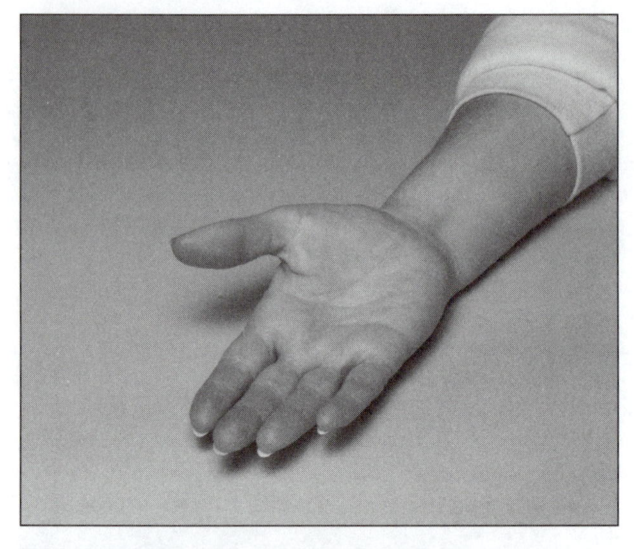

Figure 1-5-33 Start position for hand opposition.

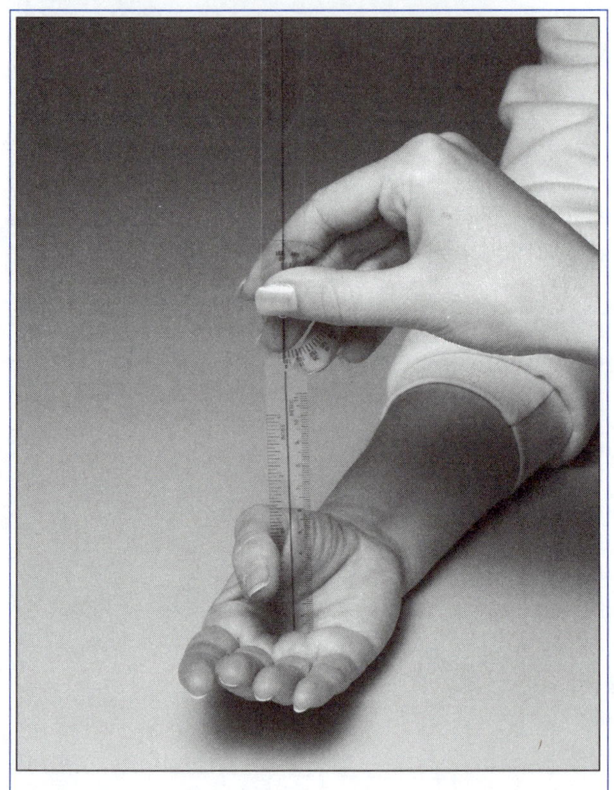

Figure 1-5-34a ASHT end position for hand opposition.

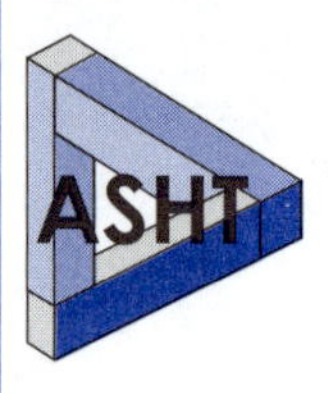

ASHT guideline recommendation for the measurement of opposition places the ruler of the goniometer from the IP joint of the thumb to the distal palmar crease over the third metacarpal (Figure 1-5-34a). Because this manual focuses on function, this measurement was not chosen as the primary testing option. (The American Society for Hand Therapists, 1992).

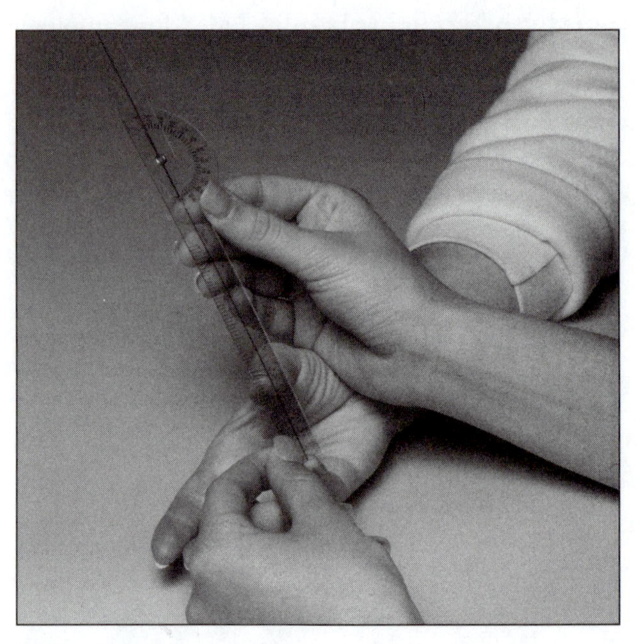

Figure 1-5-34 End position for hand opposition.

Client Position: Client is sitting with feet on the floor.

Starting—testing extremity is resting on the table with the humerus abducted to 90 degrees, elbow flexed, and forearm in supination (Figure 1-5-33).

Ending—client moves the testing extremity into opposition (Figure 1-5-34).

Therapist Position: Observe at the wrist to avoid compensation.

Goniometer Position:

The ruler measurements, which are located on one of the arms of the goniometer, are used for opposition. The measurement is taken from the tip of the fifth digit to the tip of the first digit. The measurement is recorded in the number of centimeters of opposition that is lacking. This same method can be used for opposition of the first digit to any of the digits.

SECTION 1-6: Goniometric Measurements of the Hip and Knee

Hip: *flexion*

End feel: soft

Normal ROM: 0–120 degrees

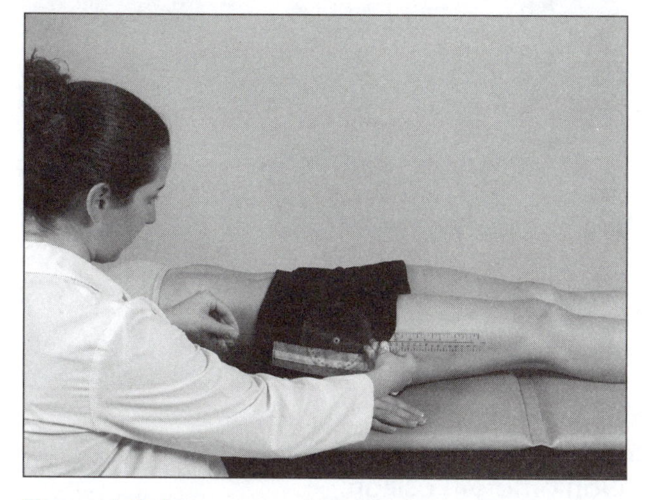

Figure 1-6-1 Start position for hip flexion.

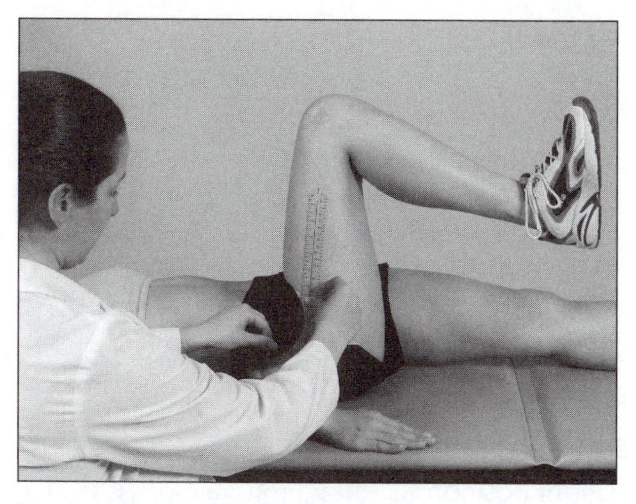

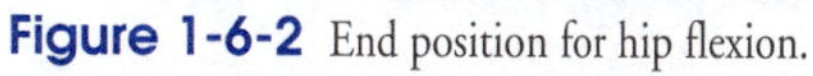

Figure 1-6-2 End position for hip flexion.

Client Position: Client is supine and pelvis stabilized on surface.

Starting—testing extremity is in 0 degrees of hip and knee extension (Figure 1-6-1).

Ending—client moves the testing extremity into maximum hip flexion, while the knee is also flexed (Figure 1-6-2).

Therapist Position: Observe at the pelvis and lumbar region to avoid compensatory movement.

Goniometer Position:

FULCRUM: lateral aspect of the greater trochanter

STABLE ARM: parallel to mid-axillary line of the trunk

MOVABLE ARM: parallel to the lateral aspect of the femur

Hip: *extension*

End feel: firm

Normal ROM: 0–30 degrees

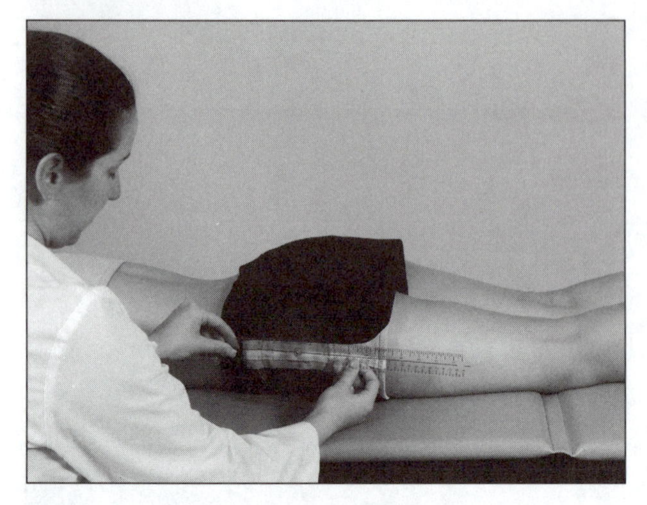

Figure 1-6-3 Start position for hip extension.

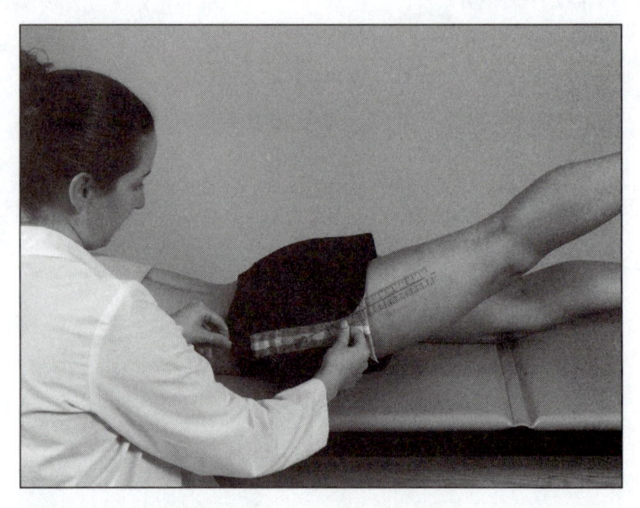

Figure 1-6-4 End position for hip extension.

Client Position: Client is prone and pelvis stabilized on surface.

Starting—testing extremity is in 0 degrees of hip and knee extension, and feet off testing surface (Figure 1-6-3).

Ending—client moves the testing extremity into maximum hip extension, while the knee remains extended (Figure 1-6-4).

Therapist Position: Observe at the pelvis and lumbar region to avoid compensatory movement.

Goniometer Position:

FULCRUM: lateral aspect of the greater trochanter

STABLE ARM: parallel to mid-axillary line of the trunk

MOVABLE ARM: parallel to the lateral aspect of the femur

Hip: *abduction*

End feel: firm

Normal ROM: 0–45 degrees

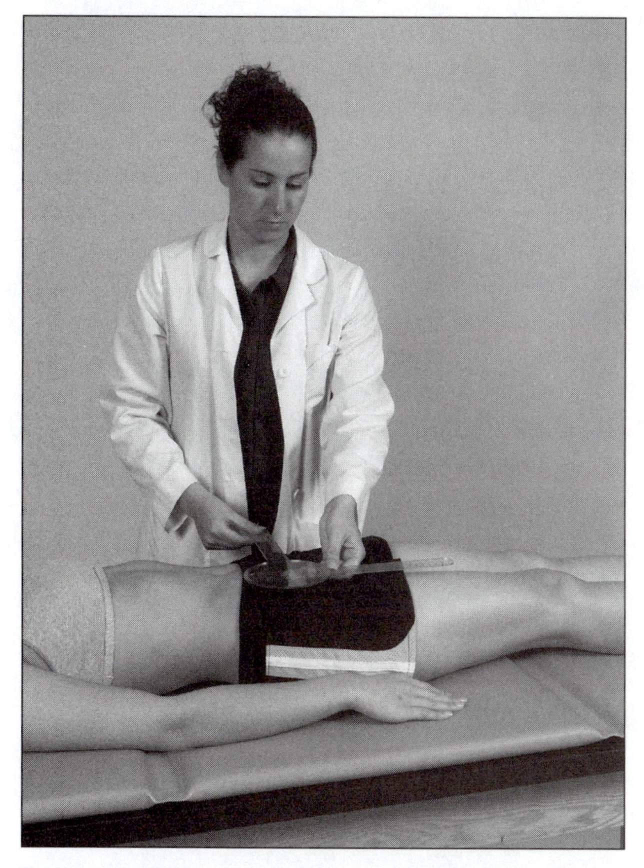

Figure 1-6-5 Start position for hip abduction.

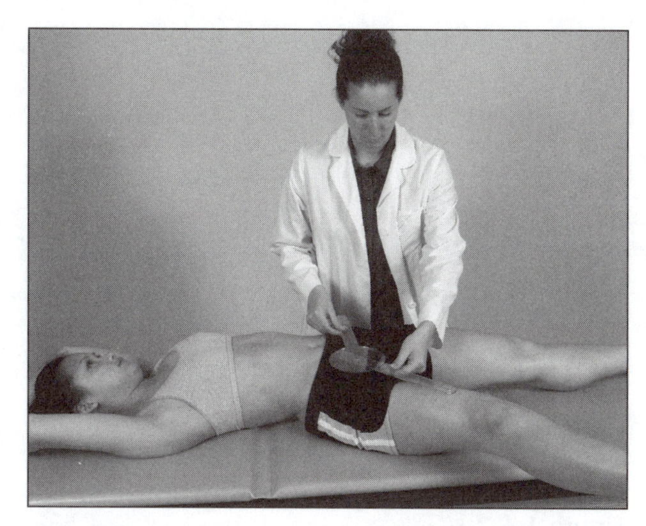

Figure 1-6-6 End position for hip abduction.

Client Position: Client is supine and pelvis stabilized on surface.

Starting—testing extremity is in 0 degrees of hip and knee extension (Figure 1-6-5).

Ending—client moves the testing extremity into maximum hip abduction (Figure 1-6-6).

Therapist Position: Observe at the pelvis and lumbar region to prevent compensatory movement.

Goniometer Position:

FULCRUM: over anterior superior iliac spine (ASIS)

STABLE ARM: horizontally between both ASIS

MOVABLE ARM: parallel to the anterior midline of the femur

Hip: *adduction*

End feel: firm

Normal ROM: 30–0 degrees

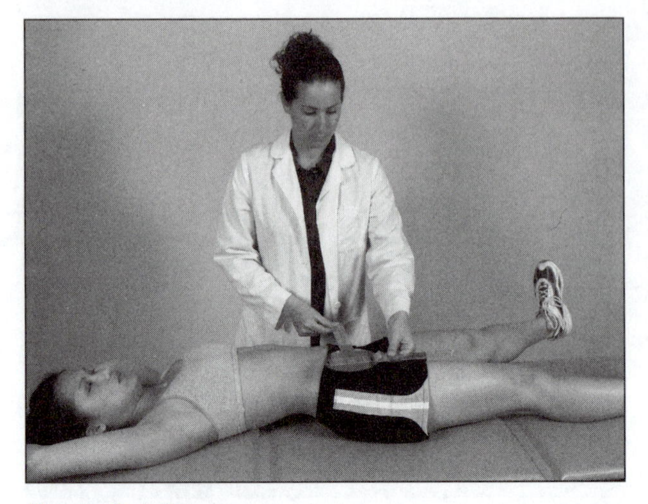

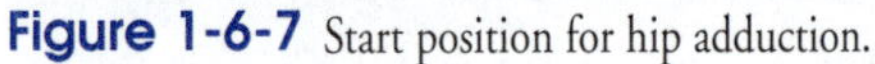

Figure 1-6-7 Start position for hip adduction.

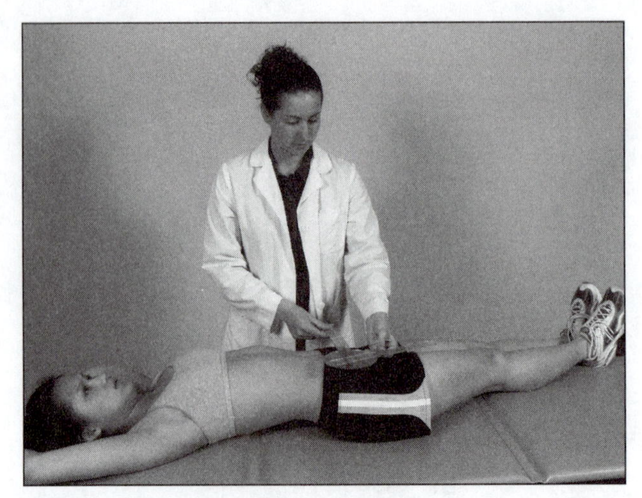

Figure 1-6-8 End position for hip adduction.

Client Position: Client is supine and pelvis stabilized on surface.

Starting—testing extremity is in hip abduction and knee extension (Figure 1-6-7).

Ending—client moves the testing extremity into maximum hip adduction (Figure 1-6-8).

Therapist Position: Observe at the pelvis and lumbar region to prevent compensatory movement.

Goniometer Position:

FULCRUM: over anterior superior iliac spine (ASIS)

STABLE ARM: horizontally between both ASIS

MOVABLE ARM: parallel to the anterior midline of the femur

Hip: *external rotation*

End feel: firm

Normal ROM: 0–45 degrees

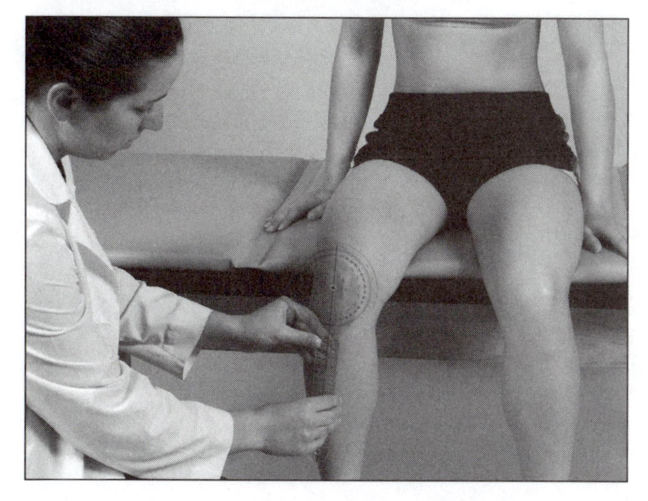

Figure 1-6-9 Start position for hip external rotation.

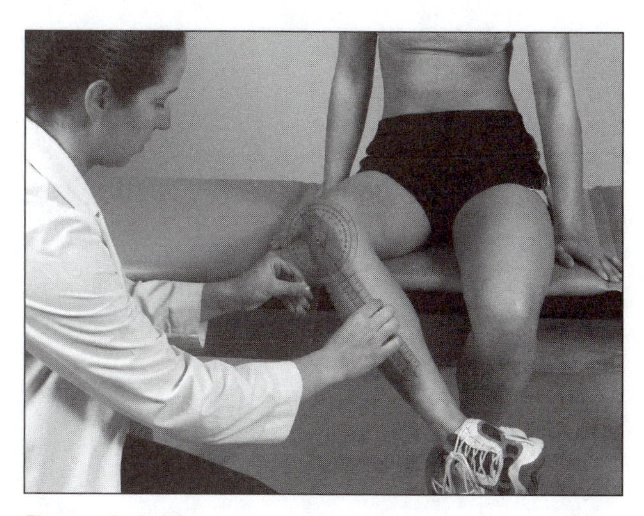

Figure 1-6-10 End position for hip external rotation.

Client Position: Client is sitting.

Starting—testing extremity is in 0 degrees of hip abduction/adduction and rotation, and 90 degrees of hip and knee flexion (Figure 1-6-9).

Ending—client moves the testing extremity into maximum hip external rotation (Figure 1-6-10).

Therapist Position: Observe at the pelvis and lumbar region to prevent compensatory movement.

Goniometer Position:

FULCRUM: over midpoint of patella

STABLE ARM: perpendicular to the floor

MOVABLE ARM: parallel to the anterior midline of the tibia midway between the two malleoli

Hip: *internal rotation*

End feel: firm

Normal ROM: 0–45 degrees

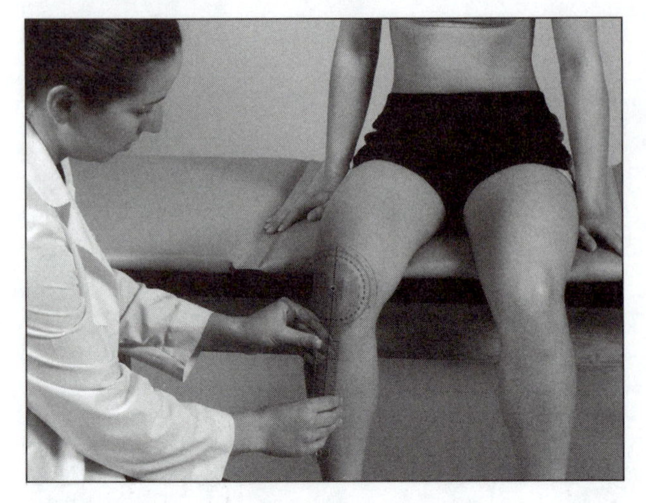

Figure 1-6-11 Start position for hip internal rotation.

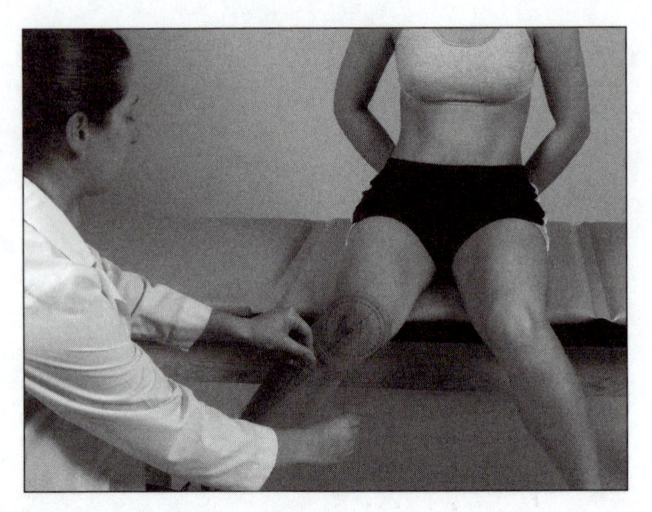

Figure 1-6-12 End position for hip internal rotation.

Client Position: Client is sitting.

Starting—testing extremity is in 0 degrees of hip abduction/adduction and rotation, and 90 degrees of hip and knee flexion (Figure 1-6-11).

Ending—client moves the testing extremity into maximum hip internal rotation (Figure 1-6-12).

Therapist Position: Observe at the pelvis and lumbar region to prevent compensatory movement.

Goniometer Position:

FULCRUM: over midpoint of patella

STABLE ARM: perpendicular to the floor

MOVABLE ARM: parallel to the anterior midline of the tibia midway between the two malleoli

Knee: *flexion*

End feel: soft

Normal ROM: 0–135 degrees

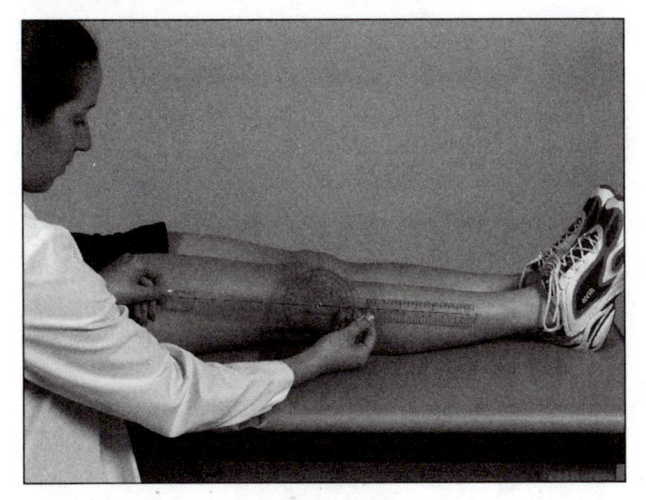

Figure 1-6-13 Start position for knee flexion.

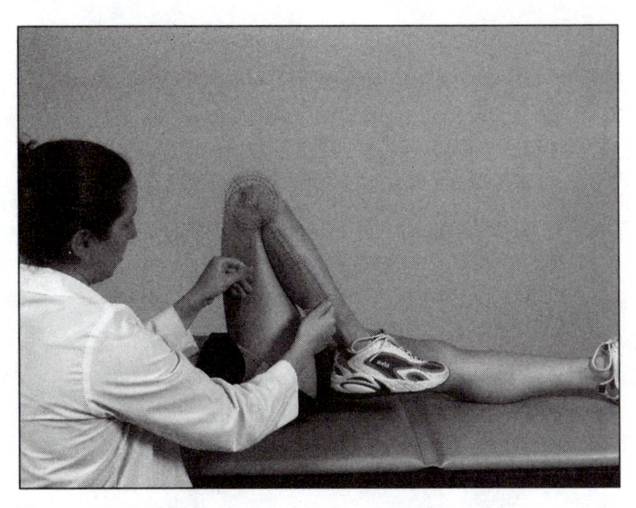

Figure 1-6-14 End position for knee flexion.

Client Position: Client is supine.

Starting—testing extremity hip is in neutral and knee extended (Figure 1-6-13).

Ending—client moves the testing extremity into maximum knee flexion (hip will also flex) (Figure 1-6-14).

Therapist Position: Observe at the femur to prevent compensatory movement.

Goniometer Position:

FULCRUM: over lateral epicondyle of femur

STABLE ARM: parallel to lateral midline of femur

MOVABLE ARM: parallel to the lateral midline of the fibula

Alternate Position

Prone (Figures 1-6-13a and 1-6-14a).

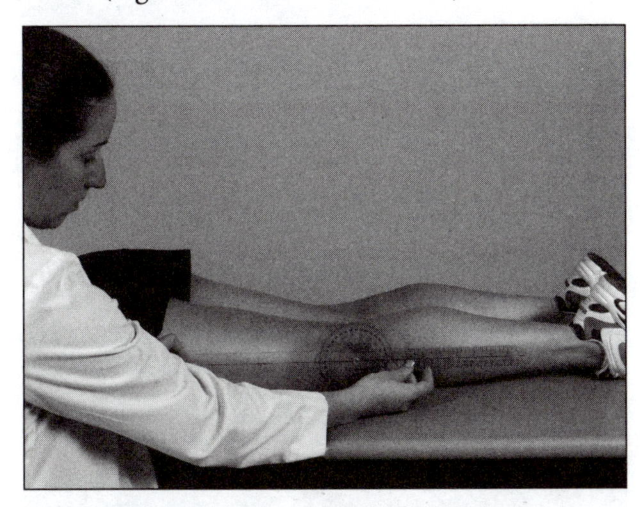

Figure 1-6-13a Alternate start position for knee flexion.

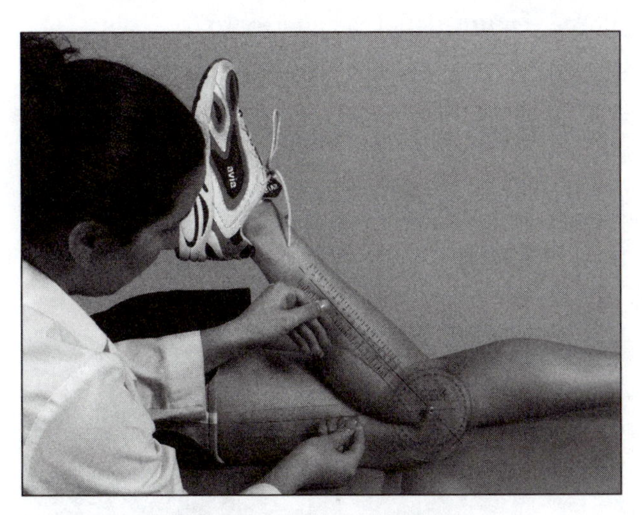

Figure 1-6-14a Alternate end position for knee flexion.

Knee: *extension*

End feel: firm

Normal ROM: 135–0 degrees

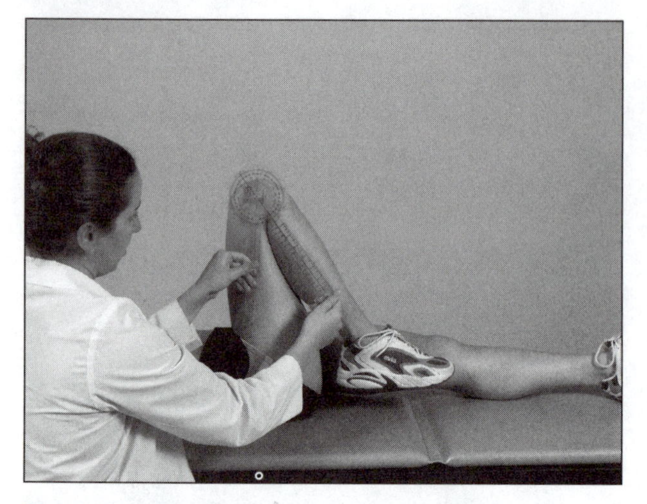

Figure 1-6-15 Start position for knee extension.

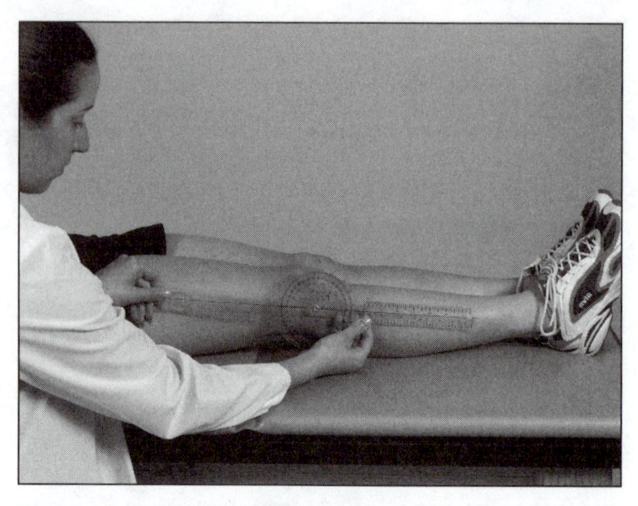

Figure 1-6-16 End position for knee extension.

Client Position: Client is supine.

Starting—testing extremity hip and knee are flexed (Figure 1-6-15).

Ending—client moves the testing extremity into maximum knee extension (hip will also extend) (Figure 1-6-16).

Therapist Position: Observe at the femur to prevent compensatory movement.

Goniometer Position:

FULCRUM: over lateral epicondyle of femur

STABLE ARM: parallel to lateral midline of femur

MOVABLE ARM: parallel to the lateral midline of the fibula

Alternate Position

Prone (Figures 1-6-15a and 1-6-16a).

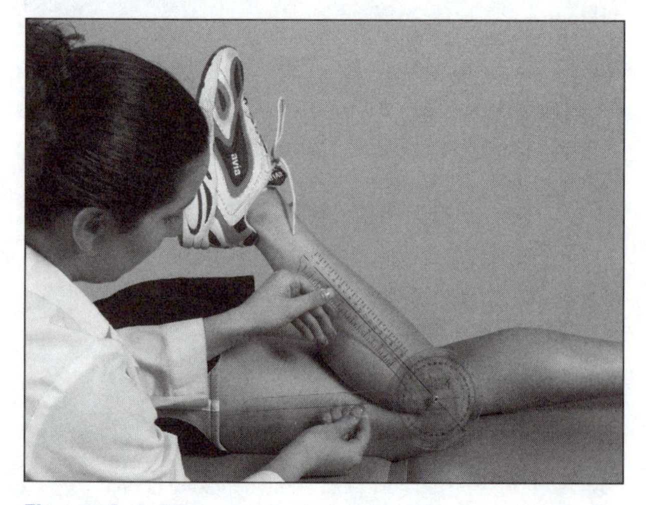

Figure 1-6-15a Alternate start position for knee extension.

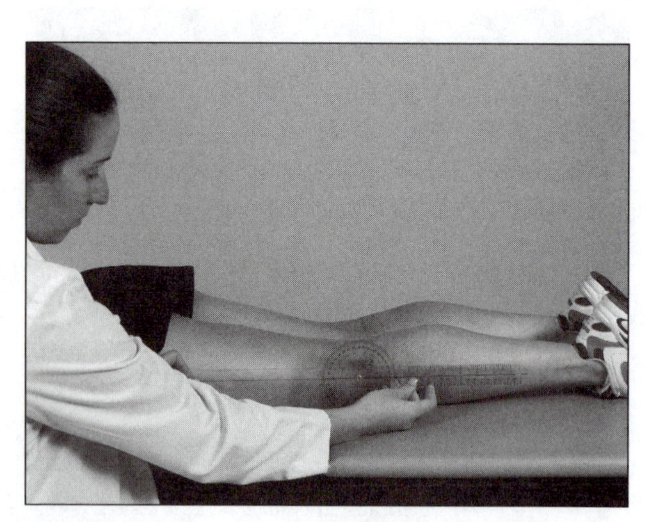

Figure 1-6-16a Alternate end position for knee extension.

SECTION 1-7: Goniometric Measurements of the Ankle and Foot

Ankle: *dorsiflexion*

End feel: firm
Normal ROM: 0–20 degrees

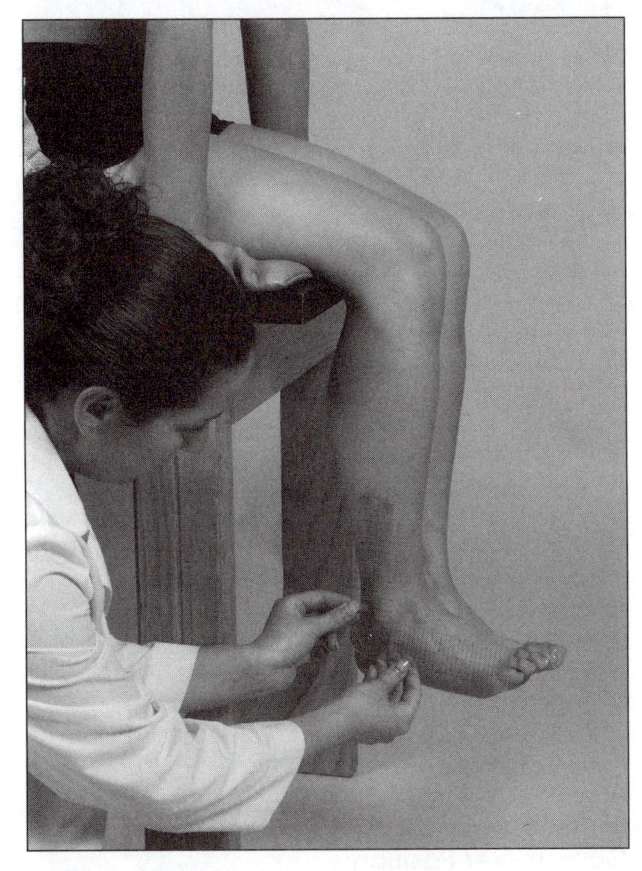

Figure 1-7-1 Start position for ankle dorsiflexion.

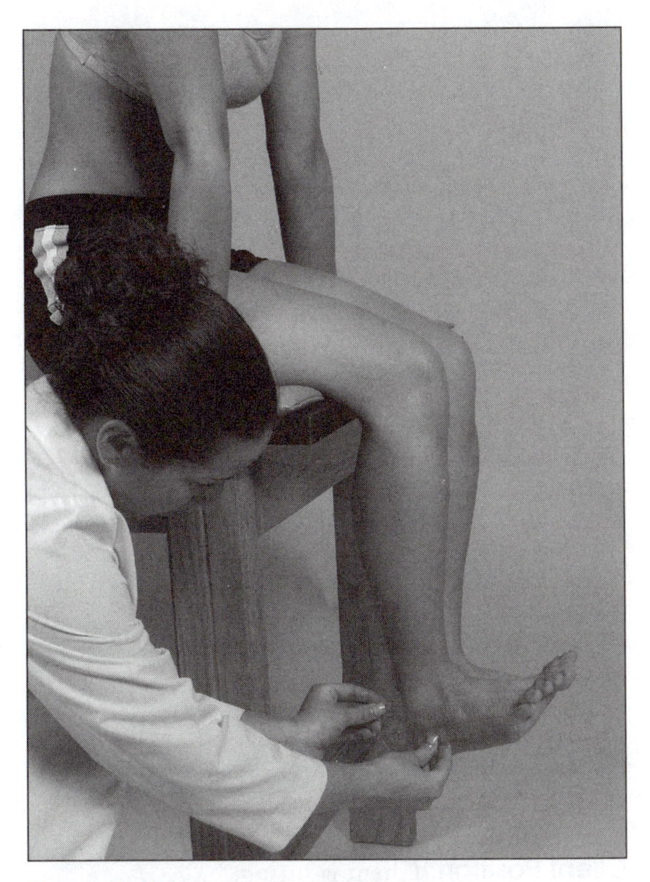

Figure 1-7-2 End position for ankle dorsiflexion.

Client Position: Client is sitting.

Starting—testing extremity is in 90 degrees of hip and knee flexion. Ankle is in neutral (Figure 1-7-1).

Ending—client moves the testing extremity into maximum ankle dorsiflexion (Figure 1-7-2).

Therapist Position: Observe at the tibia and fibula to prevent compensatory movement.

Goniometer Position:

FULCRUM: lateral aspect of lateral malleolus

STABLE ARM: parallel to lateral midline of fibula

MOVABLE ARM: parallel to the lateral midline of the 5th metatarsal

Ankle: *plantar flexion*

End feel: firm

Normal ROM: 0–50 degrees

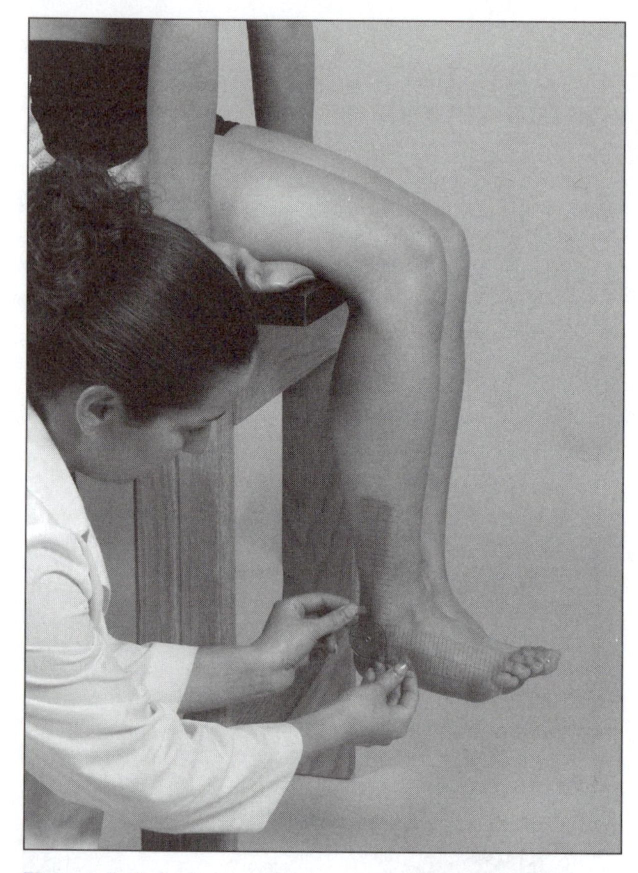

Figure 1-7-3 Start position for ankle plantar flexion.

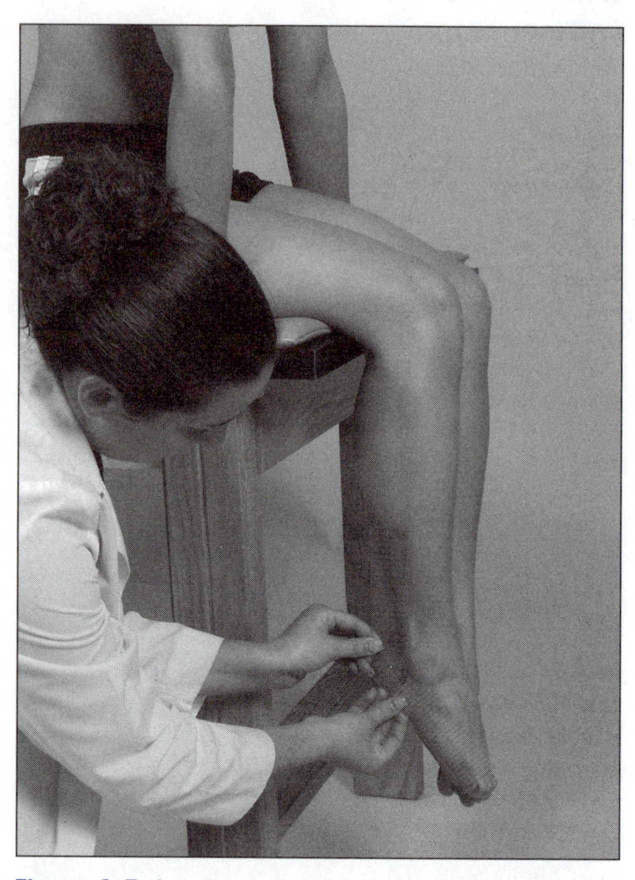

Figure 1-7-4 End position for ankle plantar flexion.

Client Position: Client is sitting.

Starting—testing extremity is in 90 degrees of hip and knee flexion. Ankle is in neutral (Figure 1-7-3).

Ending—client moves the testing extremity into maximum ankle plantar flexion (Figure 1-7-4).

Therapist Position: Observe at the tibia and fibula to prevent compensatory movement.

Goniometer Position:

FULCRUM: lateral aspect of lateral malleolus

STABLE ARM: parallel to lateral midline of fibula

MOVABLE ARM: parallel to the lateral midline of the 5th metatarsal

Ankle: *eversion (forefoot)*

End feel: hard

Normal ROM: 0–15 degrees

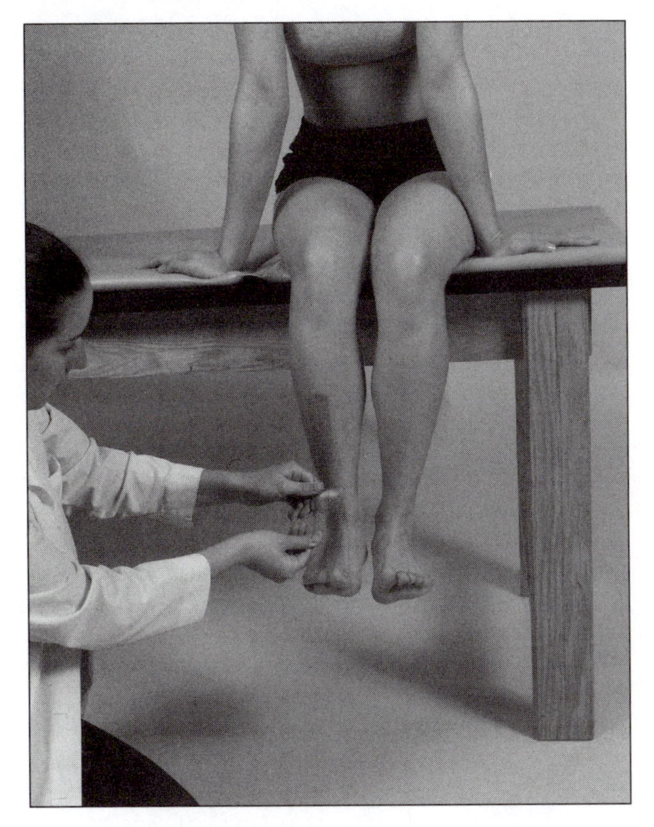

Figure 1-7-5 Start position for ankle eversion (forefoot).

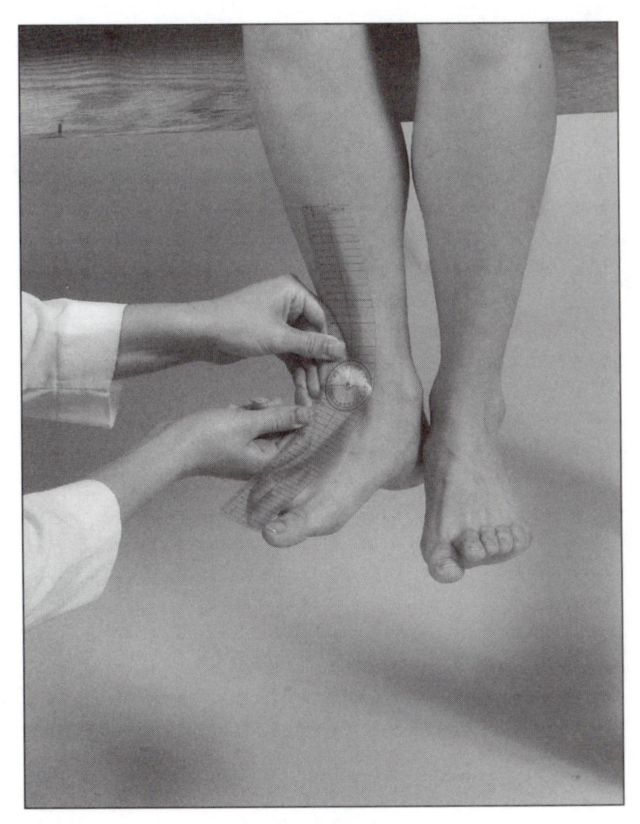

Figure 1-7-6 End position for ankle eversion (forefoot).

Client Position: Client is sitting.

Starting—testing extremity is in 90 degrees of hip and knee flexion. Ankle is in neutral (Figure 1-7-5).

Ending—client moves the testing extremity into maximum ankle eversion (Figure 1-7-6).

Therapist Position: Observe at the tibia and fibula to prevent compensatory movements.

Goniometer Position:

FULCRUM: over anterior aspect of ankle midway between malleoli

STABLE ARM: parallel to the anterior midline of lower leg

MOVABLE ARM: parallel to the anterior midline of the 2nd metatarsal

Ankle: *inversion (forefoot)*

End feel: firm

Normal ROM: 0–35 degrees

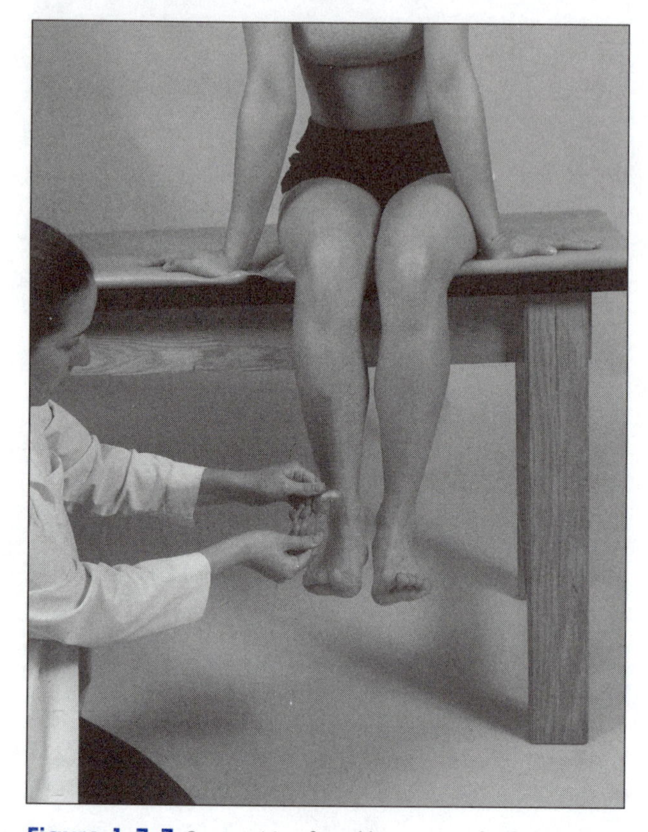

Figure 1-7-7 Start position for ankle inversion (forefoot).

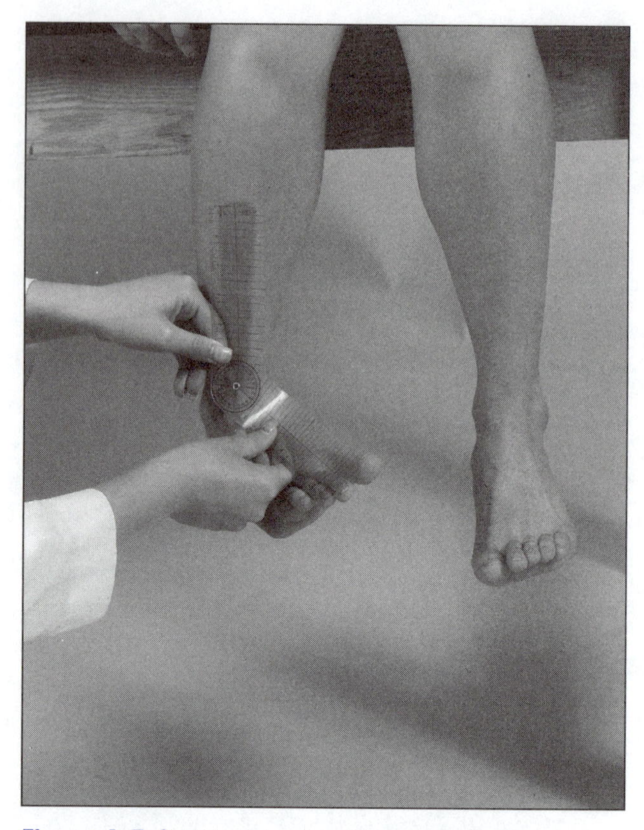

Figure 1-7-8 End position for ankle inversion (forefoot).

Client Position: Client is sitting.

Starting—testing extremity is in 90 degrees of hip and knee flexion. Ankle is in neutral (Figure 1-7-7).

Ending—client moves the testing extremity into maximum ankle inversion (Figure 1-7-8).

Therapist Position: Observe at the tibia and fibula to prevent compensatory movement.

Goniometer Position:

FULCRUM: over anterior aspect of ankle midway between the two malleoli

STABLE ARM: parallel to the anterior midline of lower leg

MOVABLE ARM: parallel to the anterior midline of the 2nd metatarsal

Ankle: *eversion (hindfoot/subtalar)*

End feel: firm/hard

Normal ROM: 0–5 degrees

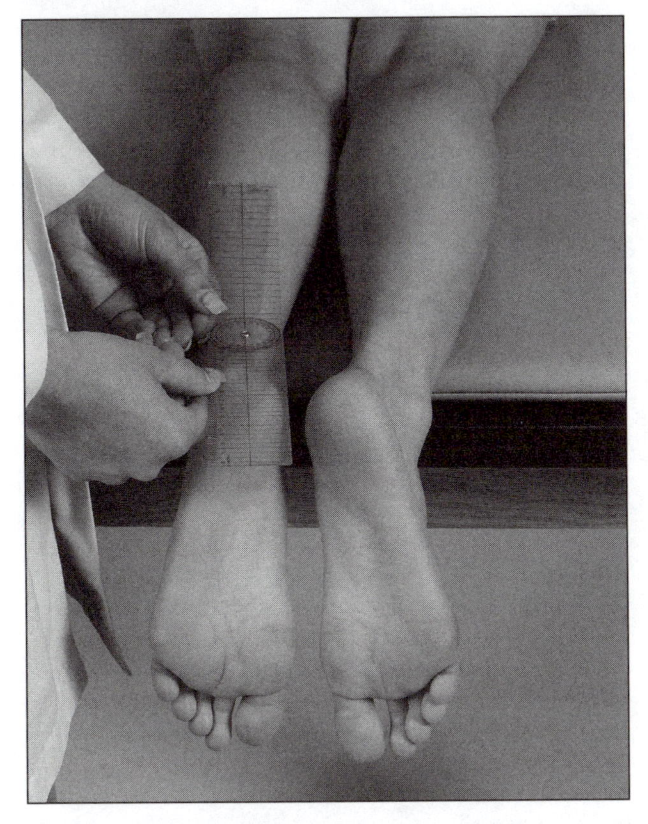

Figure 1-7-9 Start position for ankle eversion (hindfoot).

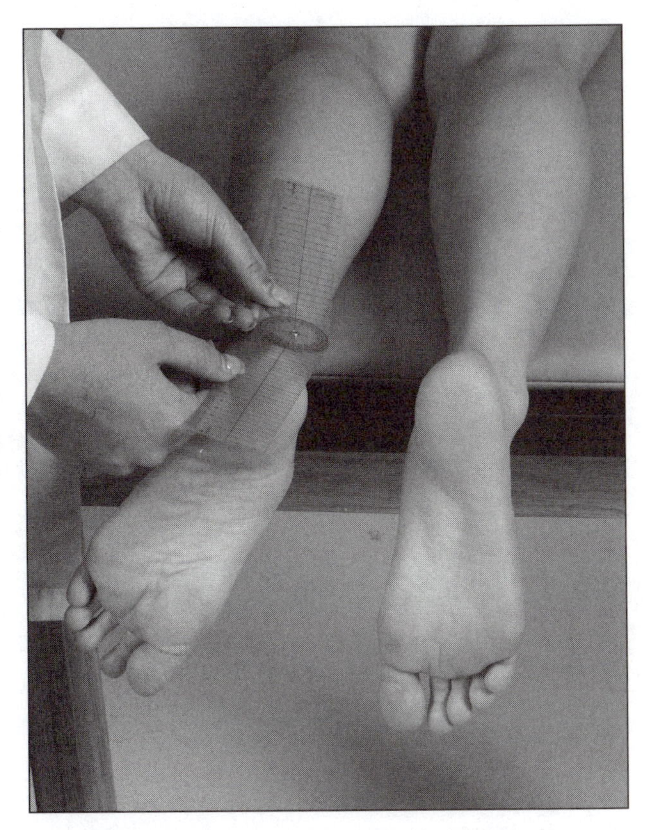

Figure 1-7-10 End position for ankle eversion (hindfoot)

Client Position: Client is prone.

Starting—testing hip and knee are in neutral. Ankle is in neutral with foot over edge of testing surface (Figure 1-7-9).

Ending-client moves the testing extremity into maximum ankle eversion (Figure 1-7-10).

Therapist Position: Observe at the tibia and fibula to prevent compensatory movement.

Goniometer Position:

FULCRUM: over posterior aspect of ankle midway between the two malleoli

STABLE ARM: parallel to the posterior midline of lower leg

MOVABLE ARM: parallel to the posterior midline of the calcaneus

Ankle: *inversion (hindfoot/subtalar)*

End feel: firm

Normal ROM: 0–5 degrees

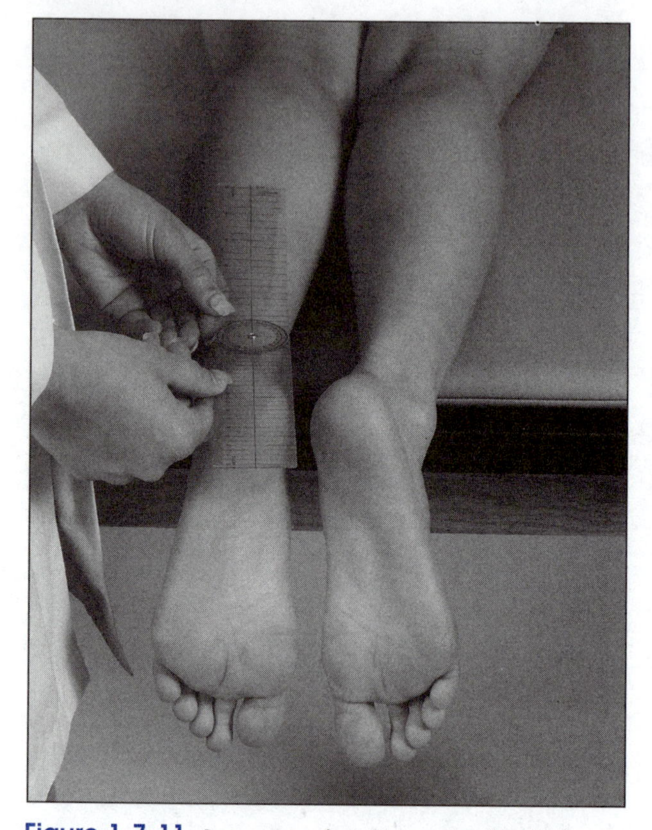

Figure 1-7-11 Start position for ankle inversion (hindfoot).

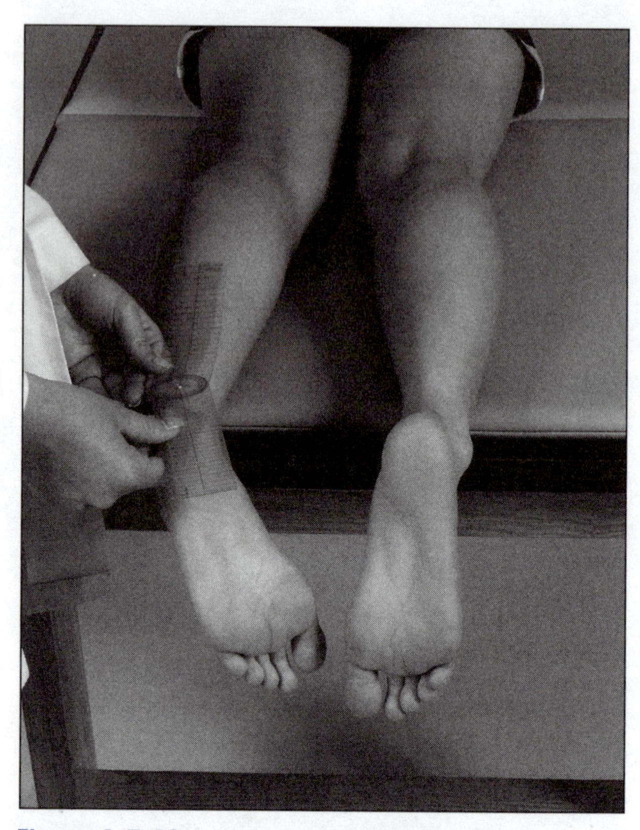

Figure 1-7-12 End position for ankle inversion (hindfoot).

Client Position: Client is prone.

Starting—testing hip and knee are in neutral. Ankle is in neutral with foot over edge of testing surface (Figure 1-7-11).

Ending—client moves the testing extremity into maximum ankle inversion (Figure 1-7-12).

Therapist Position: Observe at the tibia and fibula to prevent compensatory movement.

Goniometer Position:

FULCRUM: over posterior aspect of ankle between the two malleoli

STABLE ARM: parallel to the posterior midline of lower leg

MOVABLE ARM: parallel to the posterior midline of the calcaneus

Foot: *metatarsophalangeal (MTP) flexion*

End feel: firm

Normal ROM: great toe 0–45 degrees, toes #2 through 5, 0–40 degrees

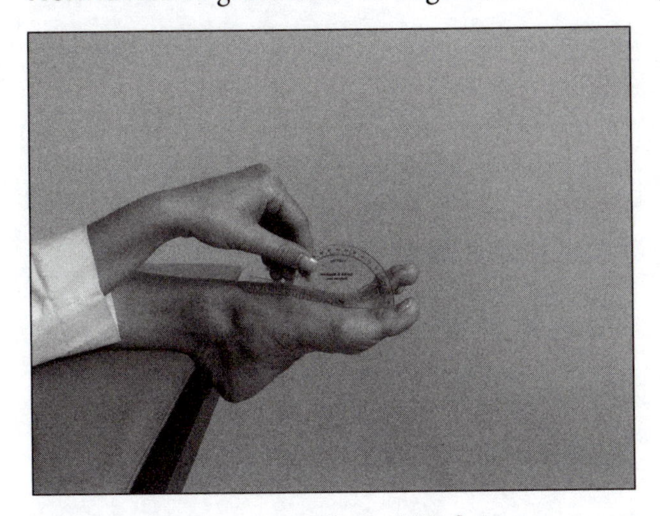

Figure 1-7-13 Start position for foot MTP flexion.

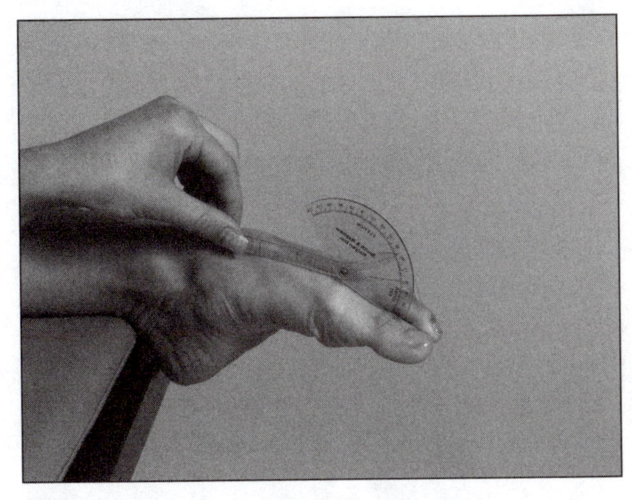

Figure 1-7-14 End position for foot MTP flexion.

Client Position: Client is supine.

Starting—testing hip and knee are in neutral. Ankle, foot, and toes in neutral with foot over edge of testing surface (Figure 1-7-13).

Ending—client moves the testing extremity into maximum MTP flexion (Figure 1-7-14).

Therapist Position: Observe at the ankle and foot to prevent compensatory movements.

Goniometer Position:

FULCRUM: over dorsum of MTP

STABLE ARM: parallel to dorsal midline of metatarsal

MOVABLE ARM: parallel to dorsal midline of proximal phalanx

Foot: *metatarsophalangeal (MTP) extension*

End feel: firm

Normal ROM: great toe 45–0, toes #2 through 5, 40–0 degrees

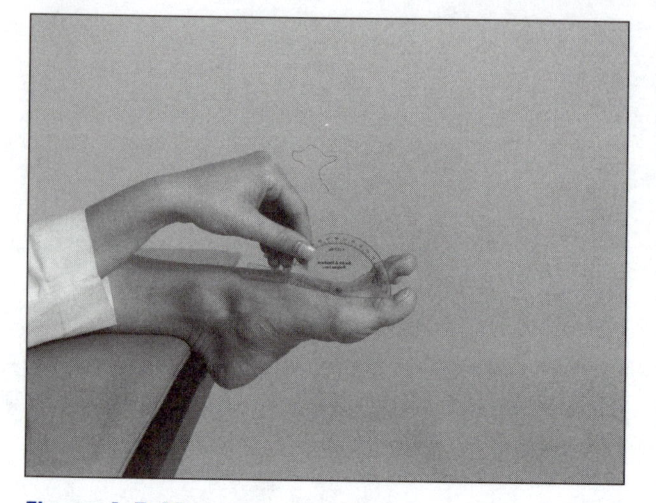

Figure 1-7-15 Start position for foot MTP extension.

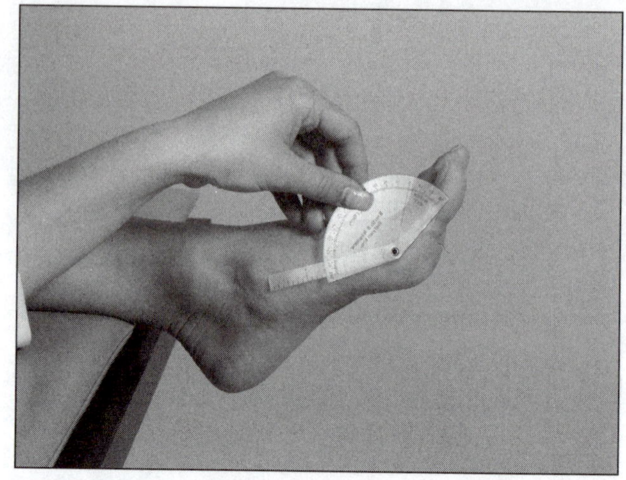

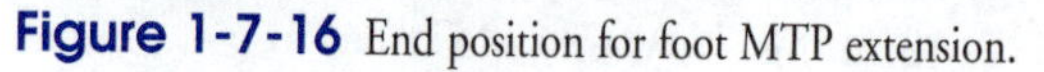

Figure 1-7-16 End position for foot MTP extension.

Client Position: Client is supine.

Starting—testing hip and knee are in neutral. Ankle, foot, and toes in neutral with foot over edge of testing surface (Figure 1-7-15).

Ending—client moves the testing extremity into maximum MTP extension (Figure 1-7-16).

Therapist Position: Observe at the ankle and foot to prevent compensatory movement.

Goniometer Position:

FULCRUM: over dorsum of MTP

STABLE ARM: parallel to dorsal midline of metatarsal

MOVABLE ARM: parallel to dorsal midline of proximal phalanx

Alternate position of goniometer: on plantar aspect of foot

Foot: *metatarsophalangeal (MTP) abduction*

End feel: firm

Normal ROM: compare to opposite side

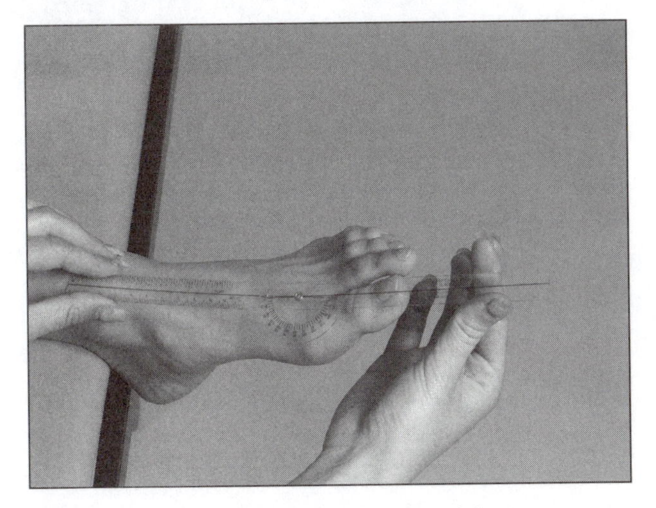

Figure 1-7-17 Start position for foot MTP abduction.

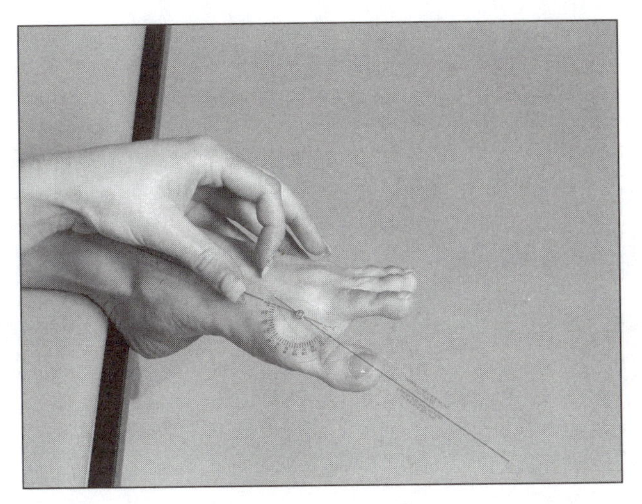

Figure 1-7-18 End position for foot MTP abduction.

Client Position: Client is supine.

Starting—testing hip and knee are in neutral. Ankle, foot, and toes in neutral with foot over edge of testing surface (Figure 1-7-17).

Ending—client moves the testing extremity into maximum MTP abduction (Figure 1-7-18).

Therapist Position: Observe at the ankle and foot to prevent compensatory movement.

Goniometer Position:

FULCRUM: over dorsum of MTP

STABLE ARM: parallel to dorsal midline of metatarsal

MOVABLE ARM: parallel to dorsal midline of proximal phalanx

Foot: *metatarsophalangeal (MTP) adduction*

End feel: firm

Normal ROM: compare to opposite side

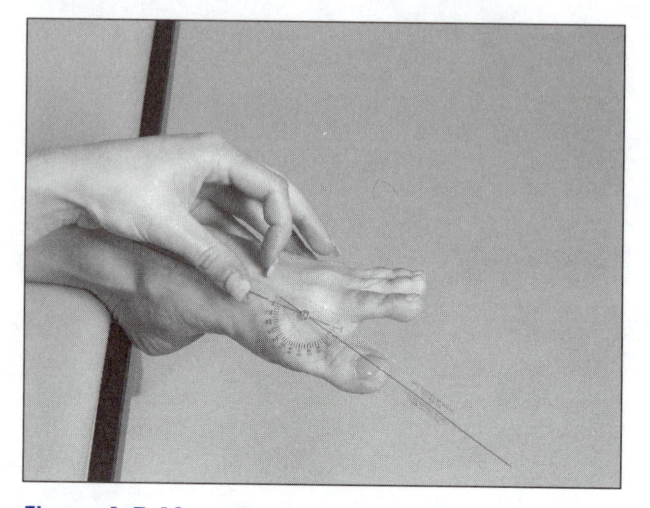

Figure 1-7-19 Start position for foot MTP adduction.

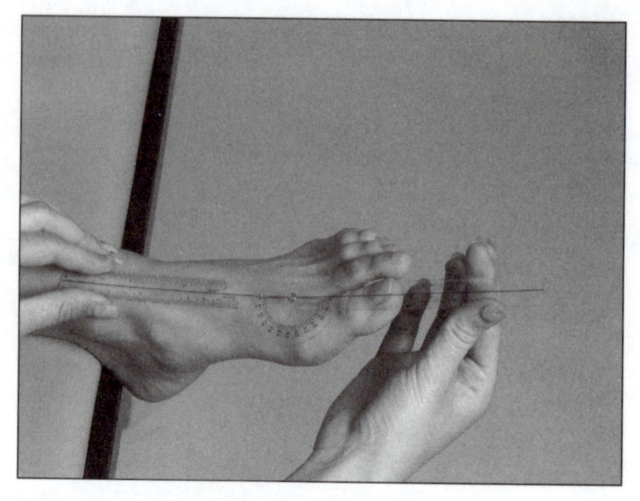

Figure 1-7-20 End position for foot MTP adduction.

Client Position: Client is supine.

Starting—testing hip and knee are in neutral. Ankle, foot, and toes in neutral with foot over edge of testing surface (Figure 1-7-19).

Ending—client moves the testing extremity into maximum MTP adduction (Figure 1-7-20).

Therapist Position: Observe at the ankle and foot to prevent compensatory movement.

Goniometer Position:

FULCRUM: over dorsum of MTP

STABLE ARM: parallel to dorsal midline of metatarsal

MOVABLE ARM: parallel to dorsal midline of proximal phalanx

Foot: *proximal interphalangeal (PIP) flexion*

End feel: soft/firm

Normal ROM: great toe 0–90 degrees, toes #2 through 5, 0–35 degrees

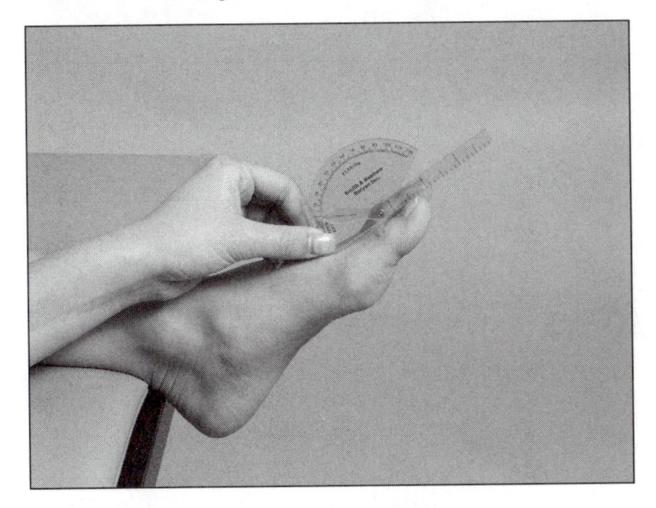

Figure 1-7-21 Start position for foot PIP flexion.

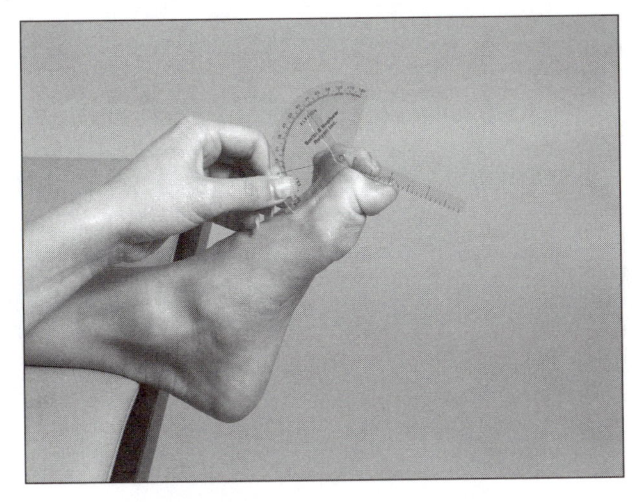

Figure 1-7-22 End position for foot PIP flexion.

Client Position: Client is supine.

Starting—testing hip and knee are in neutral. Ankle, foot, and toes in neutral with foot over edge of testing surface (Figure 1-7-21).

Ending—client moves the testing extremity into maximum PIP flexion (Figure 1-7-22).

Therapist Position: Observe at the ankle and foot to prevent compensatory movement.

Goniometer Position:

FULCRUM: over dorsum of PIP

STABLE ARM: parallel to dorsal midline of proximal phalanx

MOVABLE ARM: parallel to dorsal midline of middle phalanx

Foot: *proximal interphalangeal (PIP) extension*

End feel: firm

Normal ROM: great toe 90–0 degrees, toes #2 through 5, 35–0 degrees

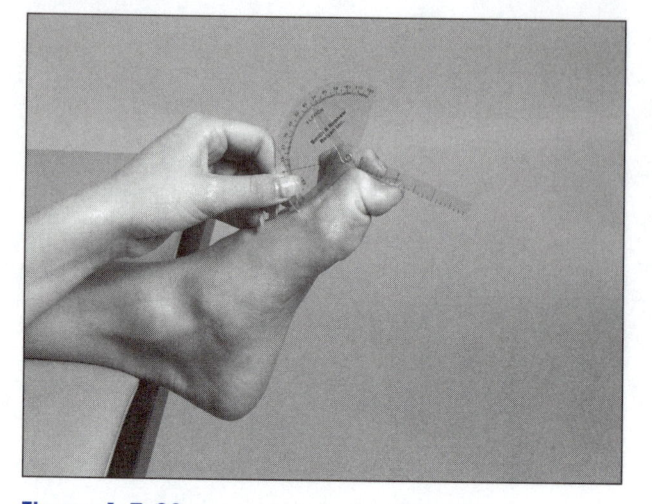

Figure 1-7-23 Start position for foot PIP extension.

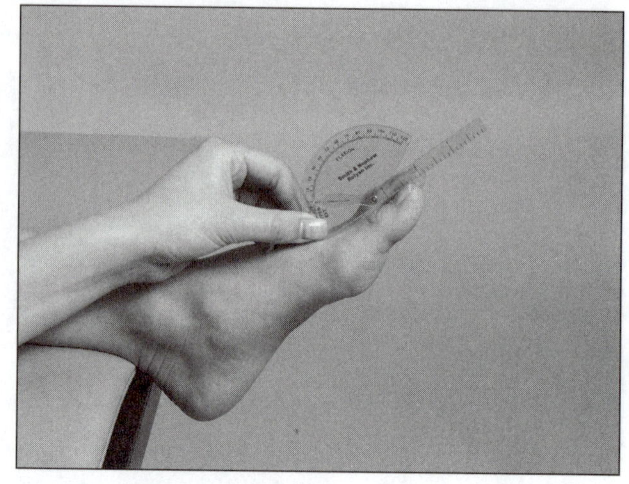

Figure 1-7-24 End position for foot PIP extension.

Client Position: Client is supine.

Starting—testing hip and knee are in neutral. Ankle, foot, and toes in neutral with foot over edge of testing surface (Figure 1-7-23).

Ending—client moves the testing extremity into maximum PIP extension (Figure 1-7-24).

Therapist Position: Observe at the ankle and foot to prevent compensatory movement.

Goniometer Position:

FULCRUM: over dorsum of PIP

STABLE ARM: parallel to dorsal midline of proximal phalanx

MOVABLE ARM: parallel to dorsal midline of middle phalanx

Foot: *distal interphalangeal (DIP) flexion*

End feel: firm

Normal ROM: 0–60 degrees

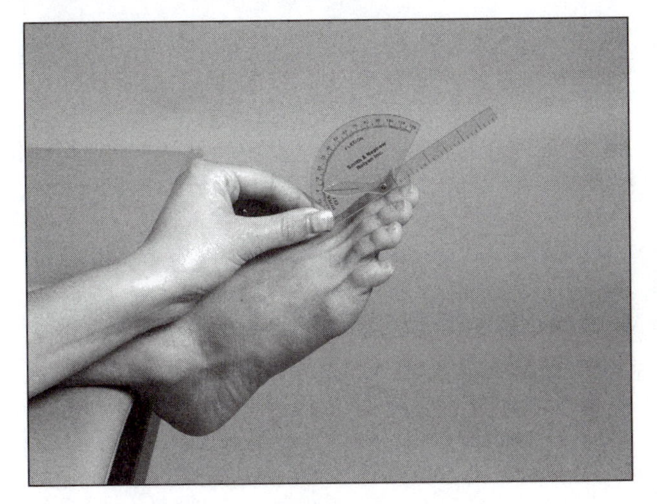

Figure 1-7-25 Start position for foot DIP flexion.

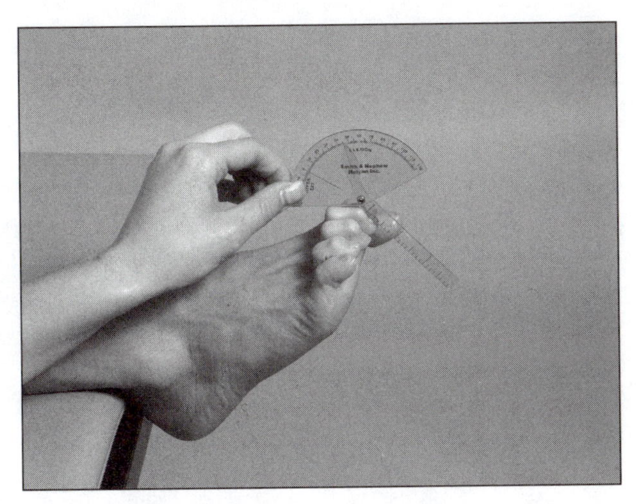

Figure 1-7-26 End position for foot DIP flexion.

Client Position: Client is supine.

Starting—testing hip and knee are in neutral. Ankle, foot, and toes in neutral with foot over edge of testing surface (Figure 1-7-25).

Ending—client moves the testing extremity into maximum DIP flexion (Figure 1-7-26).

Therapist Position: Observe at the ankle and foot to prevent compensatory movement.

Goniometer Position:

FULCRUM: over dorsum of DIP

STABLE ARM: parallel to dorsal midline of middle phalanx

MOVABLE ARM: parallel to dorsal midline of distal phalanx

Foot: *distal interphalangeal (DIP) extension*

End feel: firm

Normal ROM: compare to opposite side

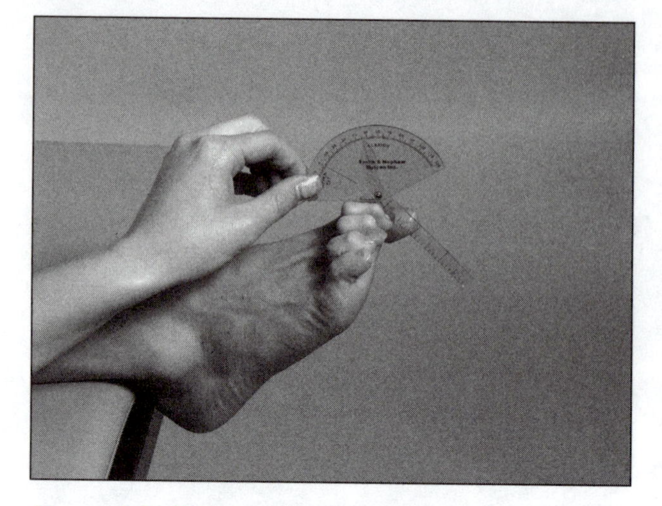

Figure 1-7-27 Start position for foot DIP extension.

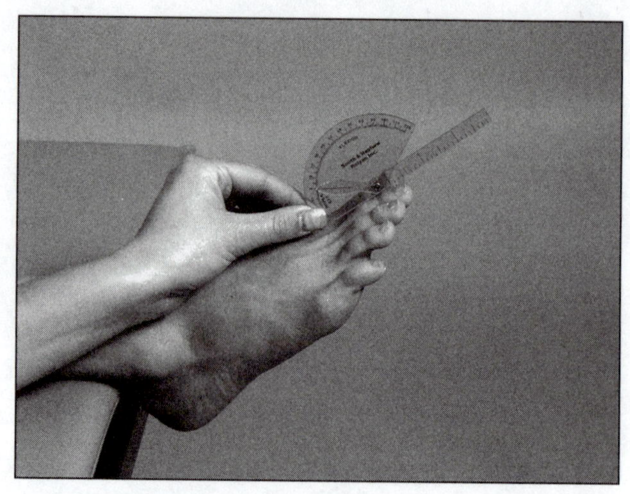

Figure 1-7-28 End position for foot DIP extension.

Client Position: Client is supine.

Starting—testing hip and knee are in neutral. Ankle, foot, and toes in neutral with foot over edge of testing surface (Figure 1-7-27).

Ending—client moves the testing extremity into maximum DIP extension (Figure 1-7-28).

Therapist Position: Observe at the ankle and foot to prevent compensatory movement.

Goniometer Position:

FULCRUM: over dorsum of DIP

STABLE ARM: parallel to dorsal midline of middle phalanx

MOVABLE ARM: parallel to dorsal midline of distal phalanx

chapter 2

Gross Manual Muscle Testing

SECTION 2-1: Introduction to Gross Manual Muscle Testing

After completing this chapter the student should be able to accomplish the following:

- define the terms functional, gross, and isolated manual muscle testing
- demonstrate the ability to perform and grade gross manual muscle testing
- demonstrate appropriate clinical reasoning to determine when gross muscle testing should progress to the more specific isolated manual muscle testing

Along with these specific skills, the student should begin practicing the use of terminology that clients can comprehend rather than medical terminology, as well as the skill of building client rapport.

DEFINITIONS

As described in chapter one of this manual, when evaluating a client's muscle strength, a therapist should first observe the client during a functional activity. This **functional observation** may be referred to as a **screening** because it is not a formal assessment but a method to allow the therapist to determine quickly which muscle groups need further testing. Often therapists today are asked to evaluate a client's skills in a limited amount of time; therefore, this observation can save time in two ways. First, if no deficits are noted, further muscle testing of those functional muscles may be eliminated depending on the client's diagnosis and the policies of the individual facility. Second, the observation can take place during another assessment, such as activities of daily living (ADL). Examples of functional activities can be found in Table 1 of this manual's introduction.

Once the muscle groups in need of testing have been determined, the therapist continues with **gross manual muscle testing**. This is a form of manual muscle testing where muscle groups are tested together. An example of a muscle group is the shoulder flexors. During gross manual muscle testing, the isolated muscles are not tested, but only the muscle group. Again, this form of muscle testing can save time not only because it can be administered quickly, but also because the therapist may only need to know which muscle groups, not which specific muscles, have deficits. The amount of specificity required for an initial therapy evaluation is determined by individual therapy facilities and the needs of the individual client.

If a more specific strength testing is required, then **isolated manual muscle testing** must be completed. This test isolates which muscle or muscles have a deficit in strength. Because each muscle is isolated for testing, this is a more time-consuming form of muscle testing than either the functional observation or the gross manual muscle testing. As noted in chapter three of this manual, some muscles cannot be isolated.

In muscle testing, the therapist must consider the effect of gravity on the client because gravity itself is a form of resistance on muscles. Normally, we do not feel the effect of gravity, but when muscles are weakened the effect can be significant. When completing both gross and isolated manual muscle testing, the therapist must have the ability to position the client **against gravity** and in a **gravity-eliminated** position. Against gravity refers to the type of movement that occurs when a client is moving the extremity or body part perpendicular to the floor because the force of gravity is exerted down toward the floor. In order to be in a gravity-eliminated position, the client moves the extremity or body part parallel to the floor (supported by the therapist, a roller board, a powder board, or some other means to hold the extremity parallel). An example of against-gravity testing is asking a client to raise his arm into shoulder flexion while standing. To change this to gravity-eliminated testing, the client would need to lie on his side and complete shoulder flexion parallel to the floor.

Once the therapist has determined which position to place the client in, the positions of both resistance and stabilization must be considered. **Resistance** is applied manually by the therapist in order to determine which muscle strength grade a client currently demonstrates. Resistance is only applied when testing in the against-gravity positions. If a client cannot move an extremity against the resistance of gravity, then manual resistance by the therapist is certainly not appropriate. When applying resistance in the against-gravity position, the therapist's hand should generally be placed just distal to the joint on which the testing muscles act. If the resistance is applied too distally, the therapist may get inaccurate results because of increased torque on the muscles and joint. In addition, if the resistance is applied too distally, a second joint may be involved which could cause inaccurate results. Using the same shoulder flexion example, resistance should be applied on the proximal humerus. If resistance is applied at the forearm, the therapist has an advantage because of the increased lever arm of resistance. In addition, if resistance is applied at the forearm there may be an influence of the elbow joint or the elbow muscles on the shoulder flexion testing. As will be seen in specific sections, it is not always possible to place the resistance just distal to the joint, but this rule should be followed as much as possible.

Stabilization is necessary in both against-gravity and gravity-eliminated positions. **Stabilization** of the joint is also applied manually by the therapist. The purpose of the stabilization is to avoid any compensation, or use of other muscles, by the client. The therapist places the stabilizing hand just proximal to the joint on which the testing muscles act to isolate the function of that joint.

Two other terms that the therapist must be knowledgeable of prior to beginning muscle testing are **passive range of motion** (PROM) and **active range of motion** (AROM). PROM is completed by the therapist alone. The therapist moves the extremity through the available arc of motion without the assistance of the client. AROM is the opposite of PROM. The client moves the extremity through the available arc of motion without the assistance of the therapist. In general, PROM is completed to assess the joint integrity, and to assess the tone or muscle tightness of the muscle groups. If abnormal tone (excessive tightness of the muscles called "hypertonicity") is found, muscle testing should not be performed. The presence of abnormal tone will lead to inaccurate results because the therapist will not be testing muscle strength, but will be testing the muscle's abnormal tone. Because the therapist is evaluating muscle strength, functional observation and manual muscle testing are completed with the client completing AROM.

PROCEDURE

As stated previously, the observation of muscle strength during functional activities is completed as a screening prior to any other testing. Once this has been completed, the therapist determines if gross, or isolated, manual muscle testing, or a combination of both are appropriate. Prior to the actual testing procedure, the therapist must complete three steps. The first step is to place the client in a comfortable position on a plinth, mat table, or in a chair. The extremity or body part must be in a position such that the muscle group will act in either an against-gravity or gravity-eliminated motion. Once the client is properly positioned, the therapist completes the second step, which is explaining the muscle testing procedures to the client and demonstrating the motion that will be requested of the client. The last step that must be completed prior to the initiation of testing is PROM. PROM is completed to assess muscle tone and joint integrity as these may both influence the accuracy of muscle testing.

The testing procedure itself also involves three steps. The first is to ask the client to complete the motion that was demonstrated by the therapist. This is completed by the client and, therefore, is AROM. This quick step not only clarifies that the client understood the directions given by the therapist, but also reinforces that the client can move the extremity in the against-gravity or gravity-eliminated position in which he has been placed by the therapist. The second step is stabilization and resistance. Recall that the stabilization hand is placed just proximal to the joint and the resistance hand is placed just distal to the joint on which the muscles act. Resistance is always applied in the opposite direction from the client's motion. For example, if the client's wrist flexors are being tested, the client moves the wrist into flexion and the resistance is applied in the direction of wrist extension. The final step of the testing procedure is to grade the muscle strength. For muscle grades, see Table 2-1-1. If testing any of the extremities, these six steps would then be completed on the contralateral side. It is important to test both sides of the body to assess for symmetry and establish the client's "normal" strength.

Upon completion of the six steps described, the results must be recorded. There are a variety of formats for recording which are generally determined by individual facilities; however, any recording must include the muscle grades for all extremities tested as well as what type of testing was completed (gross or isolated manual muscle testing). Any variations from the standard procedures that were necessary for a particular client must also be included.

TABLE 2-1-1 Muscle Grades

WORD/LETTER GRADE	# GRADE	DEFINITION
Normal (N)	5	Complete ROM, against gravity, full resistance
Good (G)	4	Complete ROM, against gravity, moderate resistance
Good minus (G–)	4–	Complete ROM, against gravity, minimum resistance
Fair plus (F+)	3+	Complete ROM, against gravity, no resistance
Fair	3	Complete ROM, against gravity, no resistance, but unable to sustain ROM
Fair minus (F–)	3–	Less than $^{1}/_{2}$ ROM, against gravity, no resistance
Poor plus (P+)	2+	Complete ROM, gravity-eliminated
Poor	2	$^{1}/_{2}$ to Full ROM, gravity-eliminated
Poor minus (P–)	2–	Less than $^{1}/_{2}$ ROM, gravity-eliminated
Trace (T)	1	Palpation of contraction only, no motion
Zero (0)	0	No muscle contraction seen or palpated

CONTRAINDICATIONS AND PRECAUTIONS

The following are contraindications to muscle testing because the therapist can cause injury to the client if muscle testing is attempted:

- inflammation
- significant pain
- recent fracture
- bone carcinoma or any fragile bone condition
- significant spasticity

Precaution should be taken when completing muscle testing if the client has a history of any of the following because injury to the client may occur:

- cardiovascular conditions
- high blood pressure
- chronic obstructive pulmonary disease
- conditions where fatigue may exacerbate condition (example: multiple sclerosis)
- arthritis

SECTION 2-2: Gross Manual Muscle Testing of the Trunk and Neck

Listed after each action in this section are the muscles that act to produce that movement. If deficits are noted during gross manual muscle testing, and isolated manual muscle testing is appropriate, the procedures for the isolated manual muscle testing of these muscles are found in Section 3-2 of this manual. It is important to note, however, that many of the trunk and neck muscles are only tested in the gross manual muscle format because it is not possible to isolate specific muscles.

Trunk: *flexion*

The trunk flexors include the following muscles: primarily rectus abdominis with assistance from internal oblique and external oblique.

Normal, Good, Fair

Client Position: Starting—client is supine with the legs supported under the knees for slight knee flexion (Figure 2-2-1).

Motion—client moves in the direction of trunk flexion (Figure 2-2-2).

Therapist Position: There is no stabilization or resistance applied in this test.

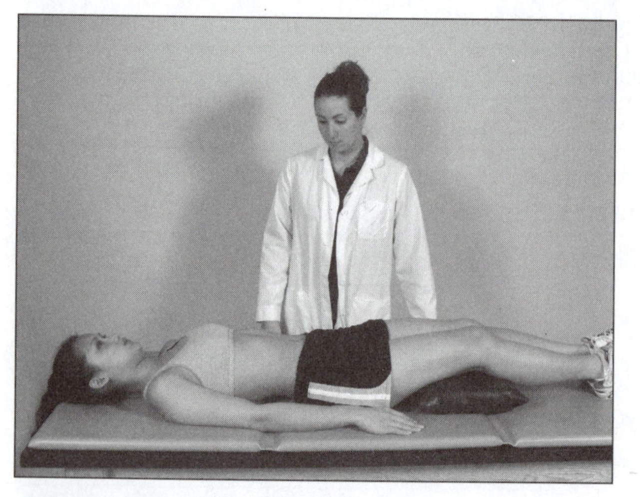

Figure 2-2-1 Start position for trunk flexion.

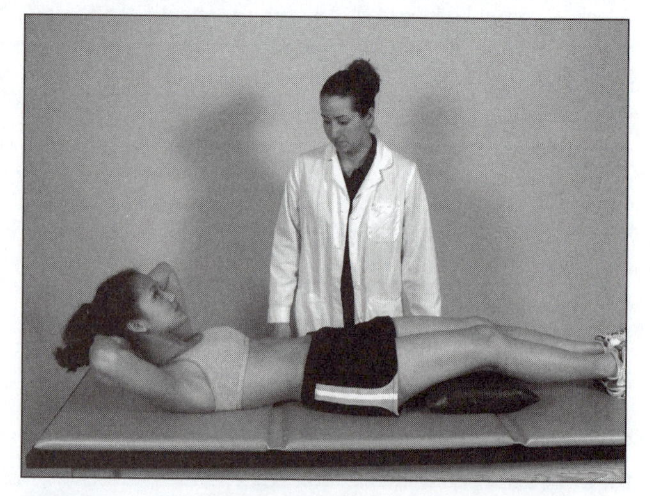

Figure 2-2-2 End position for trunk flexion with arm position for normal.

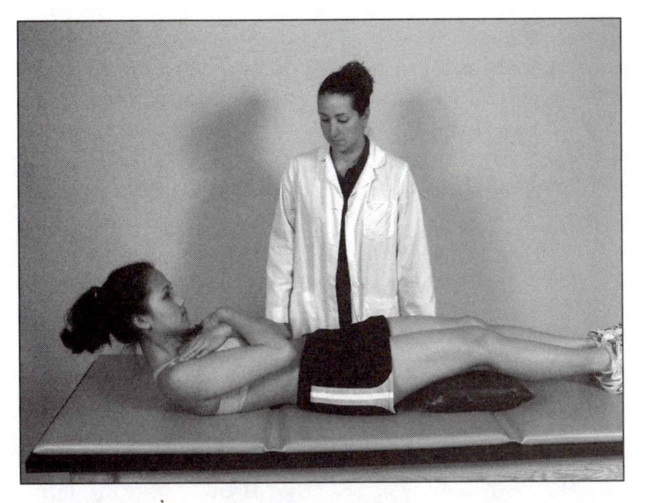

Figure 2-2-3 Arm position for good.

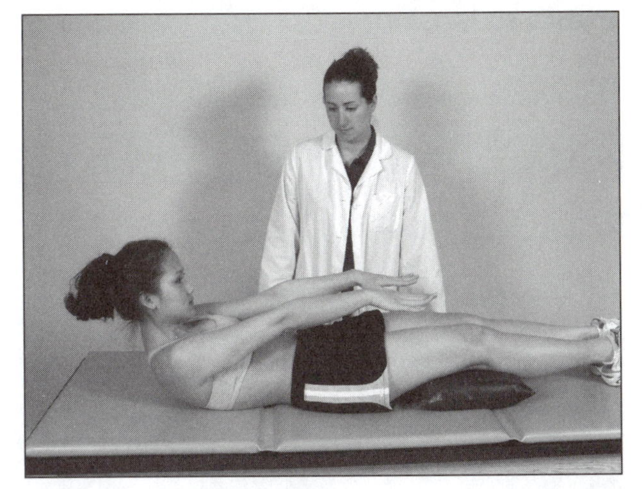

Figure 2-2-4 Arm position for fair.

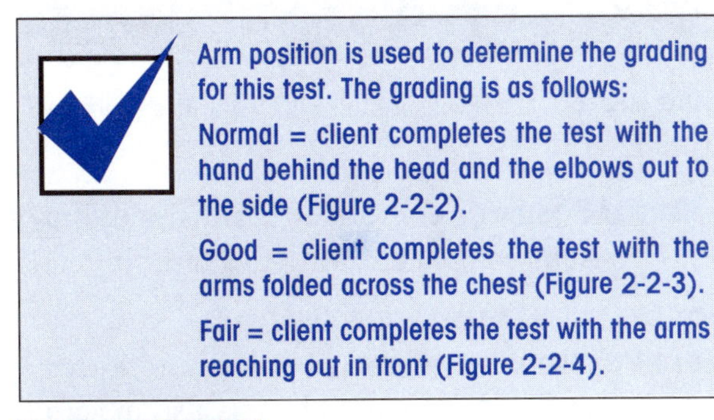

Arm position is used to determine the grading for this test. The grading is as follows:

Normal = client completes the test with the hand behind the head and the elbows out to the side (Figure 2-2-2).

Good = client completes the test with the arms folded across the chest (Figure 2-2-3).

Fair = client completes the test with the arms reaching out in front (Figure 2-2-4).

Poor

Client Position: Starting—client is supine with legs supported under the knees for slight knee flexion. Arms are at the side.

Motion—client moves in the direction of trunk flexion while the arms follow by the sides.

Therapist Position: There is no stabilization or resistance applied during this test.

Alternate Test

Client Position: Starting—client is supine with arms above head or across chest. Hips are at 90 degrees of flexion with knee extension. Back should be firm against the table (Figure 2-2-1a).

Motion—client slowly lowers the legs while maintaining the back against the table.

Leg position determines the grading as follows:

Normal = client can slowly lower the legs to the table while maintaining the back against the table.

Good= client can slowly lower the legs to a 30 degree angle from the table while maintaining the back against the table.

Fair = client can slowly lower the legs to a 60 degree angle from the table while maintaining the back against the table (Figure 2-2-4a).

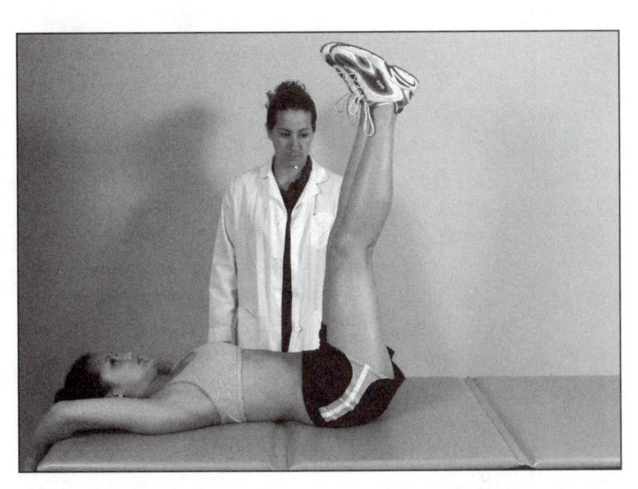

Figure 2-2-1a Alternate start position for trunk flexion.

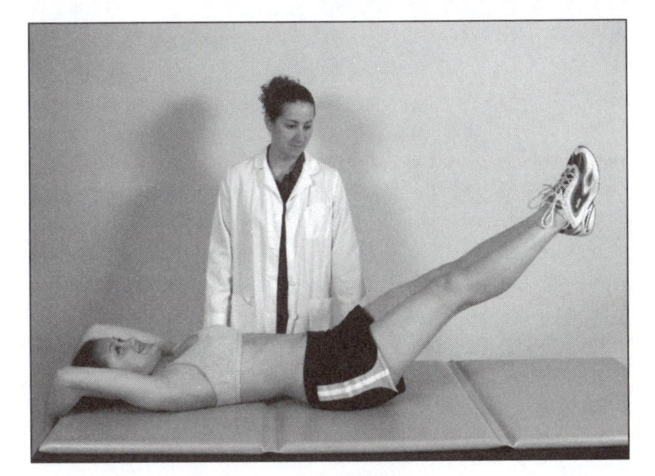

Figure 2-2-4a Alternate end position for fair.

Trunk: *extension*

The trunk extensors include the following muscles: erector spinae, interspinales, and intertransversarii, multifidi, and semispinales thoracis.

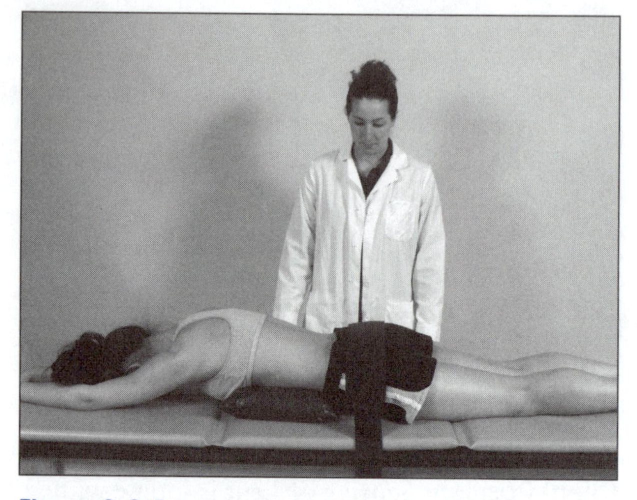

Figure 2-2-5 Start position for trunk extension.

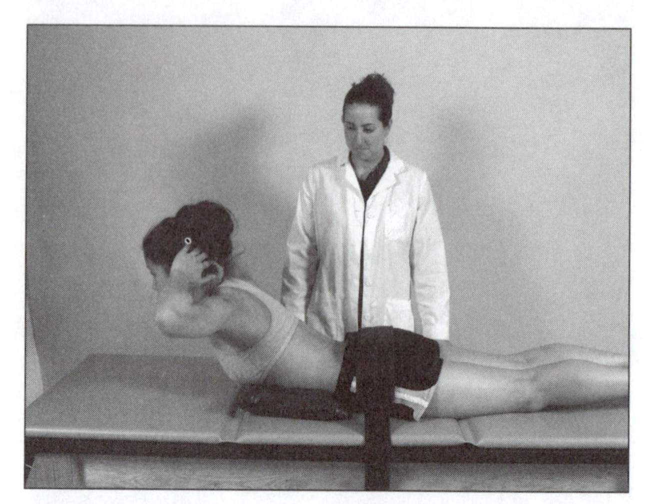

Figure 2-2-6 End position for trunk extension with arm position for normal.

Normal, Good, Fair

Client Position: Starting—client is prone with a pillow under the abdomen. (There is a strap across the pelvis for stabilization) (Figure 2-2-5).

Motion—client moves in the direction of trunk extension (Figure 2-2-6).

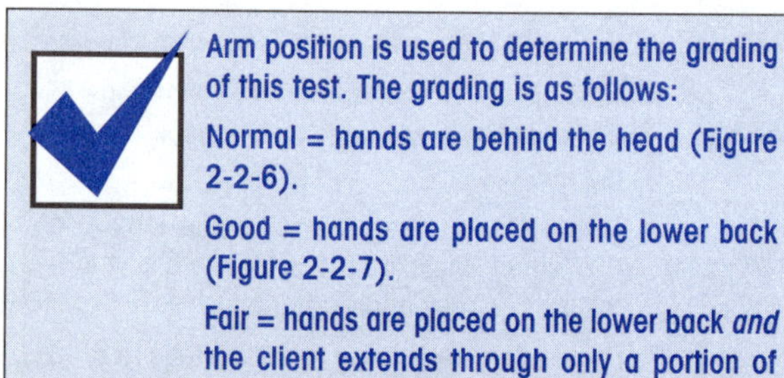

Arm position is used to determine the grading of this test. The grading is as follows:

Normal = hands are behind the head (Figure 2-2-6).

Good = hands are placed on the lower back (Figure 2-2-7).

Fair = hands are placed on the lower back *and* the client extends through only a portion of the motion (Figure 2-2-8).

Therapist Position: There is no manual stabilization or resistance applied during this test.

Poor

Client Position: Starting—client is prone with a pillow under the abdomen. (There is a strap across the pelvis for stabilization.) Arms are at the side.

Motion—client moves in the direction of trunk extension as arms follow.

Therapist Position: There is no manual stabilization or resistance applied during this test.

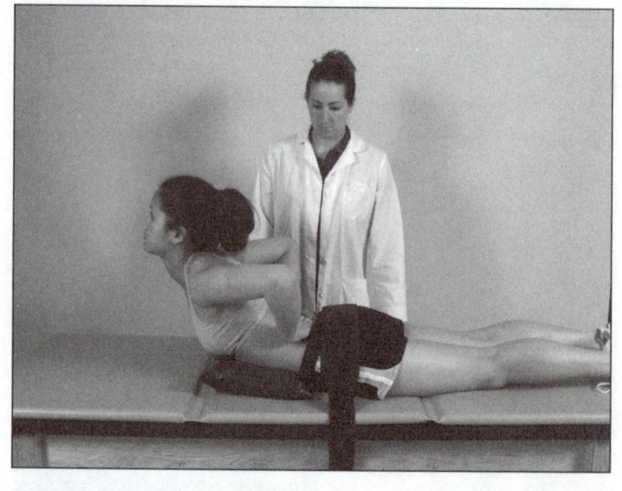

Figure 2-2-7 Arm position for good.

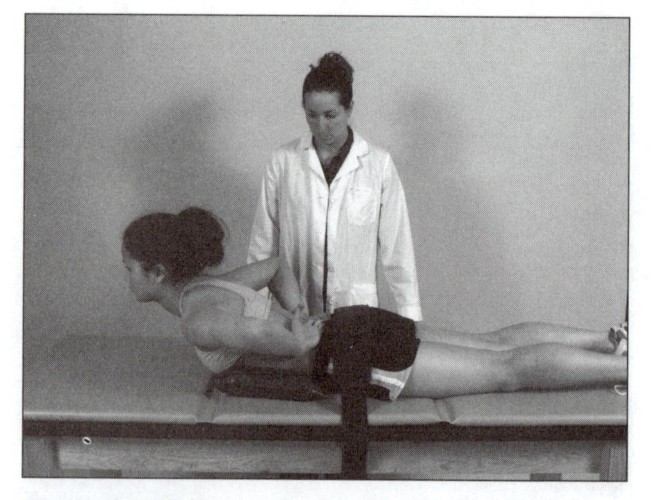

Figure 2-2-8 Arm position for fair.

Trunk: *oblique rotation*

The trunk oblique rotators include the following muscles: external oblique, internal oblique, and rectus abdominis.

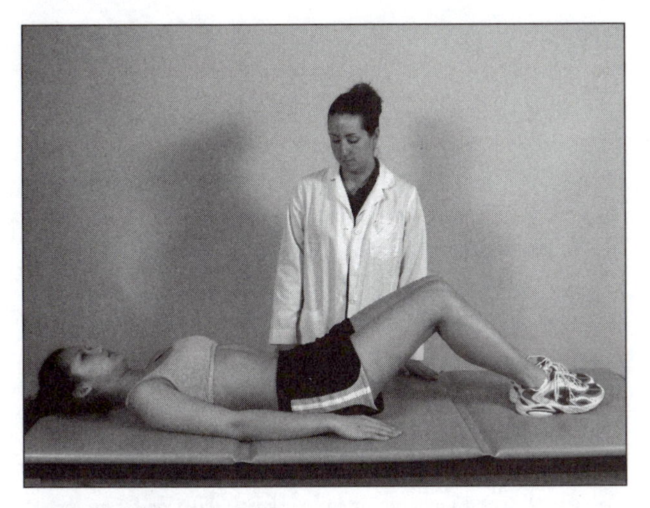

Figure 2-2-9 Start position for trunk oblique flexion.

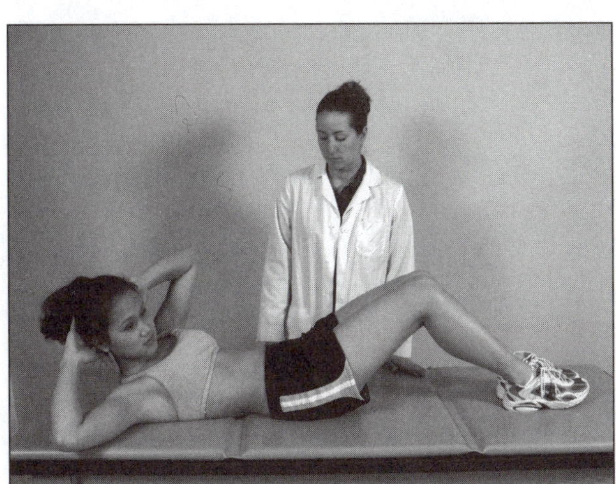

Figure 2-2-10 End position for trunk oblique flexion with arm position for normal.

Normal, Good, Fair

Client Position: Starting—client is supine with the knees flexed (Figure 2-2-9).

Motion—client moves in the direction of trunk flexion and rotation (Figure 2-2-10).

Therapist Position: Stabilize at the client's feet. No resistance is applied during this test.

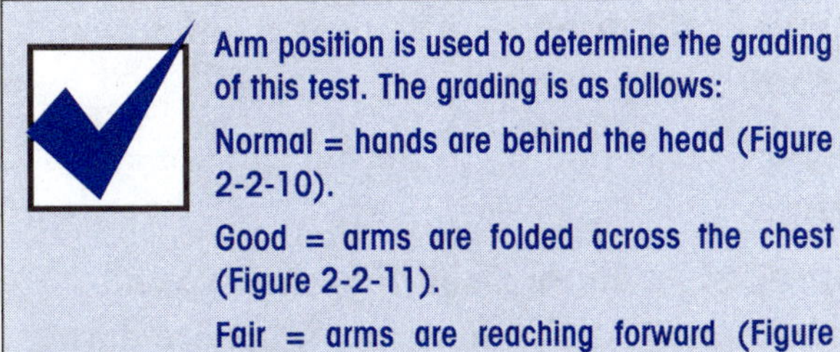

Arm position is used to determine the grading of this test. The grading is as follows:

Normal = hands are behind the head (Figure 2-2-10).

Good = arms are folded across the chest (Figure 2-2-11).

Fair = arms are reaching forward (Figure 2-2-12).

Poor

Client Position: Starting—client is sitting with arms at the side.

Motion—client moves in the direction of trunk flexion and rotation

Therapist Position: There is no stabilization or resistance applied during this test.

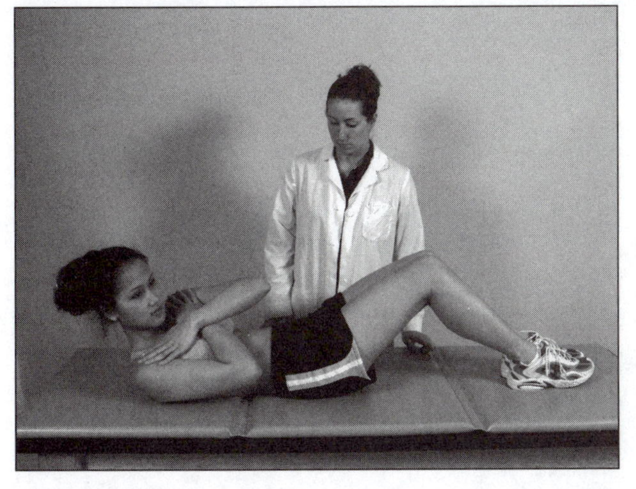

Figure 2-2-11 Arm position for good.

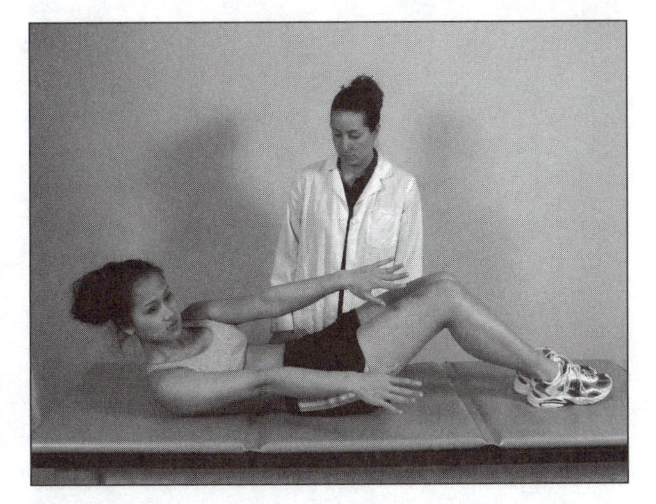

Figure 2-2-12 Arm position for fair.

Trunk: *lateral flexion*

The trunk lateral flexors include the following muscles: external oblique, internal oblique, rectus abdominis, and quadratus lumborum.

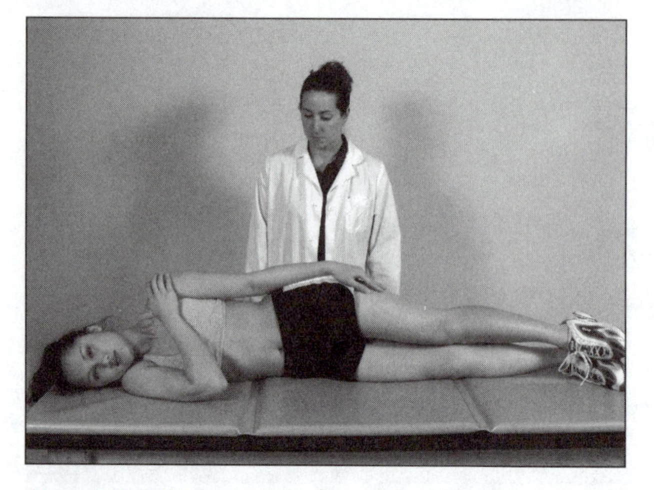

Figure 2-2-13 Start position for trunk lateral flexion.

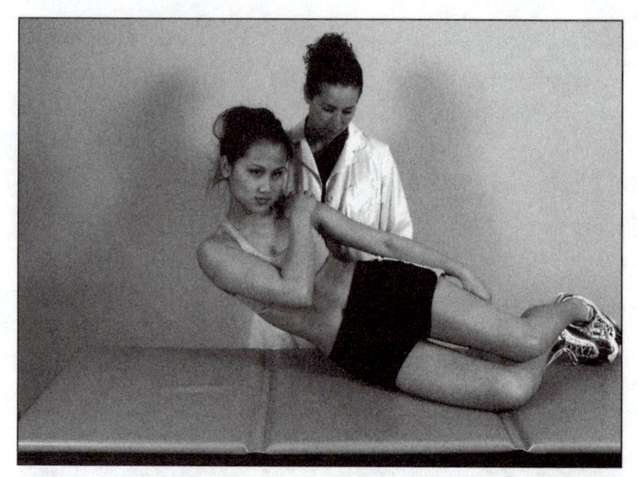

Figure 2-2-14 End position for trunk lateral flexion for normal.

Normal, Good, Fair

Client Position: Starting—client is side-lying on the nontest side. The upper extremity on the test side is at the side. The upper extremity on the nontest side is across the chest (Figure 2-2-13).

Motion—client moves in the direction of trunk lateral flexion (Figure 2-2-14).

Therapist Position: Stabilize at the hips and lower extremities. No resistance is applied during this test.

> The amount of lateral flexion off the mat determines the grading for this test. The grading is as follows:
>
> Normal = lateral flexion through the full range (Figure 2-2-14).
>
> Good = lateral flexion to approximately four inches off the mat (Figure 2-2-15).
>
> Fair = only slight lateral flexion off the mat (Figure 2-2-16).

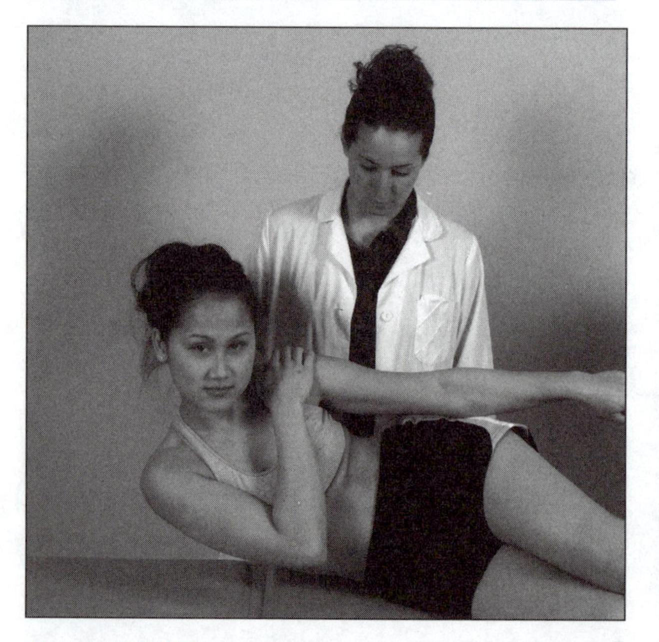

Figure 2-2-15 End position for good.

Poor

Client Position: Starting—client is supine with the arms across the chest.

Motion—client moves in the direction of lateral flexion.

Therapist Position: Stabilize at the hips and lower extremities. No resistance is applied during this test.

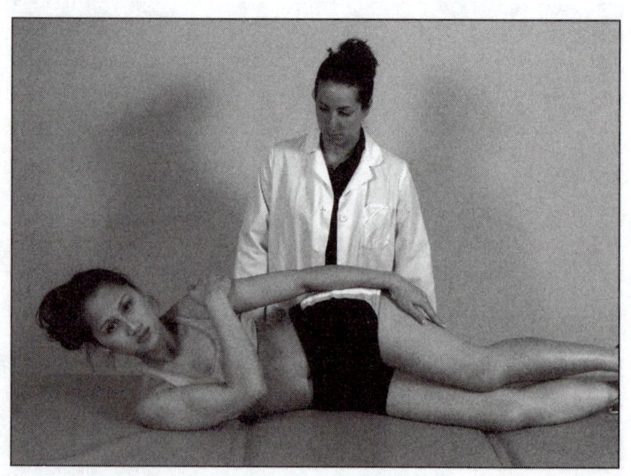

Figure 2-2-16 End position for fair.

Neck: *flexion*

The neck flexors include the following muscles: longus capitus, longus colli, rectus capitis anterior, sternocleidomastoid, and scalenus anterior.

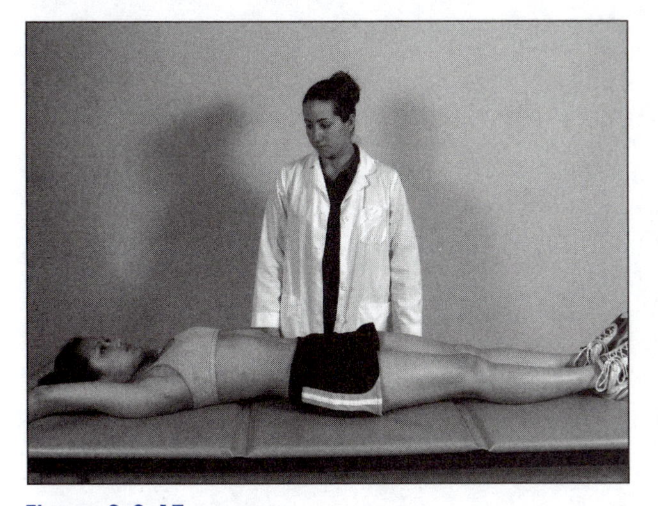

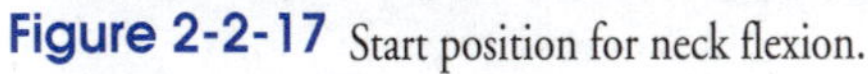

Figure 2-2-17 Start position for neck flexion.

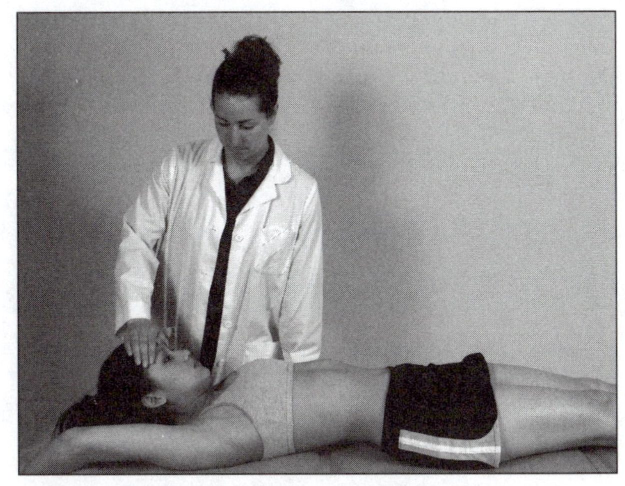

Figure 2-2-18 End position for neck flexion.

Normal, Good, Fair

Client Position: Starting—client is supine with the arms placed over the head (Figure 2-2-17).

Motion—client moves in the direction of neck flexion making sure that the chin is tucked toward the sternum (Figure 2-2-18). If the client is allowed to raise the head directly toward the ceiling, this may be an inaccurate test because of the use of alternate musculature.

Therapist Position: Resistance is applied at the forehead in the direction of neck extension when testing Normal or Good strengths. No resistance is applied when testing Fair strength. No manual stabilization is used during this test.

Poor

This test does not include Poor grading.

Neck: *extension*

The neck extensors include the following muscles: erector spinae, obliquus capitus, rectus capitis posterior, splenius capitus, splenius cervicis, semispinalis cervicis, and semispinalis capitis.

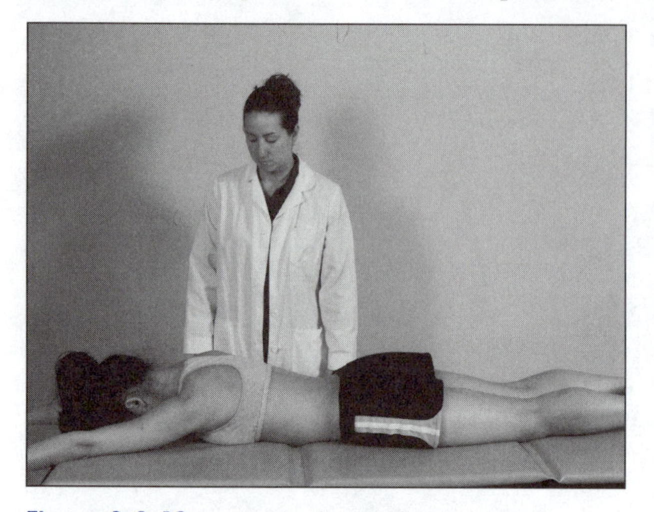
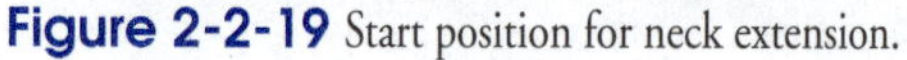

Figure 2-2-19 Start position for neck extension.

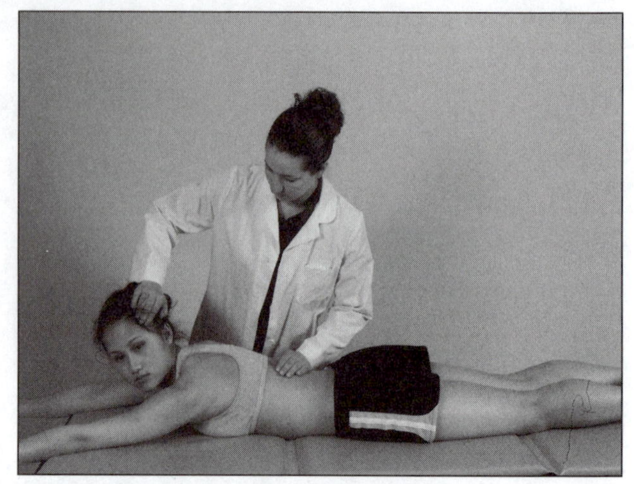

Figure 2-2-20 End position for neck extension.

Normal, Good, Fair

Note that the primary neck extensors rotate and extend the neck simultaneously. For this reason, neck extension is tested with rotation.

Client Position: Starting—client is prone with arms placed on the mat or plinth over the head (Figure 2-2-19).

Motion—client moves in the direction of neck extension while rotating toward the testing side (Figure 2-2-20).

Therapist Position: Stabilize on the posterior thoracic region to avoid compensation. Resistance is applied on the posterior-lateral aspect of the head in the directions of neck flexion and rotation toward the nontest side when testing Normal or Good strengths. No resistance is applied when testing Fair strength.

Poor

This test does not include Poor grading.

SECTION 2-3: Gross Manual Muscle Testing of the Scapula and Shoulder Complex

Listed after each action in this section are the muscles which act to produce that movement. If deficits are noted during gross manual muscle testing, and isolated manual muscle testing is appropriate, the procedures for the isolated manual muscle testing of these muscles are found in Section 3-3 of this manual.

Scapula: *elevation*

The scapula elevators include the following muscles: levator scapulae and upper trapezius.

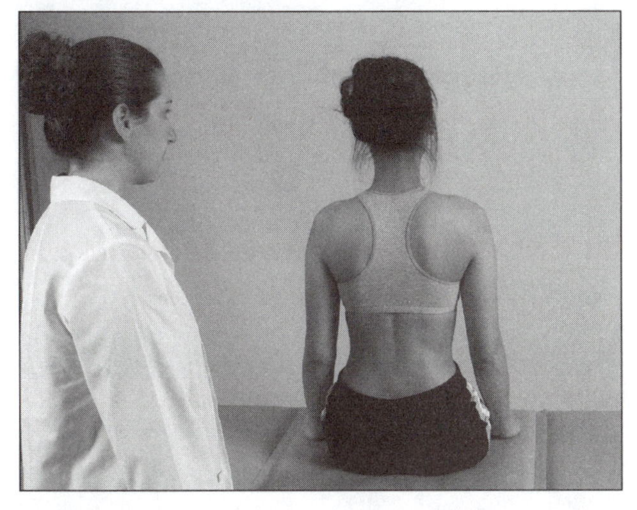

Figure 2-3-1 Start position for scapular elevation.

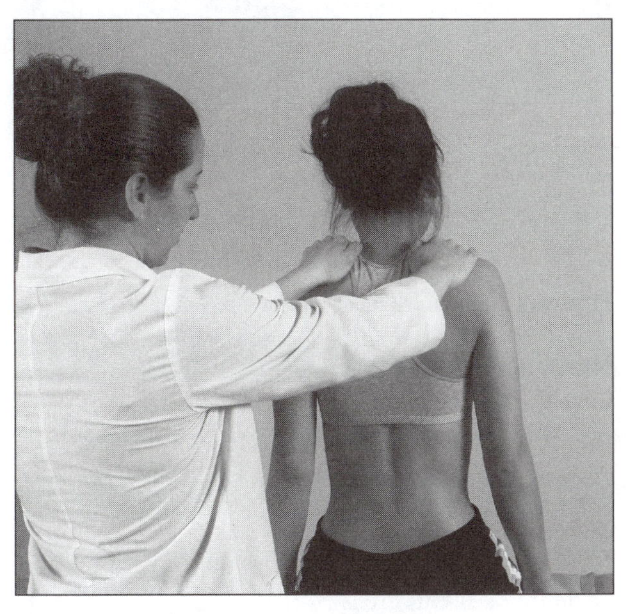

Figure 2-3-2 End position for scapular elevation.

Normal, Good, Fair

Client Position: Starting—client is sitting or standing with both upper extremities at the side (Figure 2-3-1).

Motion—client moves the scapula in the direction of elevation (Figure 2-3-2).

Therapist Position: Stabilize at the opposite shoulder. Resistance is applied on the superior and lateral shoulder in the direction of scapula depression when testing Normal or Good strengths. No resistance is applied when testing Fair strength.

Both scapulae are often tested simultaneously for elevation to help eliminate trunk motion.

Poor

Client Position: Starting—client is supine or prone with both upper extremities at the side.

Motion—client moves the scapula in the direction of elevation.

Therapist Position: Stabilize at the opposite shoulder. No resistance is applied when testing in the gravity-eliminated position.

Scapula: *depression*

The scapula depressors include the following muscles: lower trapezius.

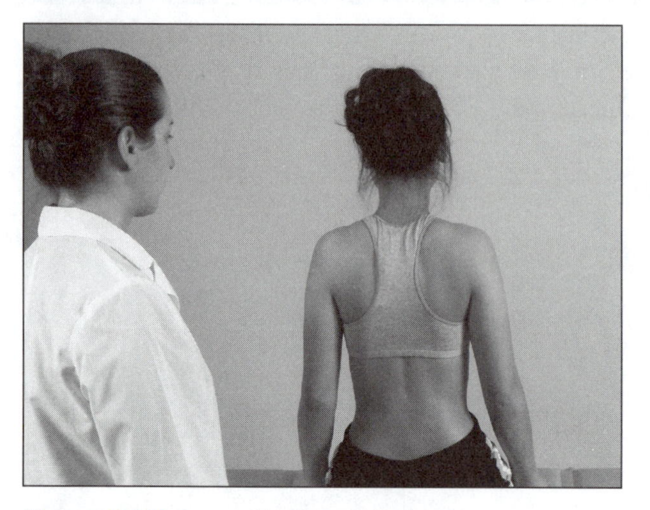

Figure 2-3-3 Start position for scapular depression.

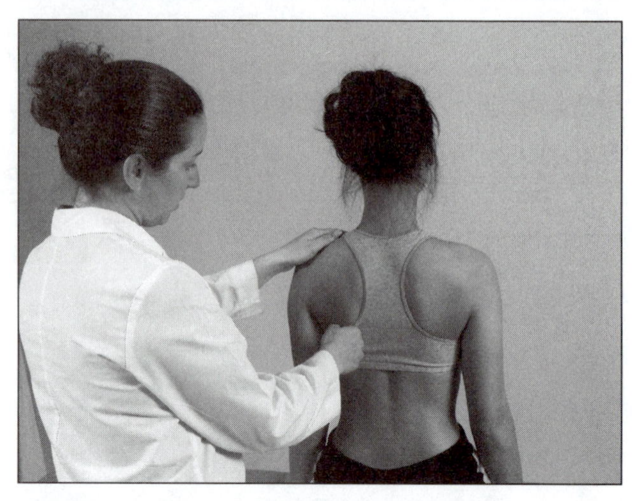

Figure 2-3-4 End position for scapular depression.

Normal, Good, Fair

Client Position: Starting—client is sitting or standing with both upper extremities at the side and the scapula is in neutral to slight elevation (Figure 2-3-3).

Motion—client moves the scapula in the direction of depression (Figure 2-3-4).

Therapist Position: Stabilize at the shoulder. Resistance is applied at the scapula inferior angle in the direction of scapula elevation when testing Normal or Good strengths. No resistance is applied when testing Fair strength.

Poor

Client Position: Starting—client is supine or prone with both upper extremities at the side.

Motion—client moves the scapula in the direction of depression.

Therapist Position: Stabilize at the shoulder. No resistance is applied when testing in the gravity-eliminated position.

Both scapulae are often tested simultaneously for depression to avoid trunk motion.

Scapula: *adduction*

The scapula adductors include the following muscles: middle trapezius and rhomboids.

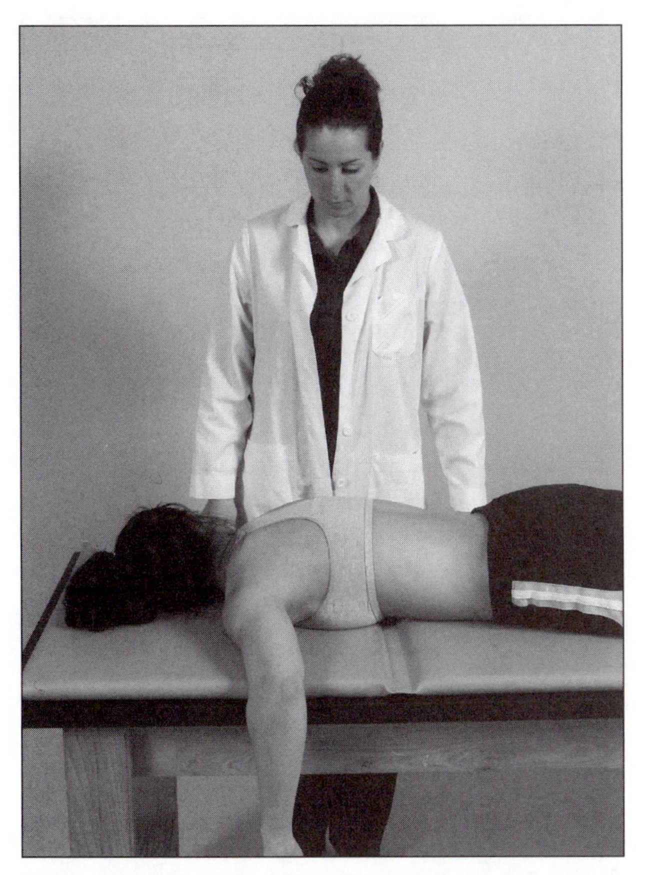

Figure 2-3-5 Start position for scapular adduction.

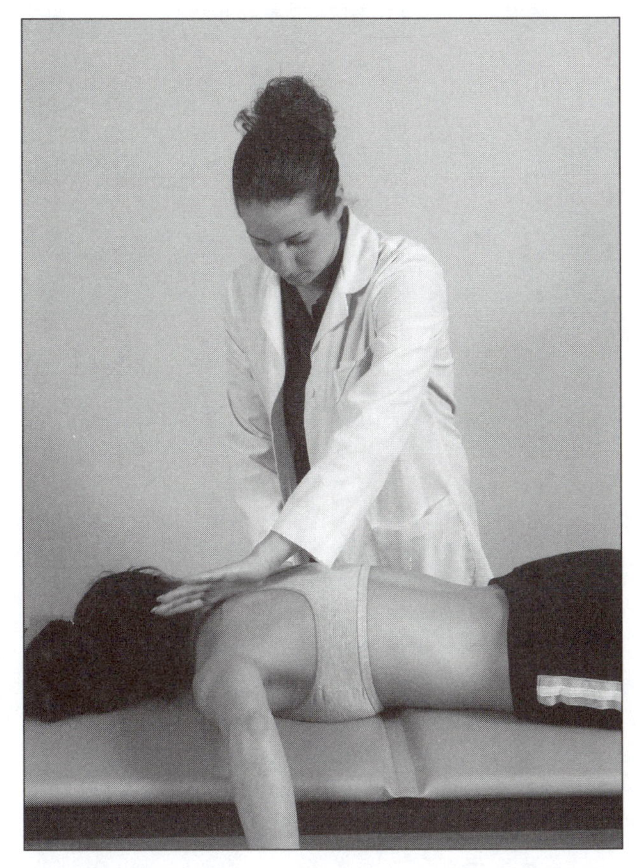

Figure 2-3-6 End position for scapular adduction.

Normal, Good, Fair

Client Position: Starting—client is prone with the testing extremity in 90 degrees of humeral abduction and elbow flexion (Figure 2-3-5).

Motion—client moves the scapula in the direction of adduction while the humerus follows (Figure 2-3-6).

Therapist Position: Stabilize at the opposite shoulder. Resistance is applied on the medial border of the scapula in the direction of scapular abduction when testing Normal or Good strengths. No resistance is applied when testing Fair strength.

Poor

Client Position: Starting—client is sitting or standing with the testing extremity supported at 90 degrees of abduction and elbow flexion.

Motion—client moves the scapula in the direction of adduction as the supported humerus follows.

Therapist Position: Stabilize at the opposite shoulder. No resistance is applied when testing in the gravity-eliminated position.

Scapula: *abduction*

The scapular abductors include the following muscles: serratus anterior and pectoralis minor.

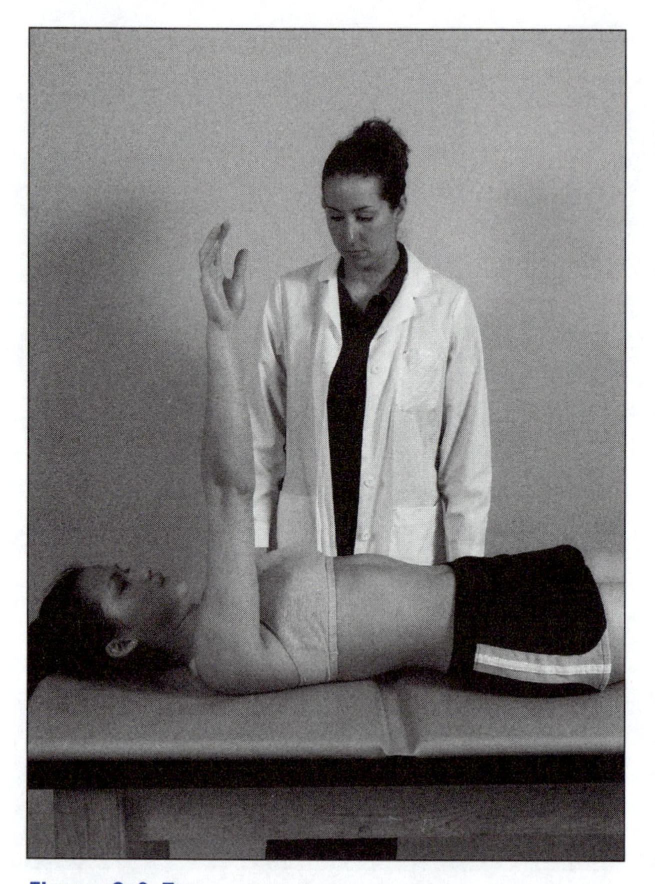

Figure 2-3-7 Start position for scapular abduction.

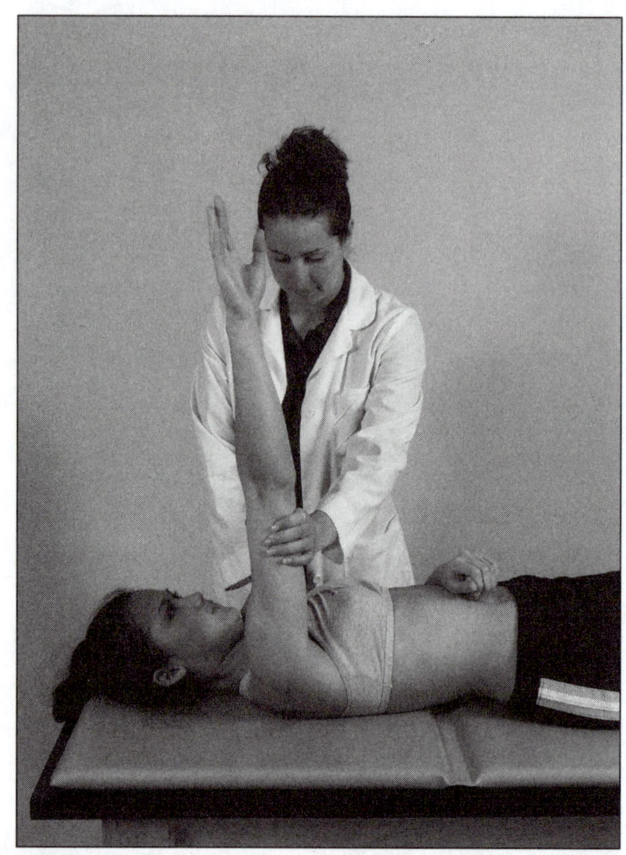

Figure 2-3-8 End position for scapular abduction.

Normal, Good, Fair

Client Position: Starting—client is supine with the testing extremity in 90 degrees of humeral flexion and complete elbow extension (Figure 2-3-7).

Motion—client moves the scapula in the direction of abduction as the humerus follows (reaching toward the ceiling) (Figure 2-3-8).

Therapist Position: Stabilize at the opposite shoulder. Resistance is applied at the proximal humerus in the direction of scapula adduction when testing Normal or Good strengths. No resistance is applied when testing Fair strength.

Poor

Client Position: Starting—client is sitting or standing with the testing extremity supported at 90 degrees of flexion.

Motion—client moves the scapula in the direction of abduction as the humerus follows (reaching forward).

Therapist Position: Stabilize at the opposite shoulder. No resistance is applied when testing in the gravity-eliminated position.

Shoulder: *humeral flexion*

The humeral flexors include the following muscles: coracobrachialis, anterior deltoid, and pectoralis major (clavicular head).

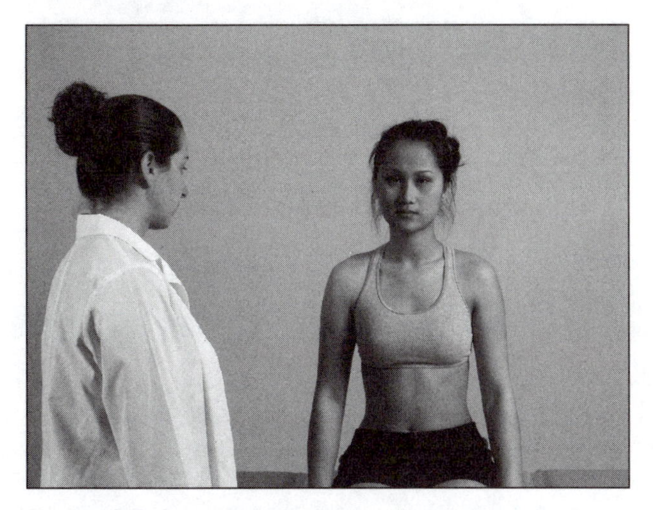

Figure 2-3-9 Start position for humeral flexion.

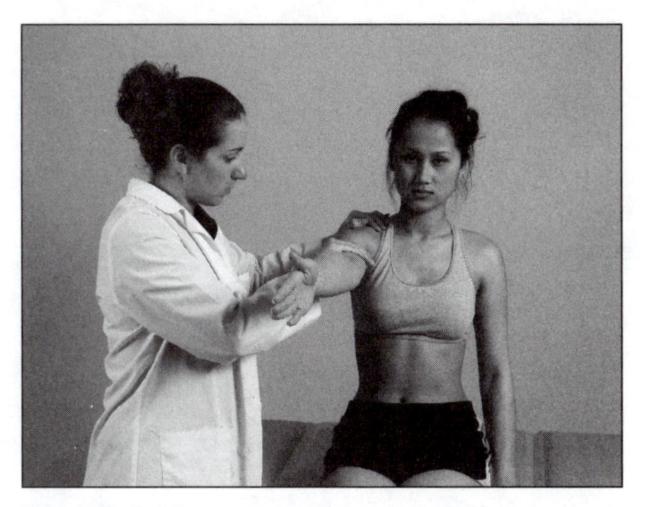

Figure 2-3-10 End position for humeral flexion.

Normal, Good, Fair

Client Position: Starting—client is sitting or standing with the testing extremity in 0 degrees of humeral flexion. The elbow is slightly flexed and the forearm is pronated (Figure 2-3-9).

Motion—client moves the extremity in the direction of humeral flexion (Figure 2-3-10).

Therapist Position: Stabilize the shoulder to avoid scapular compensation. Resistance is applied at the humerus, in the direction of humeral extension when testing Normal or Good strengths. No resistance is applied when testing Fair strength.

Poor

Client Position: Starting—client is lying on his/her side with the testing extremity positioned at the client's side, supported by a powder board or the therapist.

Motion—client moves the testing extremity in the direction of humeral flexion.

Therapist Position: Stabilize at the shoulder to avoid scapular compensation. Support the testing extremity to eliminate gravity; however, do not assist the motion. No resistance is applied when testing in the gravity-eliminated position.

Shoulder: *humeral extension/hyperextension*

The humeral extensors include the following muscles: teres major, latissimus dorsi, pectoralis major (sternal head), and posterior deltoid.

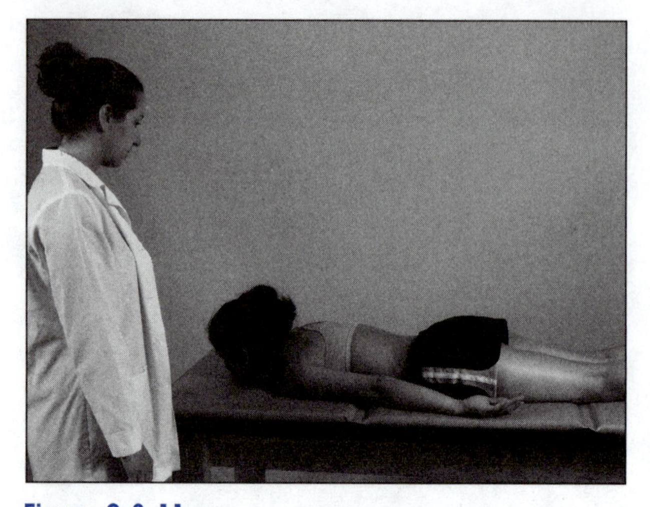

Figure 2-3-11 Start position for humeral extension/hyperextension.

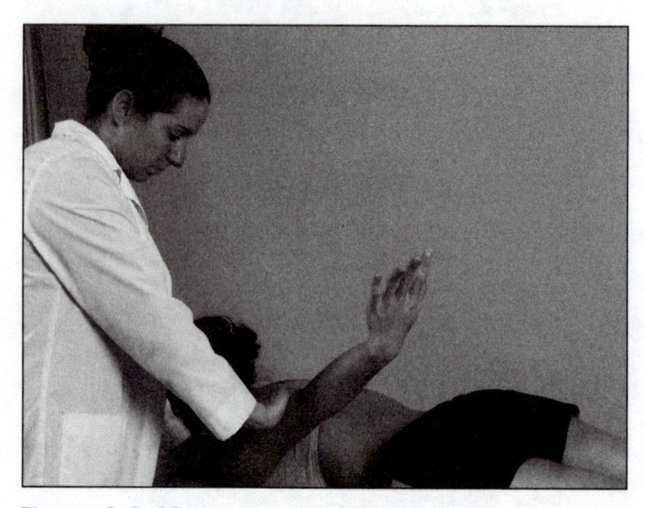

Figure 2-3-12 End position for humeral extension/hyperextension.

Normal, Good, Fair

Client Position: Starting—client is prone with the testing extremity at the side and in full humeral internal rotation (palm facing toward the ceiling) (Figure 2-3-11).

Motion—client moves the testing extremity in the direction of humeral hyperextension (Figure 2-3-12).

Therapist Position: Stabilize at the scapula to avoid compensation of scapular elevation. Resistance is applied at the proximal humerus in the direction of humeral flexion when testing Normal or Good strengths. No resistance is applied when testing Fair strength.

Poor

Client Position: Starting—client is lying on his/her side with the testing extremity positioned in neutral, at the client's side, and supported by the therapist.

Motion—Client moves the testing extremity in the direction of humeral extension.

Therapist Position: Stabilize at the scapula to avoid compensation of scapular elevation. Support the testing extremity to eliminate gravity; however, do not assist the motion. No resistance is applied when testing in the gravity-eliminated position.

Shoulder: ***humeral abduction***

The humeral abductors include the following muscles: middle deltoid and supraspinatus.

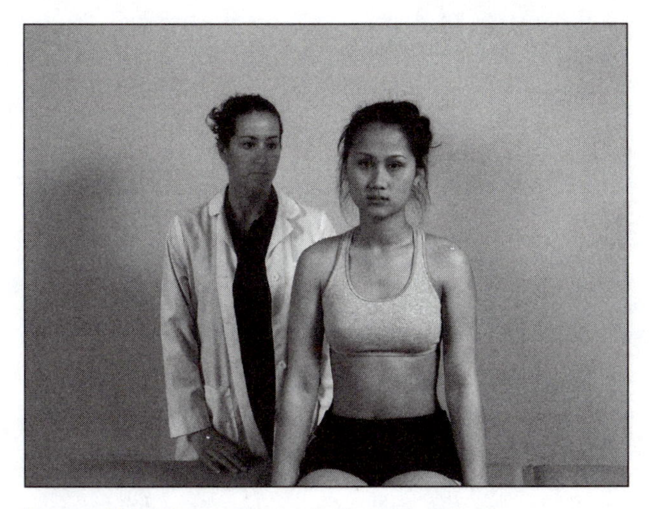

Figure 2-3-13 Start position for humeral abduction.

Figure 2-3-14 End position for humeral abduction.

Normal, Good, Fair

Client Position: Starting—client is sitting or standing with the testing extremity at the side (Figure 2-3-13).

Motion—client moves the testing extremity in the direction of humeral abduction (Figure 2-3-14).

Therapist Position: Stabilize at the shoulder to avoid compensation of scapular elevation. Resistance is applied at the humerus in the direction of humeral adduction when testing Normal or Good strengths. No resistance is applied when testing Fair strength.

Poor

Client Position: Starting—client is supine with the testing extremity at the side and supported by the therapist.

Motion—client moves the testing extremity in the direction of humeral abduction.

Therapist Position: Stabilize at the shoulder to avoid compensation of scapular elevation. Support the testing extremity to eliminate gravity; however, do not assist the motion. No resistance is applied when testing in the gravity-eliminated position.

Shoulder: *humeral adduction*

The humeral adductors include the following muscles: pectoralis major (clavicular head), teres major, and latissimus dorsi.

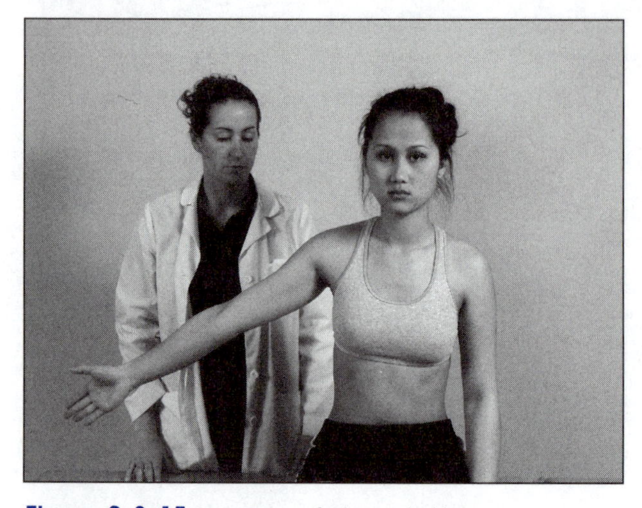

Figure 2-3-15 Start position for humeral adduction.

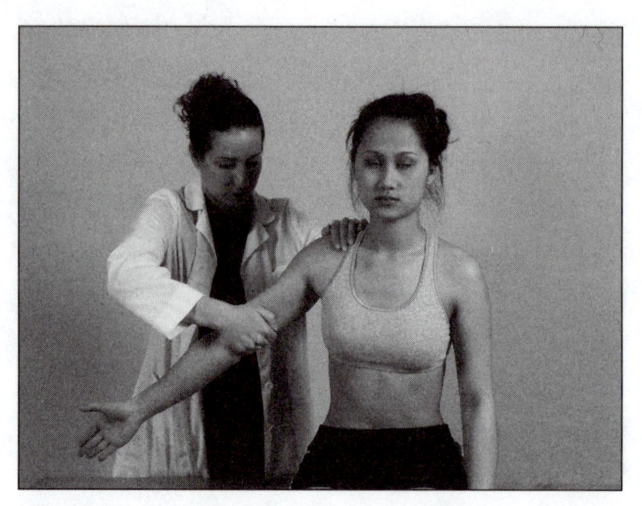

Figure 2-3-16 End position for humeral adduction.

Normal, Good, Fair

Client Position: Starting—client is sitting or standing with the testing extremity at 30 degrees humeral abduction (Figure 2-3-15).

Motion—client moves the testing extremity in the direction of humeral adduction (Figure 2-3-16).

Therapist Position: Stabilize at the shoulder to avoid compensation of scapular depression. Resistance is applied at the humerus in the direction of abduction when testing Normal or Good strengths. No resistance is applied when testing Fair strength.

Poor

Client Position: Starting—client is supine with the testing extremity at 30 degrees humeral abduction, and supported by the therapist.

Motion—client moves the testing extremity in the direction of humeral adduction.

Therapist Position: Stabilize at the shoulder to avoid compensation of scapular depression. Support the testing extremity to eliminate gravity; however, do not assist the motion. No resistance is applied when testing in the gravity-eliminated position.

Shoulder: *humeral external rotation*

The humeral external rotators include the following muscles: teres minor, infraspinatus, and posterior deltoid.

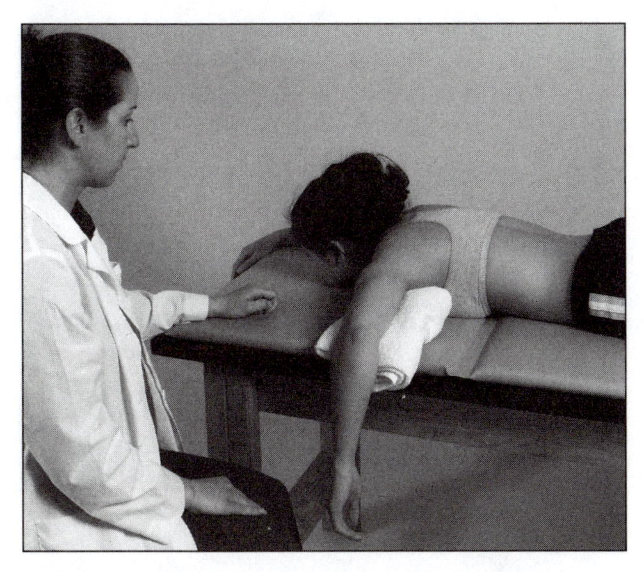

Figure 2-3-17 Start position for humeral external rotation.

Normal, Good, Fair

Client Position: Starting—client is prone with the testing extremity in 90 degrees of humeral abduction. The elbow is off the plinth and flexed to 90 degrees. A support towel is placed under the humerus (Figure 2-3-17).

Motion—client moves the testing extremity in the direction of humeral external rotation (Figure 2-3-18).

Therapist Position: Stabilize at the scapula to avoid compensation. Resistance is applied at the forearm in the direction of humeral internal rotation when testing Normal or Good strengths. No resistance is applied when testing Fair strength.

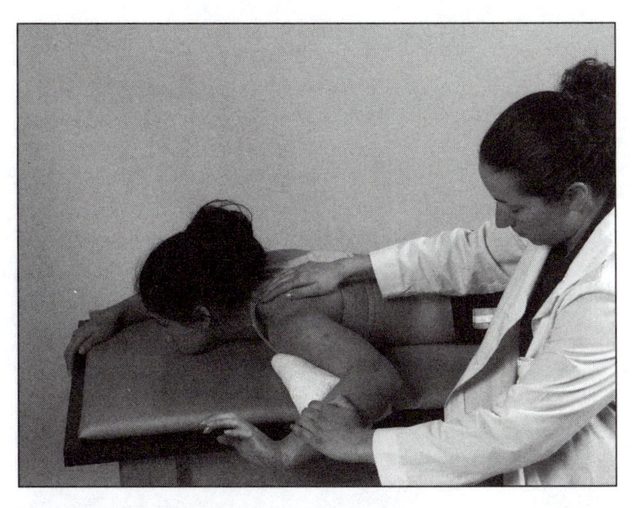

Figure 2-3-18 End position for humeral external rotation.

Poor

Client Position: Starting—client is prone with the testing extremity in neutral, and off the plinth (fingers point toward floor).

Motion—client moves the testing extremity in the direction of humeral external rotation (LUE = counter-clockwise, RUE = clockwise).

Therapist Position: Stabilize at the scapula to avoid compensation. No resistance is applied when testing in the gravity-eliminated position.

You must observe humeral rotation, not just forearm supination.

Alternate Position

Client Position: Starting—client is sitting with the testing extremity in humeral adduction, and elbow flexion to 90 degrees.

Motion—client moves the testing extremity in the direction of humeral external rotation (hands move away from the body).

Shoulder: *humeral internal rotation*

The humeral internal rotators include the following muscles: subscapularis, pectoralis major, latissimus dorsi, teres major, and anterior deltoid.

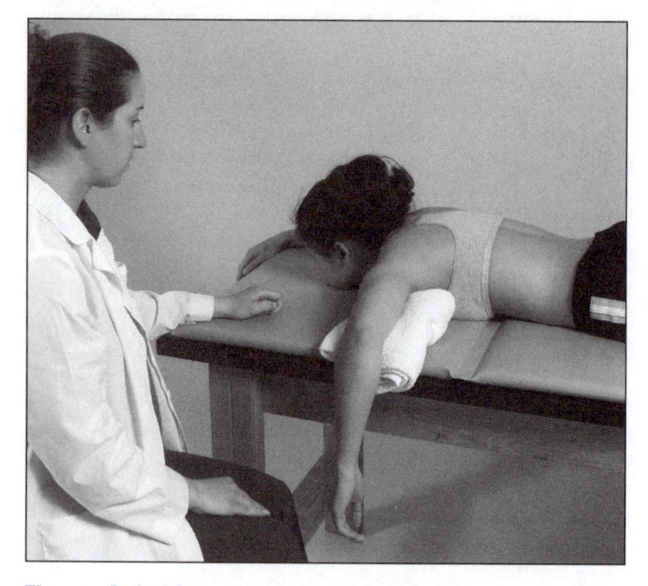

Figure 2-3-19 Start position for humeral internal rotation.

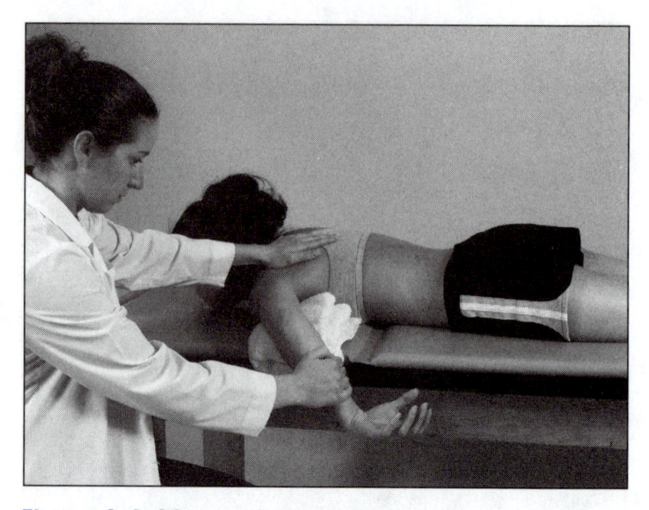

Figure 2-3-20 End position for humeral internal rotation.

Normal, Good, Fair

Client Position: Starting—client is prone with the testing extremity in 90 degrees of humeral abduction. The elbow is off the plinth and flexed to 90 degrees. A support towel is placed under the humerus (Figure 2-3-19).

Motion—client moves the testing extremity in the direction of humeral internal rotation (Figure 2-3-20).

Therapist Position: Stabilize at the scapula to avoid compensation. Resistance is applied at the forearm in the direction of humeral external rotation when testing Normal or Good strengths. No resistance is applied when testing Fair strength.

Poor

Client Position: Starting—client is prone with the testing extremity in neutral and off the plinth (fingers point toward floor).

Motion—client moves the testing extremity in the direction of humeral internal rotation (LUE = clockwise, RUE = counter-clockwise).

Therapist Position: Stabilize at the scapula to avoid compensation. No resistance is applied when testing in the gravity-eliminated position.

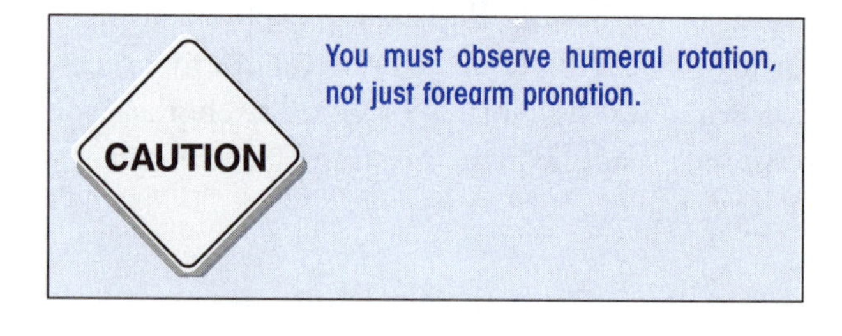

Alternate Position

Client Position: Starting—client is sitting with the testing extremity in humeral adduction, and elbow flexion to 90 degrees.

Motion—client moves the testing extremity in the direction of humeral internal rotation (hand moves toward the body).

Shoulder: *humeral horizontal abduction*

The humeral horizontal abductors include the following muscles: posterior deltoid, teres minor, and infraspinatus.

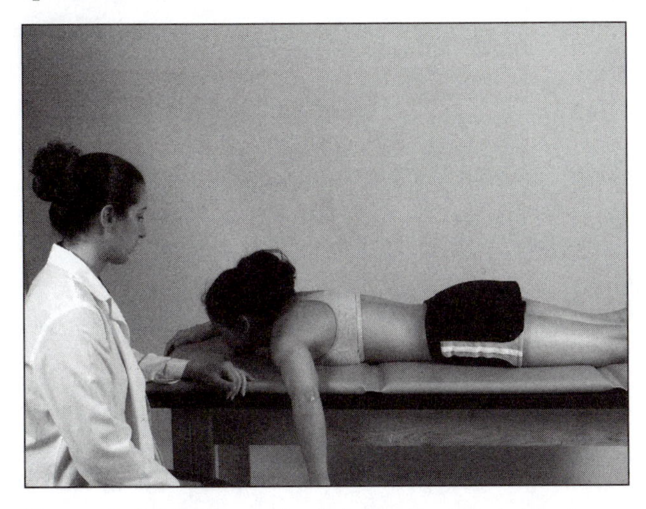

Figure 2-3-21 Start position for humeral horizontal abduction.

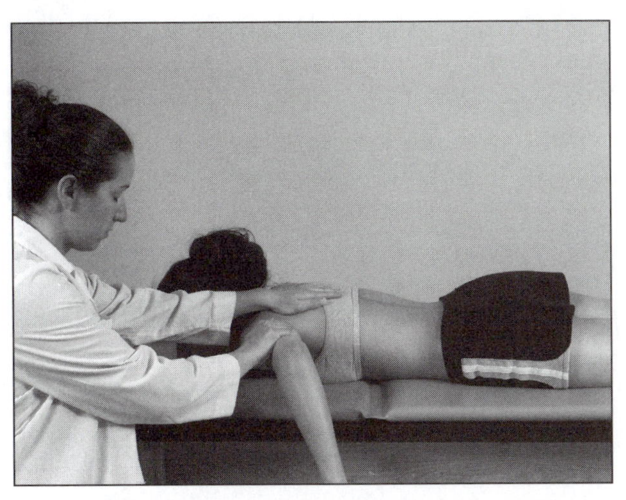

Figure 2-3-22 End position for humeral horizontal abduction.

Normal, Good, Fair

Client Position: Starting—client is prone with the testing extremity in 90 degrees of humeral abduction and the elbow flexed to 90 degrees (fingers toward the floor) (Figure 2-3-21).

Motion—client moves the testing extremity in the direction of humeral horizontal abduction (Figure 2-3-22).

Therapist Position: Stabilize at the posterior shoulder/scapula to avoid compensation by the middle trapezius and rhomboids. Resistance is applied at the humerus when testing Normal or Good strengths. No resistance is applied when testing Fair strength.

Poor

Client Position: Starting—client is sitting with the testing extremity at 90 degrees humeral abduction and 90 degrees elbow flexion, supported on a table or by the therapist.

Motion—client moves the testing extremity in the direction of humeral horizontal abduction.

Therapist Position: Stabilize at the posterior shoulder/scapula to avoid compensation. Support the extremity to eliminate gravity; however, do not assist the motion. No resistance is applied when testing in the gravity-eliminated position.

Shoulder: *humeral horizontal adduction*

The humeral horizontal adductors include the following muscles: anterior deltoid and pectoralis major (both heads).

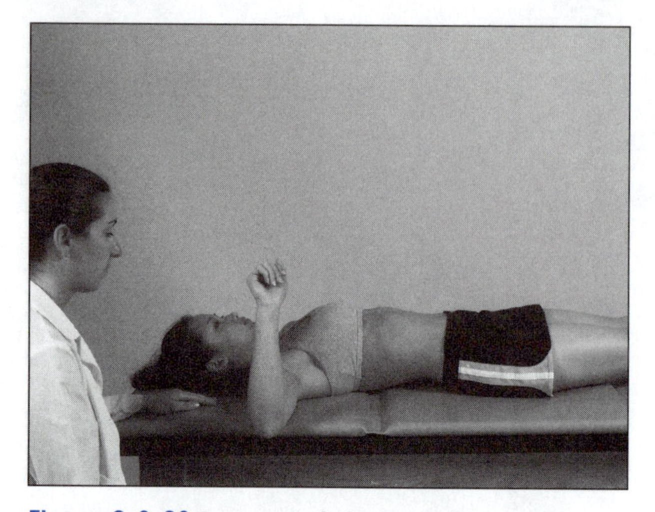

Figure 2-3-23 Start position for humeral horizontal adduction.

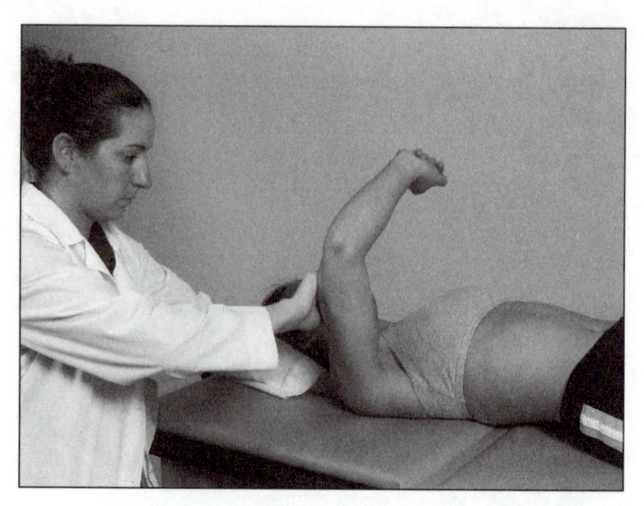

Figure 2-3-24 End position for humeral horizontal adduction.

Normal, Good, Fair

Client Position: Starting—client is supine with the testing extremity in 90 degrees of humeral abduction and elbow flexed to 90 degrees (fingers toward the ceiling) (Figure 2-3-23).

Motion—client moves the testing extremity in the direction of humeral horizontal adduction (Figure 2-3-24).

Therapist Position: Stabilize at the shoulder to avoid compensation. Resistance is applied at the humerus in the direction of horizontal abduction when testing Normal or Good strengths. No resistance is applied when testing Fair strength.

Poor

Client Position: Starting—client is sitting with the testing extremity at 90 degrees humeral abduction and 90 degrees elbow flexion, supported on a table or by therapist.

Motion—client moves the testing extremity in the direction of humeral horizontal adduction.

Therapist Position: Stabilize at the shoulder to avoid compensation. Support the testing extremity to eliminate gravity; however, do not assist the motion. No resistance is applied when testing in the gravity-eliminated position.

SECTION 2-4: Gross Manual Muscle Testing of the Elbow and Forearm

Listed after each action in this section are the muscles which act to produce that movement. If deficits are noted during gross manual muscle testing, and isolated manual muscle testing is appropriate, the procedures for the isolated manual muscle testing of these muscles are found in Section 3-4 of this manual.

Elbow: *flexion*

The elbow flexors include the following muscles: biceps brachii, brachialis, and brachioradialis.

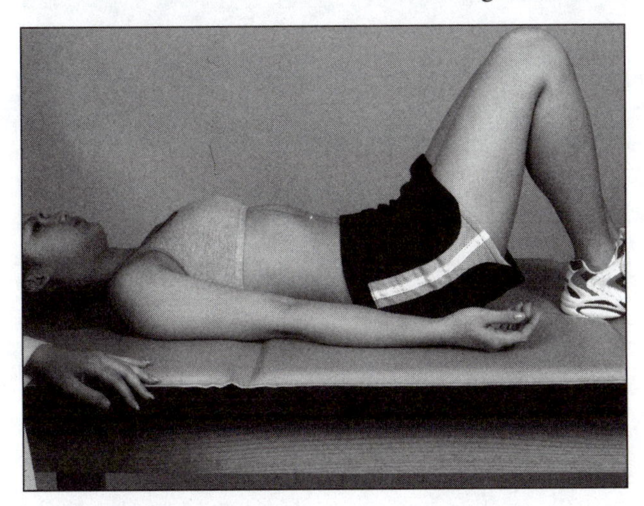

Figure 2-4-1 Start position for elbow flexion.

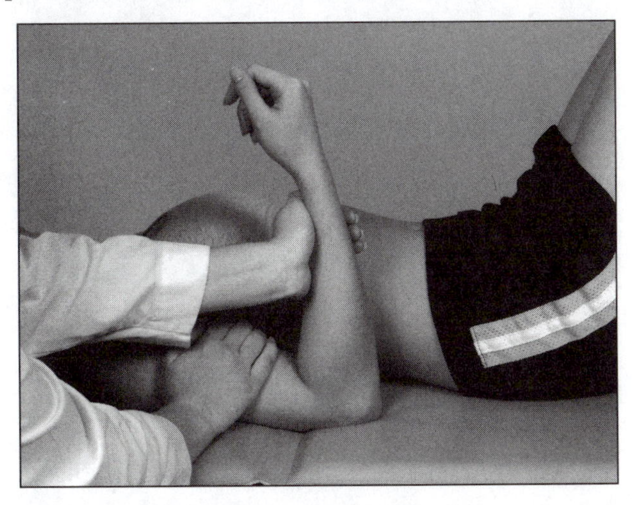

Figure 2-4-2 End position for elbow flexion.

Normal, Good, Fair

Client Position: Starting—client is supine with the knees flexed or sitting. The testing extremity is in humeral adduction, elbow extension, and forearm supination (Figure 2-4-1).

Motion—client moves the testing extremity in the direction of elbow flexion (Figure 2-4-2).

Therapist Position: Stabilize at the humerus to avoid compensation. Resistance is applied at the distal/volar forearm in the direction of elbow extension when testing Normal or Good strengths. No resistance is applied when testing Fair strength.

Poor

Client Position: Starting—client is sitting with the testing extremity at 90 degrees humeral flexion, elbow extension, and the forearm in neutral, supported on a table or by the therapist.

Motion—client moves the testing extremity in the direction of elbow flexion.

Therapist Position: Stabilize at the humerus to avoid compensation. Support the testing extremity to eliminate gravity; however, do not assist the motion. No resistance is applied when testing in the gravity-eliminated position.

Elbow: *extension*

The elbow extensors include the following muscle: triceps and anconeus.

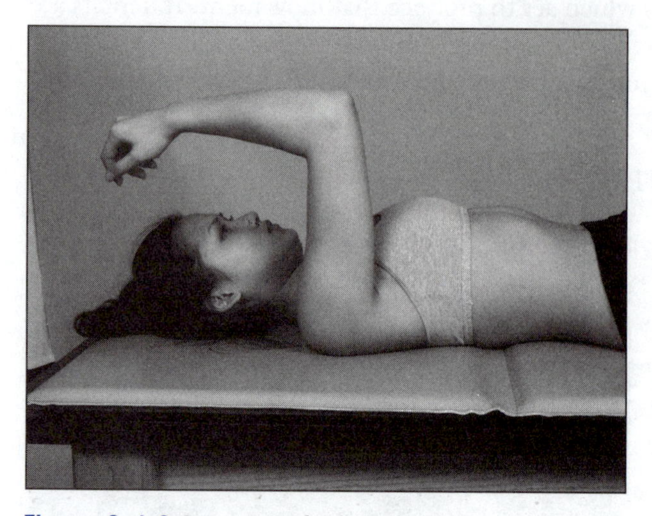

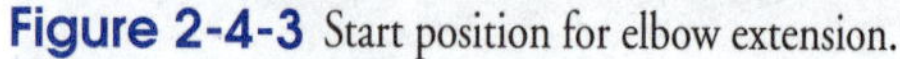

Figure 2-4-3 Start position for elbow extension.

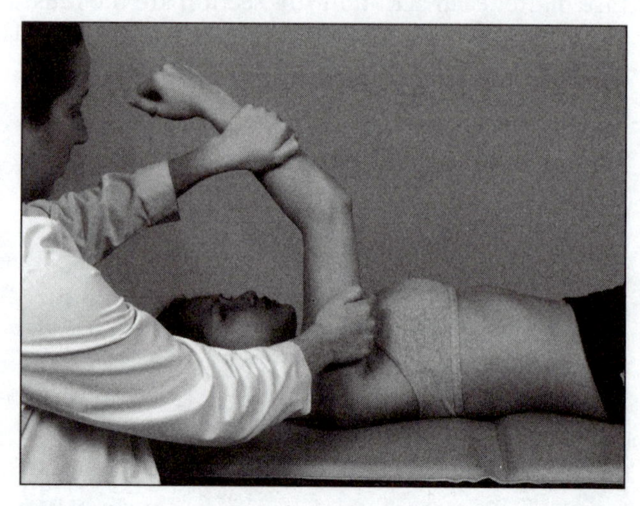

Figure 2-4-4 End position for elbow extension.

Normal, Good, Fair

Client Position: Starting—client is supine with the knees flexed. The testing extremity is at 90 degrees of humeral and elbow flexion (Figure 2-4-3).

Motion—client moves the testing extremity in the direction of elbow extension (Figure 2-4-4).

Therapist Position: Stabilize at the humerus to avoid compensation. Resistance is applied at the distal forearm, in the direction of elbow flexion when testing Normal or Good strengths. No resistance is applied when testing Fair strength.

Poor

Client Position: Starting—client is sitting with the testing extremity at 90 degrees humeral flexion and elbow flexed, supported on a table or by the therapist.

Motion—client moves the testing extremity into elbow extension.

Therapist Position: Stabilize at the humerus to avoid compensation. Support the testing extremity to eliminate gravity; however, do not assist the motion. No resistance is applied when testing in the gravity-eliminated position.

Alternate Position

Client Position: Starting—client is standing or sitting with the testing extremity in 180 degrees of humeral flexion and elbow is flexed.

Forearm: *supination*

The forearm supinators include the following muscles: supinator and biceps brachii.

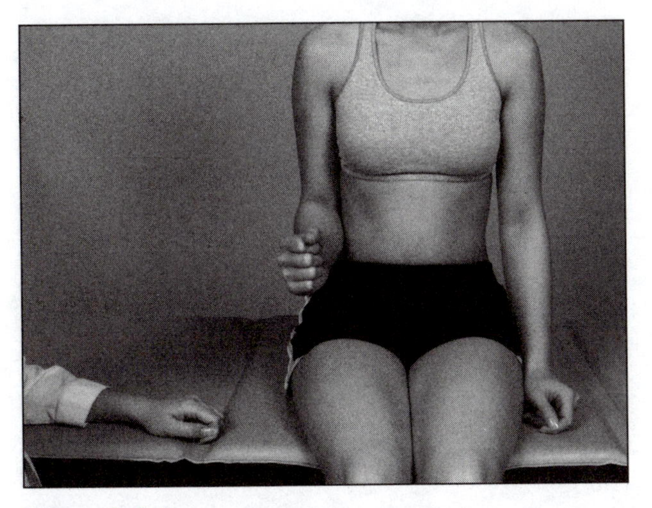

Figure 2-4-5 Start position for forearm supination.

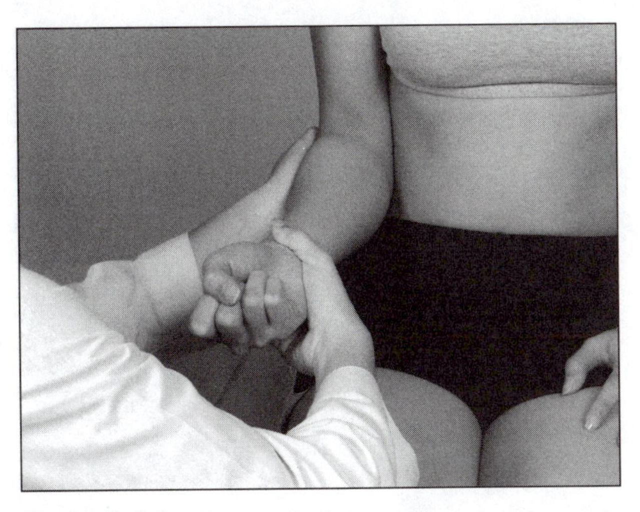

Figure 2-4-6 End position for forearm supination.

Normal, Good, Fair

Client Position: Starting—client is sitting with the testing extremity in humeral adduction, elbow flexed to 90 degrees and forearm in neutral (Figure 2-4-5).

Motion—client moves the testing extremity in the direction of forearm supination (Figure 2-4-6).

Therapist Position: Stabilize at the elbow. Resistance is applied at the distal forearm, in the direction of pronation when testing Normal or Good strengths. No resistance is applied when testing Fair strength.

Poor

Client Position: Starting—client is sitting with the humerus flexed to 90 degrees (elbow placed on table), elbow flexed to 90 degrees (fingers toward ceiling), and the forearm in neutral, supported by the therapist.

Motion—client moves the testing extremity in the direction of forearm supination.

Therapist Position: Stabilize at the forearm to avoid compensation without impeding motion. No resistance is applied when testing in the gravity-eliminated position.

Forearm: *pronation*

The forearm pronators include the following muscles: pronator teres and pronator quadratus.

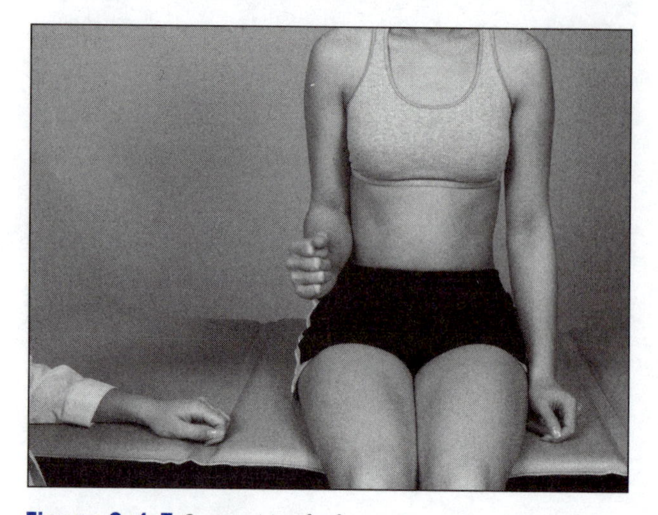

Figure 2-4-7 Start position for forearm pronation.

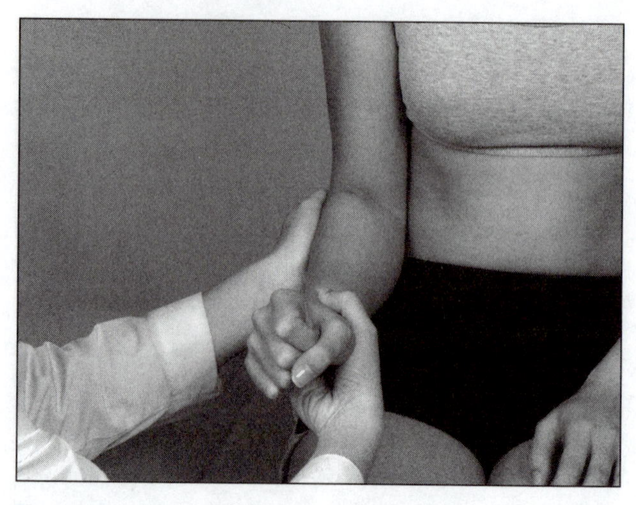

Figure 2-4-8 End position for forearm pronation.

Normal, Good, Fair

Client Position: Starting—client is sitting with the testing extremity in humeral adduction, elbow flexed to 90 degrees and forearm in neutral (Figure 2-4-7).

Motion—client moves the testing extremity in the direction of forearm pronation (Figure 2-4-8).

Therapist Position: Stabilize at the elbow to avoid compensation. Resistance is applied at the distal forearm, in the direction of supination when testing Normal or Good strengths. No resistance is applied when testing Fair strength.

Poor

Client Position: Starting—client is sitting with the humerus flexed to 90 degrees (elbow on the table), elbow flexed to 90 degrees (fingers toward ceiling), and forearm in neutral, supported by the therapist.

Motion—client moves the testing extremity in the direction of forearm pronation.

Therapist Position: Stabilize at the forearm to avoid compensation without impeding motion. No resistance is applied when testing in the gravity-eliminated position.

SECTION 2-5: Gross Manual Muscle Testing of the Wrist and Hand

Listed after each action in this section are the muscles which act to produce that movement. If deficits are noted during gross manual muscle testing, and isolated manual muscle testing is appropriate, the procedures for the isolated manual muscle testing of these muscles are found in Section 3-5 of this manual.

Wrist: *flexion*

The wrist flexors include flexor carpi ulnaris, flexor carpi radialis, and the palmaris longus.

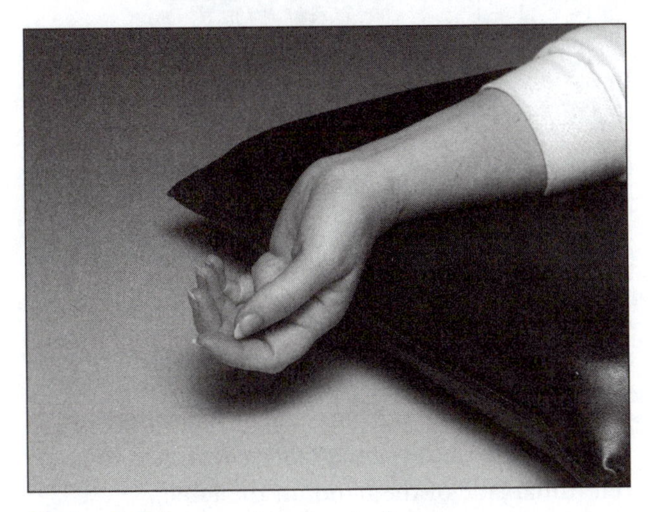

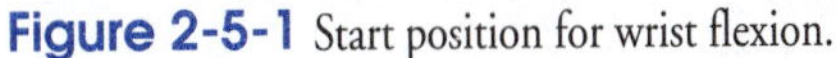

Figure 2-5-1 Start position for wrist flexion.

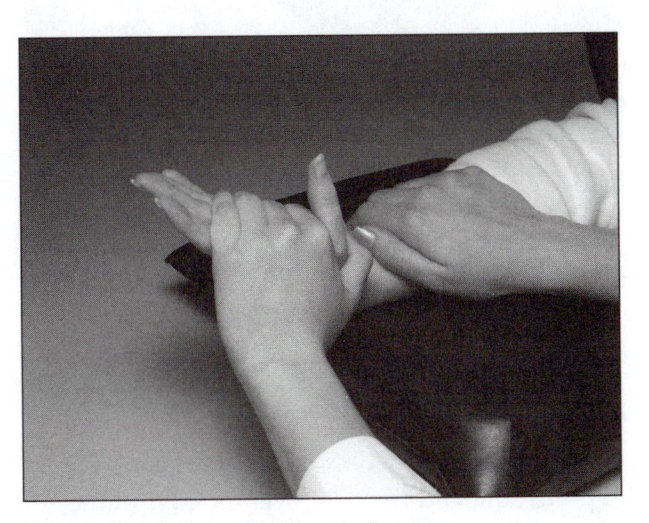

Figure 2-5-2 End position for wrist flexion.

Normal, Good, Fair

Client Position: Starting—client is sitting with the testing extremity on a table in forearm supination, and the wrist over the edge of the table in slight extension (Figure 2-5-1).

Motion—client moves the testing extremity in the direction of wrist flexion (Figure 2-5-2).

Therapist Position: Stabilize at the distal forearm to avoid compensation. Resistance is applied to the palm of the hand in the direction of wrist extension when testing Normal or Good strengths. No resistance is applied when testing Fair strength.

Poor

Client Position: Starting—client is sitting with the testing extremity on a table, forearm is in neutral (ulnar side of the hand on the table).

Motion—client moves the testing extremity in the direction of wrist flexion.

Therapist Position: Stabilize at the distal forearm to avoid compensation. No resistance is applied when testing in the gravity-eliminated position.

Wrist: *extension*

The wrist extensors include extensor carpi radialis longus, extensor carpi radialis brevis, and extensor carpi ulnaris.

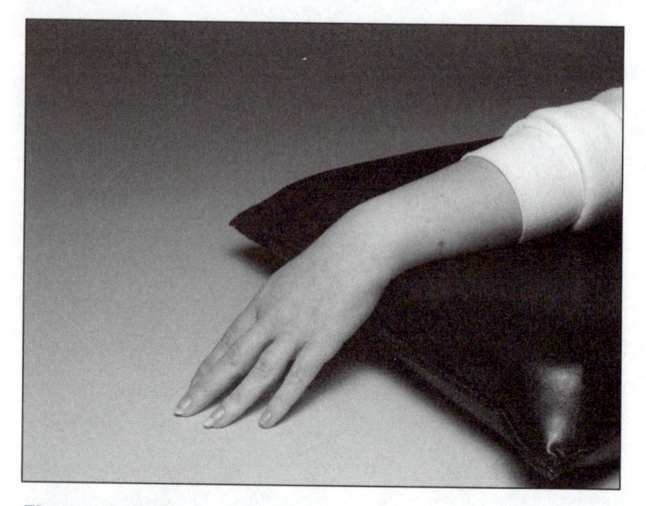

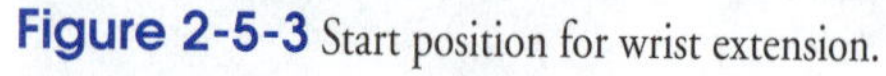

Figure 2-5-3 Start position for wrist extension.

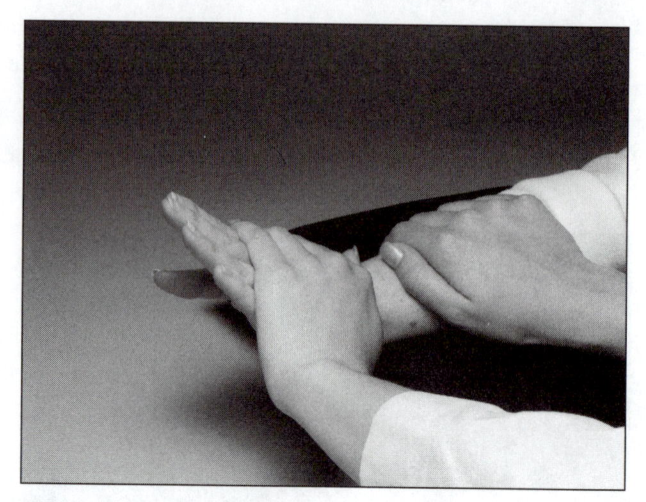

Figure 2-5-4 End position for wrist extension.

Normal, Good, Fair

Client Position: Starting—client is sitting with the testing extremity on a table with the forearm in pronation, and the wrist over the edge of the table in slight flexion (Figure 2-5-3).

Motion—client moves the testing extremity in the direction of wrist extension (Figure 2-5-4).

Therapist Position: Stabilize at the distal forearm to avoid compensation. Resistance is applied on the dorsum of the hand in the direction of wrist flexion when testing Normal or Good strengths. No resistance is applied when testing Fair strength.

Poor

Client Position: Starting—client is sitting with the testing extremity on a table, forearm is in neutral (ulnar side of the hand on the table).

Motion—client moves the testing extremity in the direction of wrist extension.

Therapist Position: Stabilize at the distal forearm to avoid compensation. No resistance is applied when testing in the gravity-eliminated position.

Wrist: *radial deviation*

The wrist radial deviators include flexor carpi radialis, extensor carpi radialis longus, and extensor carpi radialis brevis.

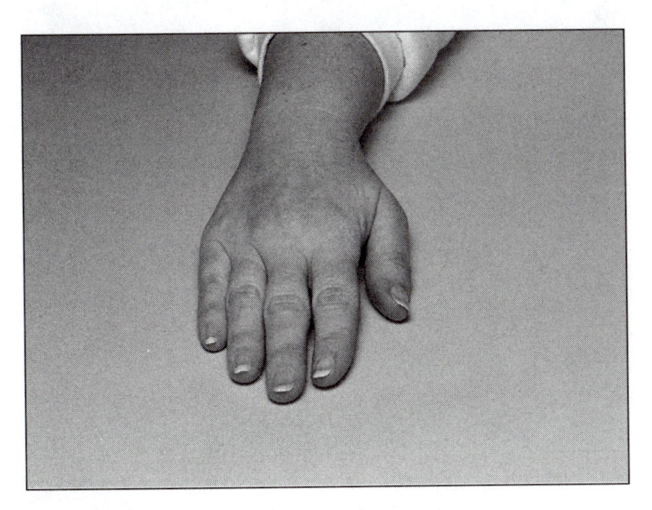

Figure 2-5-5 Start position for wrist radial deviation.

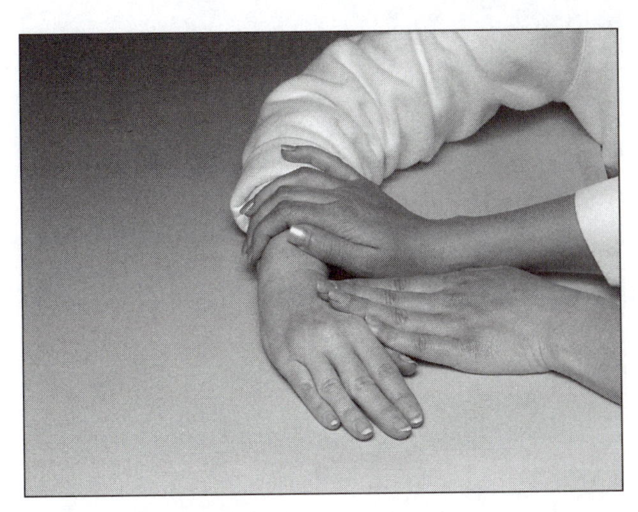

Figure 2-5-6 End position for wrist radial deviation.

Normal, Good, Fair

Client Position: Starting—client is sitting with the testing extremity placed on a table, forearm is in pronation (Figure 2-5-5).

Motion—client moves the testing extremity in the direction of wrist radial deviation (Figure 2-5-6).

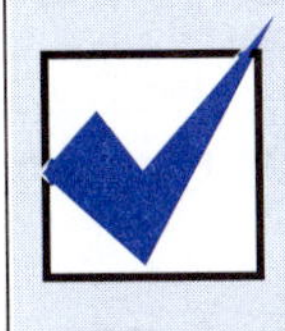

In this position the client is functioning in a gravity-eliminated plane. This position is appropriate because it is too awkward to position the client against gravity for radial and ulnar deviation.

Therapist Position: Stabilize at the distal forearm to avoid compensation. Resistance is applied at the second metacarpal in the direction of ulnar deviation when testing Normal or Good strengths. No resistance is applied when testing Fair strength.

Poor

Client Position: Starting—client is sitting with the testing extremity placed on a table, forearm is in pronation.

Motion—client moves the testing extremity in the direction of wrist radial deviation.

Therapist Position: Stabilize at the distal forearm to avoid compensation. No resistance is applied when testing in the gravity-eliminated position.

Wrist: *ulnar deviation*

The wrist ulnar deviators include flexor carpi ulnaris and extensor carpi ulnaris.

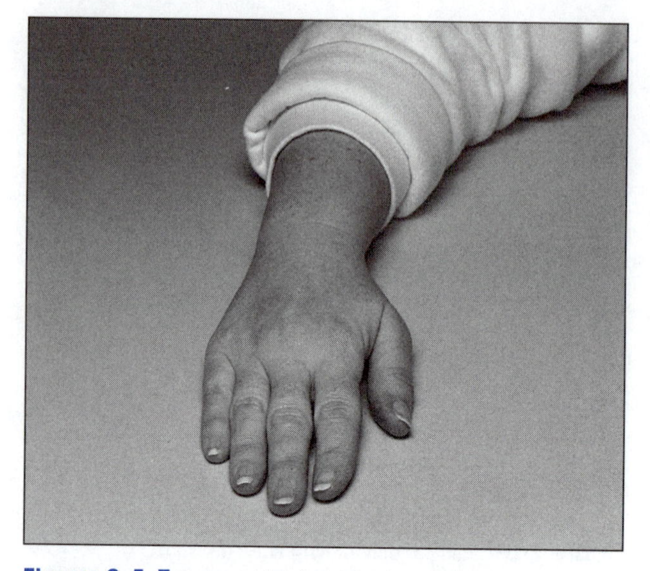

Figure 2-5-7 Start position for wrist ulnar deviation.

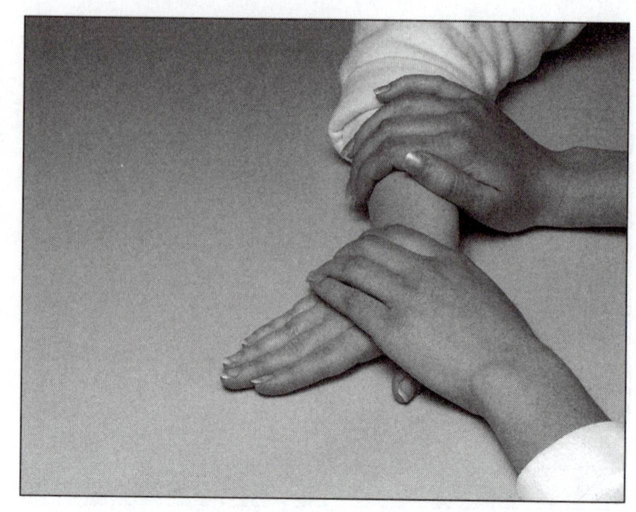

Figure 2-5-8 End position for wrist ulnar deviation.

Normal, Good, Fair

Client Position: Starting—client is sitting with the testing extremity placed on a table, forearm is in pronation (Figure 2-5-7).

Motion—client moves the testing extremity in the direction of wrist ulnar deviation (Figure 2-5-8).

In this position the client is functioning in a gravity-eliminated plane. This position is appropriate because it is too awkward to position the client against gravity for radial and ulnar deviation.

Therapist Position: Stabilize at the distal forearm to avoid compensation. Resistance is applied at the fifth metacarpal in the direction of wrist radial deviation when testing Normal or Good strengths. No resistance is applied when testing Fair strength.

Poor

Client Position: Starting—client is sitting with the testing extremity placed on a table, forearm is in pronation.

Motion—client moves the testing extremity in the direction of wrist ulnar deviation.

Therapist Position: Stabilize at the distal forearm to avoid compensation. No resistance is applied when testing in the gravity-eliminated position.

Digit: *MCP flexion*

The MCP flexors include the flexor digitorum superficialis, flexor digitorum profundus when these muscles are acting on the PIP and DIP joints, respectively, and the lumbricals acting on MCP in combination with PIP/DIP extension. Flexor digiti minimi acts on the fifth digit MCP.

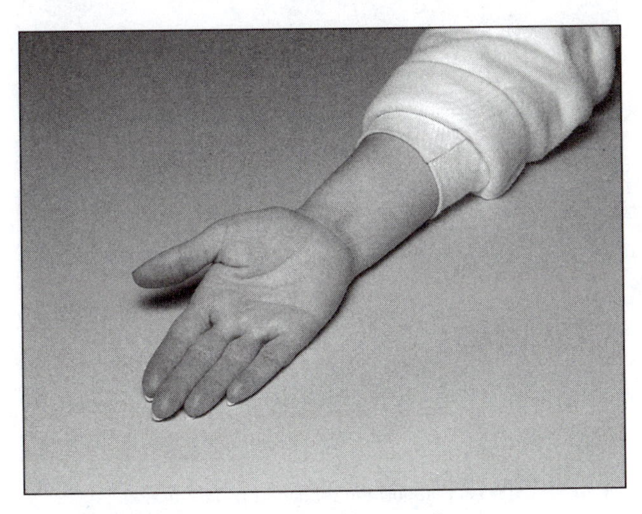

Figure 2-5-9 Start position for hand MCP flexion.

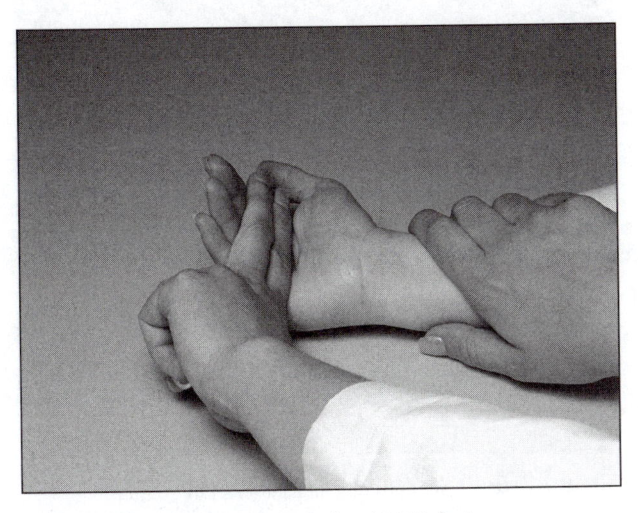

Figure 2-5-10 End position for hand MCP flexion.

Normal, Good, Fair

Client Position: Starting—client is sitting with the testing extremity in forearm supination and MCP extension (Figure 2-5-9).

Motion—client moves the testing extremity in the direction of MCP flexion. Simultaneous PIP/DIP flexion is acceptable (Figure 2-5-10).

Therapist Position: Stabilize proximal to the MCP joints at the metacarpals to avoid compensation. Resistance is applied with one or two fingers at the proximal phalanges in the direction of MCP extension when testing Normal or Good strengths. No resistance is applied when testing Fair strength.

Poor

Client Position: Starting—client is sitting with the testing extremity in neutral forearm rotation and MCP extension.

Motion—client moves the testing extremity in the direction of MCP flexion. Simultaneous PIP/DIP flexion is acceptable.

Therapist Position: Stabilize proximal to the MCP joints at the metacarpals to avoid compensation. No resistance is applied when testing in the gravity-eliminated position.

Digit: *PIP/DIP flexion*

The PIP flexor is flexor digitorum superficialis, and the DIP flexor is flexor digitorum profundus. During gross muscle testing these muscles are tested together.

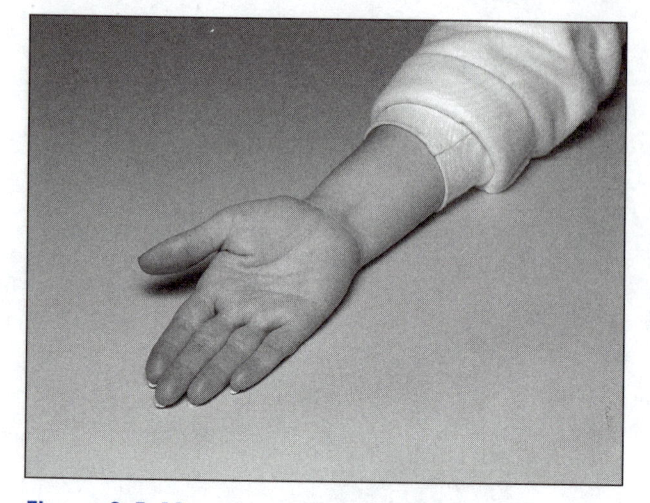

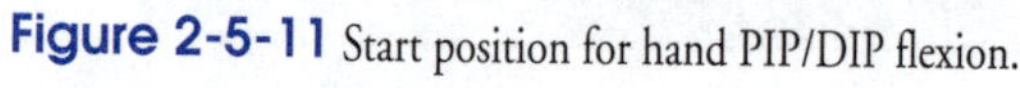

Figure 2-5-11 Start position for hand PIP/DIP flexion.

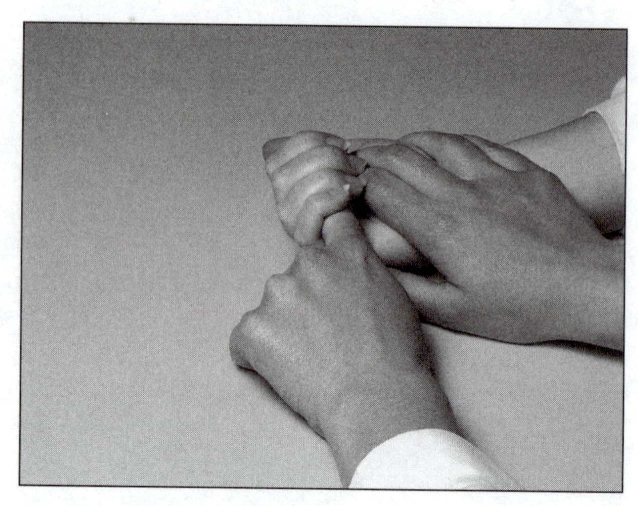

Figure 2-5-12 End position for hand PIP/DIP flexion.

Normal, Good, Fair

Client Position: Starting—client is sitting with the testing extremity in forearm supination and digit extension (Figure 2-5-11).

Motion—client moves the testing extremity in the direction of PIP/DIP flexion while keeping the MCPs in extension (not hyperextension) (Figure 2-5-12).

Therapist Position: Stabilize at the MCP joints to avoid compensation of hyperextension. Resistance is applied with one or two fingers at both the middle and distal phalanges in the direction of PIP/DIP extension when testing Normal or Good strengths. No resistance is applied when testing Fair strength.

Poor

Client Position: Starting—client is sitting with the testing extremity in neutral forearm rotation and digit extension.

Motion—client moves the testing extremity in the direction of PIP/DIP flexion.

Therapist Position: Stabilize at the MCP joints to avoid compensation. No resistance is applied when testing in the gravity-eliminated position.

Digit: *MCP/PIP/DIP extension (hyperextension)*

The hand MCP/PIP/DIP extensors are extensor digitorum, extensor indicis, and extensor digiti minimi. PIP/DIP extensors also include the lumbricales.

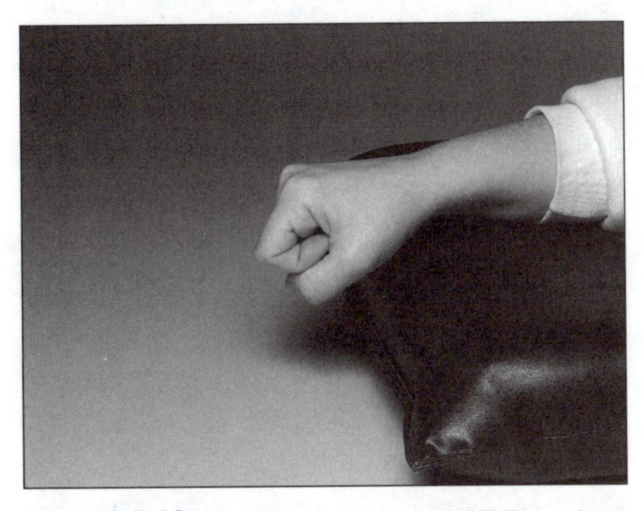

Figure 2-5-13 Start position for hand MCP/PIP/DIP extension (hyperextension).

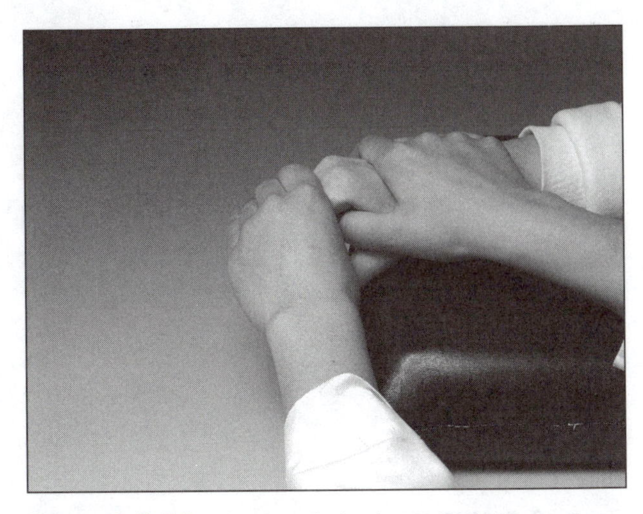

Figure 2-5-14 End position for hand MCP/PIP/DIP extension (hyperextension).

Normal, Good, Fair

Client Position: Starting—client is sitting with the testing extremity in forearm pronation and digit flexion (Figure 2-5-13).

Motion—client moves the testing extremity in the direction of MCP/PIP/DIP extension (Figure 2-5-14).

Therapist Position: Stabilize proximal to the MCP joints at the metacarpals to avoid compensation. Resistance is applied at the proximal, middle, and distal phalanges in the direction of MCP/PIP/DIP flexion when testing Normal or Good strengths. No resistance is applied when testing Fair strength.

Poor

Client Position: Starting—client is sitting with the testing extremity in neutral forearm rotation and digit flexion.

Motion—client moves the testing extremity in the direction of MCP/PIP/DIP extension.

Therapist Position: Stabilize proximal to the MCP joints at the metacarpals to avoid compensation. No resistance is applied when testing in the gravity-eliminated position.

Digit: *MCP abduction/adduction*

The MCP abductors are dorsal interossei and abductor digiti minimi. The MCP adductors are palmar interossei.

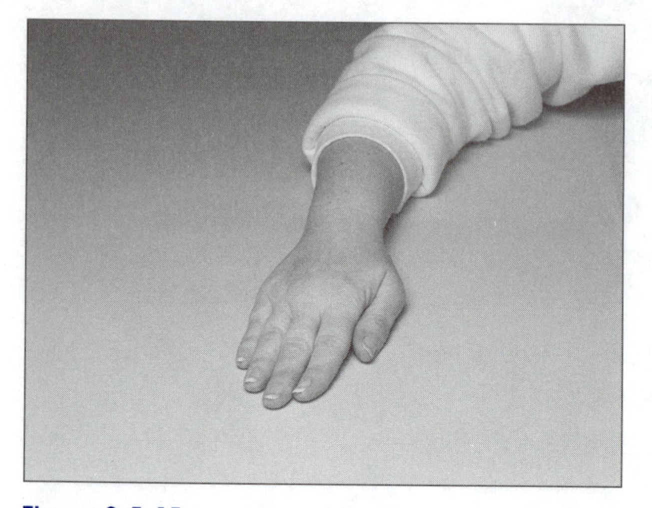

Figure 2-5-15 Start position for hand MCP abduction (adduction is opposite).

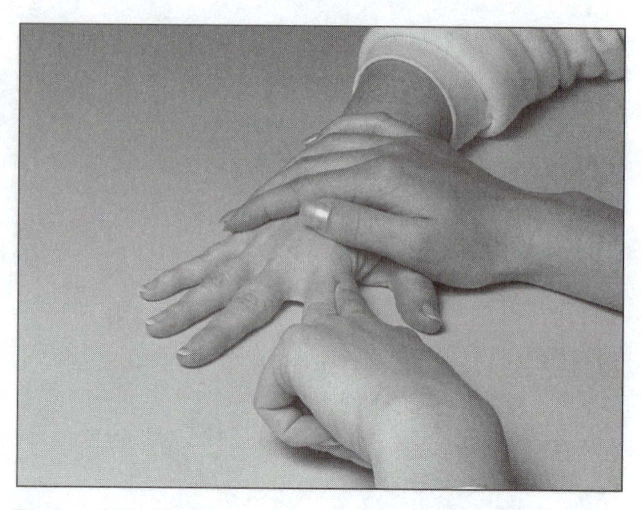

Figure 2-5-16 End position for hand MCP abduction (adduction is opposite).

Normal, Good, Fair

Client Position: Starting—client is sitting with testing extremity in forearm pronation and digit extension. For MCP abduction the digits are adducted (Figure 2-5-15), and for MCP adduction the digits are abducted.

Motion—client moves the digits in the direction of MCP abduction (Figure 2-5-16), or adduction depending on the test.

Therapist Position: Stabilize at the metacarpals. Resistance is applied to each finger for MCP abduction in the direction of adduction and for MCP adduction in the direction of abduction when testing Normal or Good strengths. For adduction, no resistance is applied to the third digit; however, for abduction, the third digit is tested on both sides. No resistance is applied when testing Fair strength.

Poor

Poor grading is not completed for this test.

Digit and thumb: *opposition*

The hand (hypothenar) muscle for opposition is opponens digiti minimi, and the thumb (thenar) muscle for opposition is opponens pollicis.

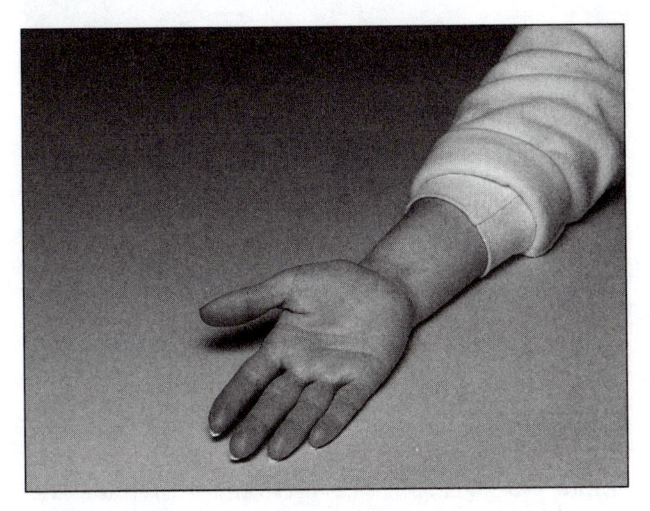

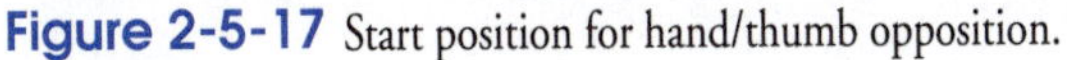

Figure 2-5-17 Start position for hand/thumb opposition.

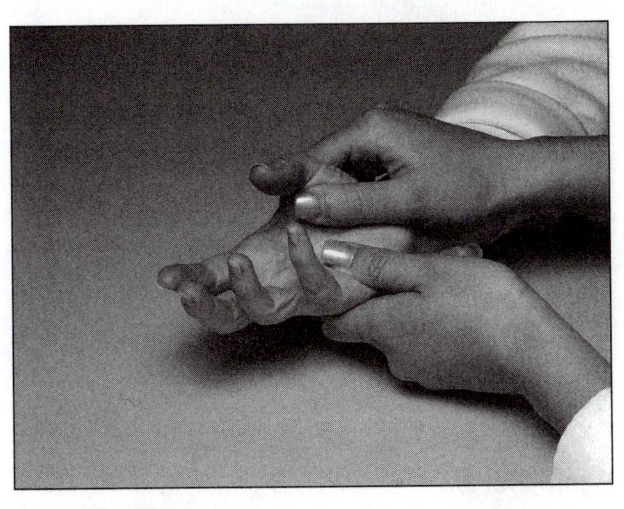

Figure 2-5-18 End position for hand/thumb opposition.

Normal, Good, Fair

Client Position: Starting—client is sitting with the testing extremity in forearm supination and the digits extended (Figure 2-5-17).

Motion—client moves in the direction of hand/thumb opposition of first and fifth digit (Figure 2-5-18).

Therapist Position: Stabilize at the wrist. Resistance is applied at both the fifth and first digits away from opposition when testing Normal or Good strengths. No resistance is applied when testing Fair strength. (All digits can be tested separately if desired.)

Poor

Poor grading is not completed for this test.

Thumb: *MCP flexion/extension*

The thumb MCP flexor is flexor pollicis brevis, and the thumb MCP extensor is extensor pollicis brevis.

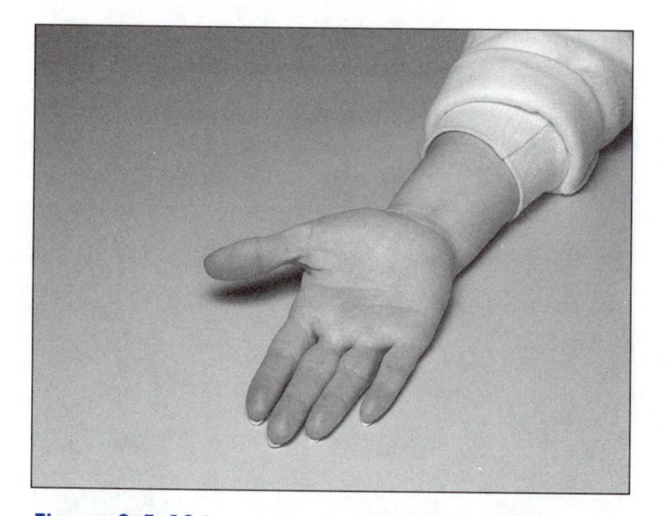

Figure 2-5-19 Start position for thumb MCP flexion (extension is opposite).

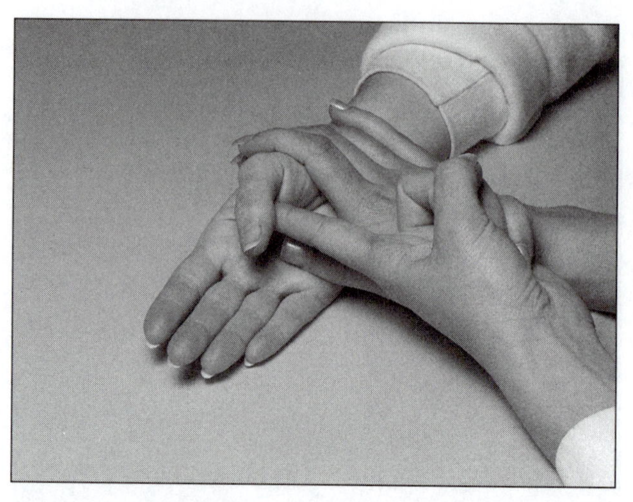

Figure 2-5-20 End position for thumb MCP flexion (extension is opposite).

Normal, Good, Fair

Client Position: Starting—client is sitting with the testing extremity in forearm supination and digits 2–5 extended. For thumb MCP flexion the thumb is in extension (Figure 2-5-19); for thumb MCP extension, the thumb is in flexion.

Motion—client moves the thumb MCP in the direction of flexion (Figure 2-5-20), or extension depending on the test.

Therapist Position: Stabilize at the thumb metacarpal. Resistance is applied at the proximal phalange for MCP flexion in the direction of extension, and for MCP extension in the direction of flexion, when testing Normal or Good strengths. No resistance is applied when testing Fair strength.

Poor

Poor grading is not completed for this test.

Thumb: *CMC flexion/extension*

The thumb CMC flexor is flexor pollicis brevis, and the thumb CMC extensors are extensor pollicis brevis and abductor pollicis longus.

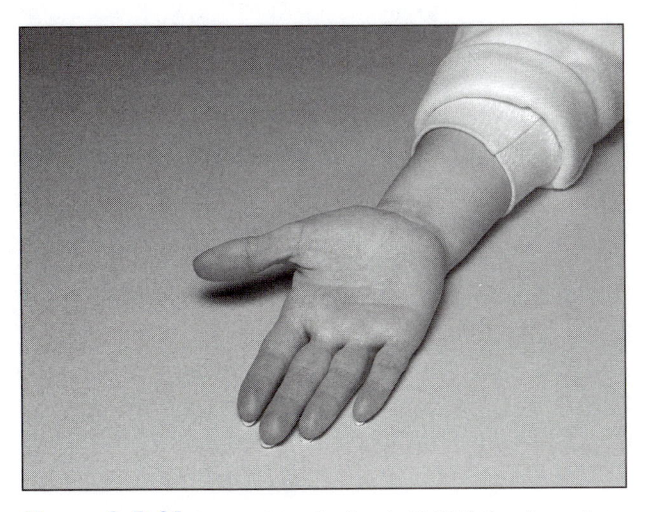

Figure 2-5-21 Start position for thumb CMC flexion (extension is opposite).

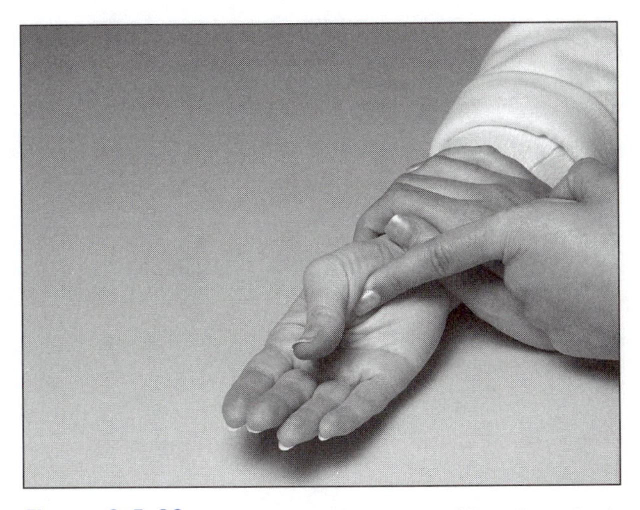

Figure 2-5-22 End position for thumb CMC flexion (extension is opposite).

Normal, Good, Fair

Client Position: Starting—client is sitting with the forearm in supination and digits 2–5 in extension. For thumb CMC flexion the thumb is in extension (Figure 2-5-21); for thumb CMC extension, the thumb is in flexion.

Motion—client moves the thumb CMC in the direction of flexion (Figure 2-5-22), or extension depending on the test.

Therapist Position: Stabilize at the wrist. Resistance is applied at the metacarpal for CMC flexion in the direction of extension, and for CMC extension in the direction of flexion when testing Normal or Good strengths. No resistance is applied when testing Fair strength.

Poor

Poor grading is not completed for this test.

Thumb: *CMC abduction/adduction*

The thumb CMC abductors are abductor pollicis brevis and abductor pollicis longus, and the thumb CMC adductor is adductor pollicis.

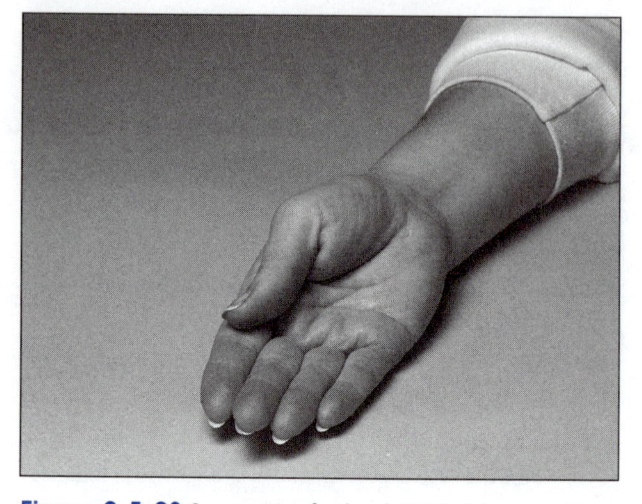

Figure 2-5-23 Start position for thumb CMC abduction (adduction is opposite).

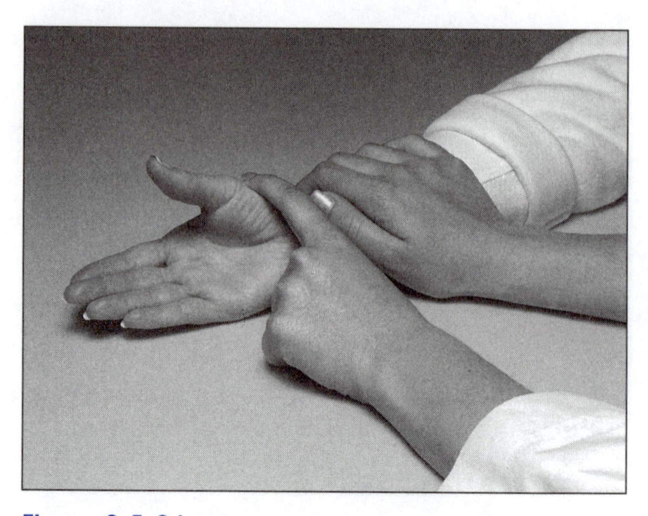

Figure 2-5-24 End position for thumb CMC abduction (adduction is opposite).

Normal, Good, Fair

Client Position: Starting—client is sitting with the forearm in supination and digits 2–5 extended. For thumb CMC abduction, the thumb is adducted (Figure 2-5-23); for CMC adduction, the thumb is abducted.

Motion—client moves the thumb CMC in the direction of abduction (Figure 2-5-24), or adduction, depending on the test.

Therapist Position: Stabilize at the wrist. Resistance is applied at the first metacarpal for CMC abduction in the direction of adduction, and for CMC adduction in the direction of abduction, when testing Normal or Good strengths. No resistance is applied when testing Fair strength.

Poor

Poor grading is not completed for this test.

Thumb: *IP flexion/extension*

The thumb IP flexor is flexor pollicis longus and the thumb IP extensor is extensor pollicis longus.

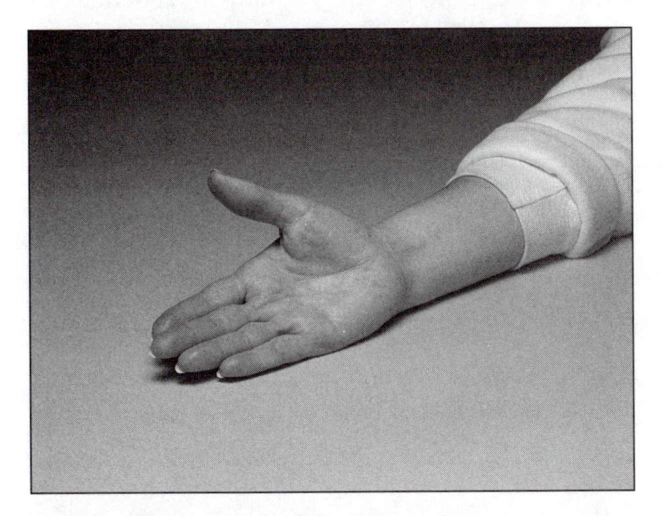

Figure 2-5-25 Start position for thumb IP flexion (extension is opposite).

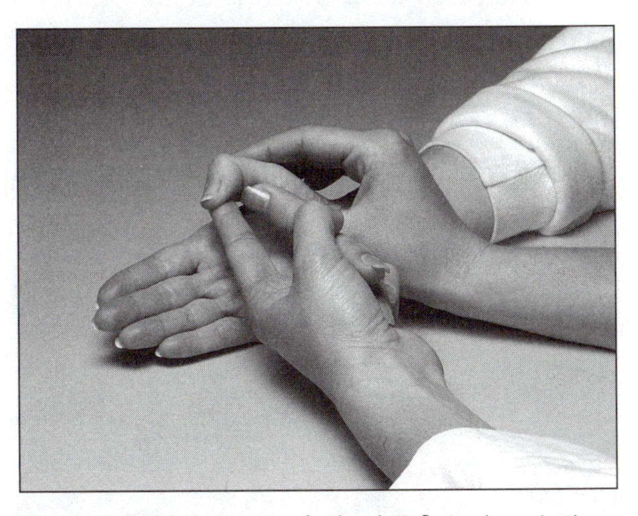

Figure 2-5-26 End position for thumb IP flexion (extension is opposite).

Normal, Good, Fair

Client Position: Starting—client is sitting with the forearm in supination. For thumb IP flexion, the joint is extended (Figure 2-5-25); for thumb IP extension, the joint is flexed.

Motion—client moves the thumb IP in the direction of flexion (Figure 2-5-26) or extension, depending on the test.

Therapist Position: Stabilize at the thumb proximal phalange. Resistance is applied for IP flexion in the direction of extension, and for IP extension in the direction of flexion, when testing Normal or Good strengths. No resistance is applied when testing Fair strength.

Poor

Poor grading is not completed for this test.

Section 2-6: Gross Manual Muscle Testing of the Hip and Knee

Listed after each action in this section are the muscles which act to produce that movement. If deficits are noted during gross manual muscle testing, and isolated manual muscle testing is appropriate, the procedures for the isolated manual muscle testing of these muscles are found in Section 3-6 of this manual.

Hip: *flexion*

The hip flexors include the following muscles: iliopsoas, sartorius, tensor fascia latae, and rectus femoris.

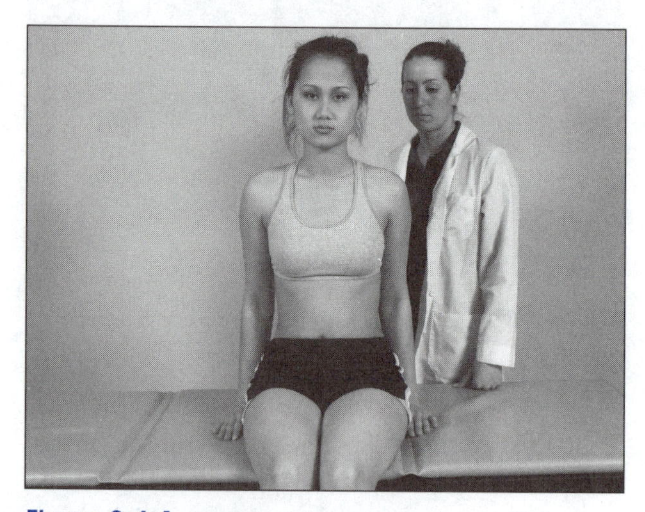

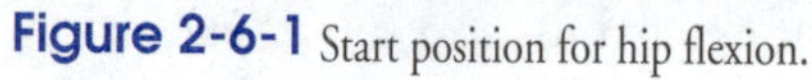

Figure 2-6-1 Start position for hip flexion.

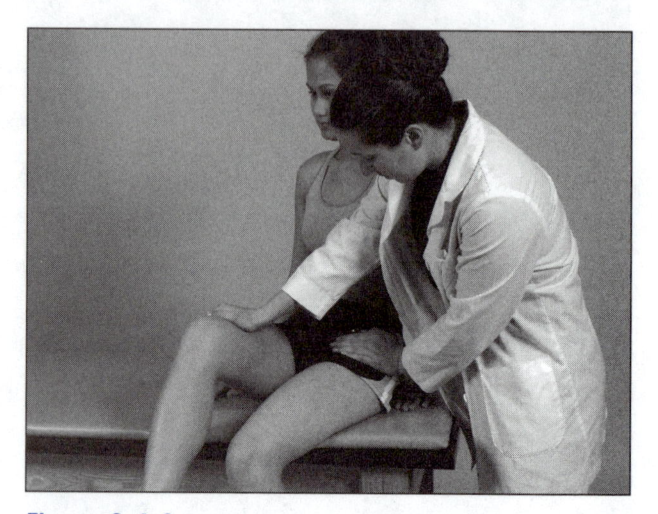

Figure 2-6-2 End position for hip flexion.

Normal, Good, Fair

Client Position: Starting—client is sitting with lower leg over edge of testing surface. The knee is flexed and foot unsupported (Figure 2-6-1).

Motion—client moves the testing extremity in the direction of hip flexion while allowing the knee to follow into slight flexion (Figure 2-6-2).

Therapist Position: Stabilize at the contralateral iliac crest of the pelvis. Resistance is applied over the anterior aspect of the thigh proximal to the knee in the direction of hip extension when testing Normal or Good strengths. No resistance is applied when testing Fair strength.

Poor

Client Position: Starting—client is lying on nontest side. Client holds nontest extremity in maximal hip and knee flexion.

Motion—client moves the testing extremity into maximal hip flexion.

Therapist Position: While standing behind the client, stabilize the side-lying position and the pelvis. Therapist supports the testing extremity to eliminate gravity without assisting the motion. No resistance is applied in the gravity-eliminated position.

Hip: *extension*

The hip extensors include the following muscles: gluteus maximus and semimembranosus, and semitendinosus when knee is flexed.

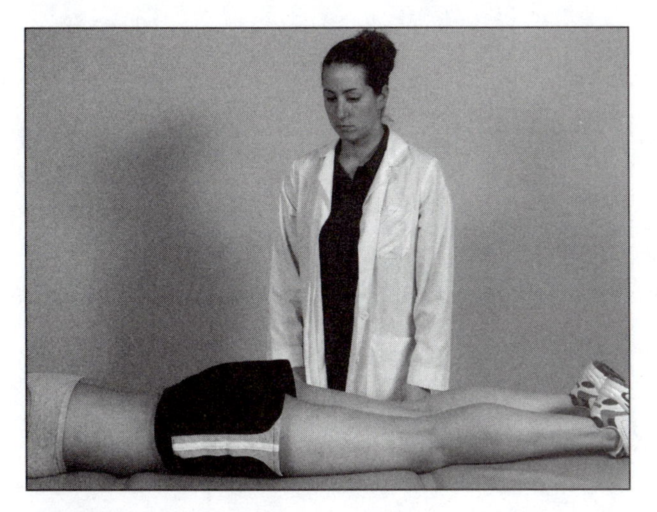

Figure 2-6-3 Start position for hip extension.

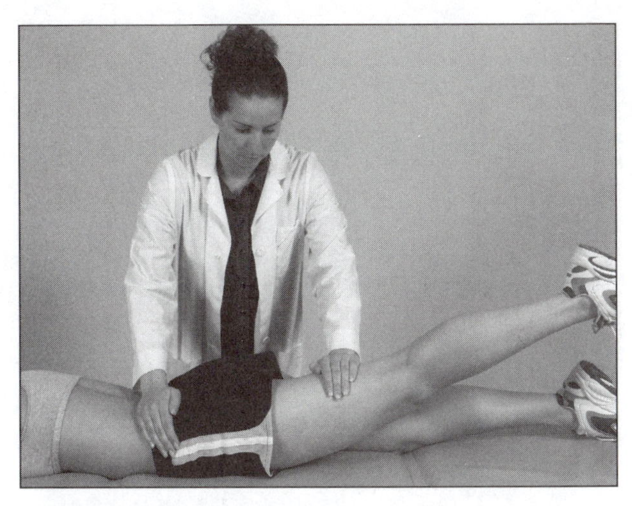

Figure 2-6-4 End position for hip extension.

Normal, Good, Fair

Client Position: Starting—client is prone with both legs extended and resting on testing surface. Client is asked to hold onto edge of testing surface as resistance is applied (Figure 2-6-3).

Motion—client moves the testing extremity in the direction of hip extension while knee remains extended (Figure 2-6-4).

Therapist Position: Stabilize at the pelvis. Resistance is applied over the posterior aspect of the thigh proximal to the knee in the direction of hip flexion when testing Normal or Good strengths. No resistance is applied when testing Fair strength.

Poor

Client Position: Starting—client is lying on nontest side. The client holds the nontest extremity in maximal hip and knee flexion. Testing hip is in neutral and knee is flexed.

Motion—client moves the testing extremity into maximal hip extension.

Therapist Position: While standing behind the client, stabilize the side-lying position and the pelvis. Therapist supports the testing extremity to eliminate gravity without assisting the motion. No resistance is applied in the gravity-eliminated position.

Alternate Position

If hip flexors are tight, client may stand with trunk flexed and trunk in prone position, resting on testing surface.

Hip: *abduction*

The hip abductors include the following muscles: sartorius, gluteus medius, gluteus minimus, and tensor fascia latae.

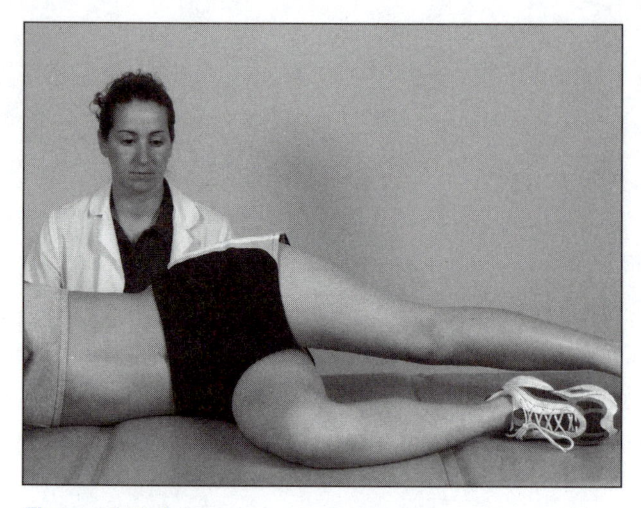

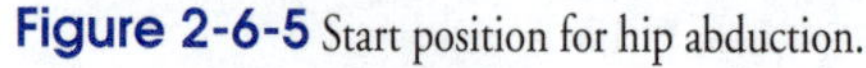

Figure 2-6-5 Start position for hip abduction.

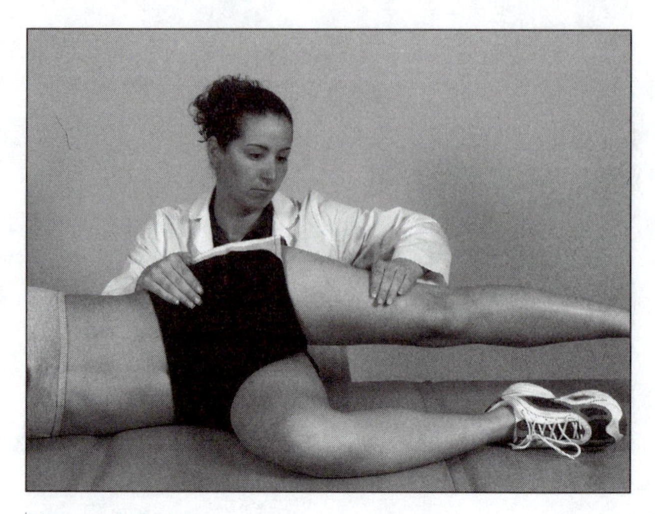

Figure 2-6-6 End position for hip abduction.

Normal, Good, Fair

Client Position: Starting—client is lying on nontest side. Client holds nontest extremity in maximal hip and knee flexion. Testing extremity is in slight hip extension, neutral rotation, and knee extension (Figure 2-6-5).

Motion—client moves the testing extremity in the direction of hip abduction (Figure 2-6-6).

Therapist Position: Stabilize at the pelvis. Resistance is applied over the lateral aspect of the thigh proximal to the knee in the direction of adduction when testing Normal or Good strengths. No resistance is applied when testing Fair strength.

Poor

Client Position: Starting—client is supine with hip and knees extended resting on testing surface.

Motion—client moves the testing extremity into maximal hip abduction.

Therapist Position: Stabilize the pelvis. Therapist supports the testing extremity to eliminate gravity without assisting the motion. No resistance is applied in the gravity-eliminated position.

Hip: *adduction*

The hip adductors include the following muscles: pectineus, adductor magnus, gracilis, adductor longus, and adductor brevis.

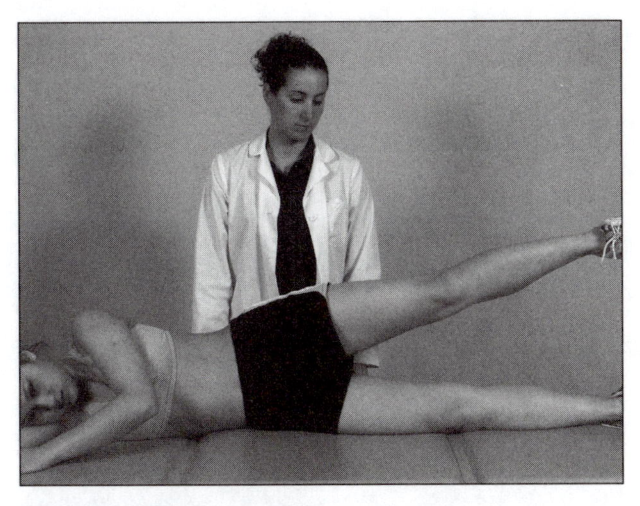

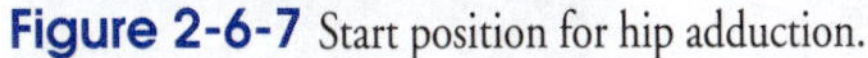

Figure 2-6-7 Start position for hip adduction.

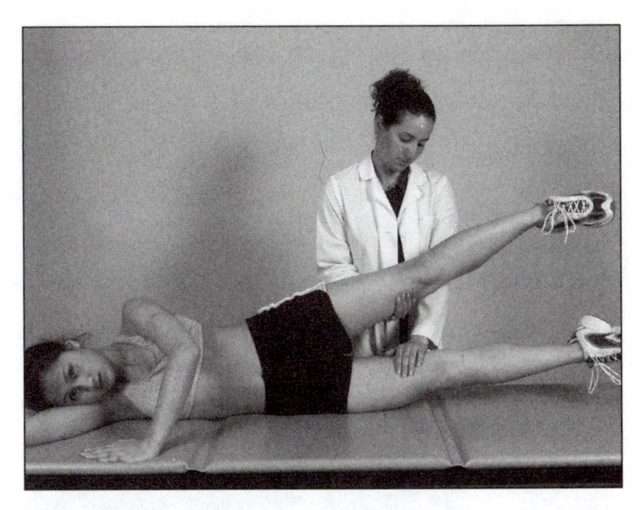

Figure 2-6-8 End position for hip adduction.

Normal, Good, Fair

Client Position: Starting—client is lying on his/her side on testing extremity, with hip in neutral and knee extended on testing surface. Nontest extremity is in abduction and knee is extended (Figure 2-6-7).

Motion—client moves the testing extremity in the direction of hip adduction toward the nontest extremity (Figure 2-6-8).

Therapist Position: Support the nontest extremity in hip abduction. Resistance is applied over the medial aspect of the thigh proximal to the knee in the direction of abduction when testing Normal or Good strengths. No resistance is applied when testing Fair strength.

Poor

Client Position: Starting—client is supine with hip in neutral and abduction, and knee extended on testing surface.

Motion—client moves the testing extremity into maximal hip adduction.

Therapist Position: Stabilize the pelvis. Therapist supports the testing extremity to eliminate gravity without assisting the motion. No resistance is applied in the gravity-eliminated position.

Hip: *external rotation*

The hip external rotators include the following muscles: piriformis, quadratus femoris, obturator femoris, obturator internis, obturator externus, gemellus superior, and gemellus inferior.

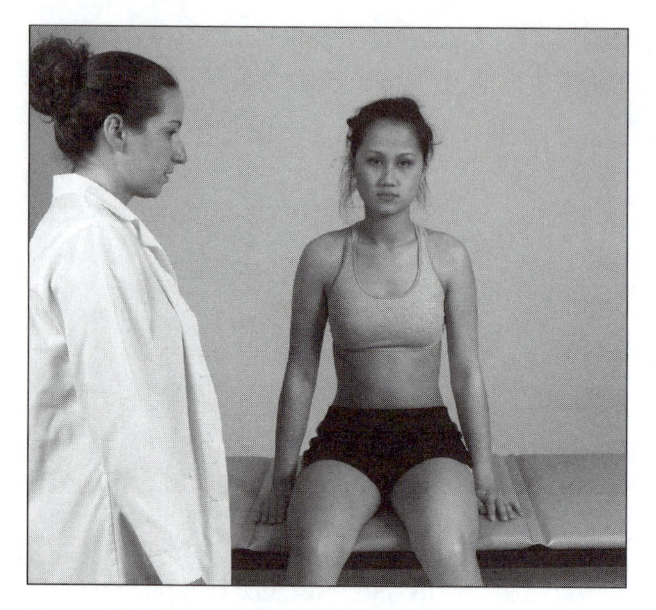

Figure 2-6-9 Start position for hip external rotation.

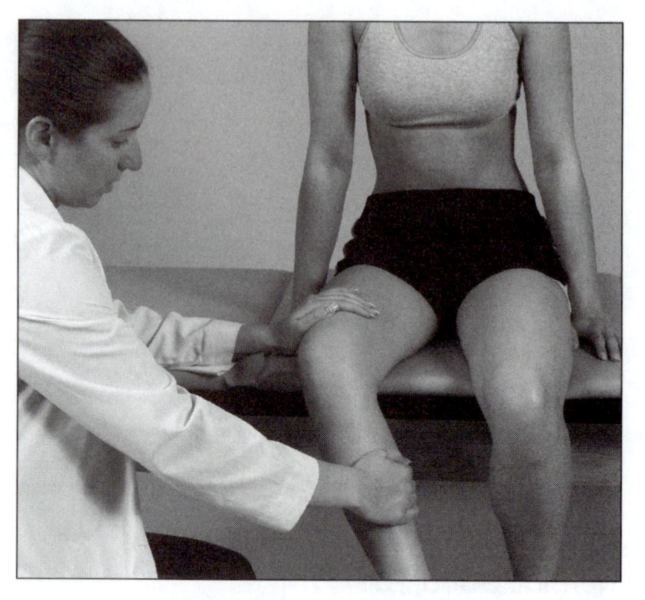

Figure 2-6-10 End position for hip external rotation.

Normal, Good, Fair

Client Position: Starting—client is sitting with testing hip in 90 degrees of flexion, knees flexed at edge of testing surface. The midpoint of patella is aligned with the anterior superior iliac spine (ASIS) (Figure 2-6-9).

Motion—client moves the testing extremity in the direction of hip external rotation (Figure 2-6-10).

Therapist Position: Stabilize at the anterolateral aspect of the distal thigh. Resistance is applied over the medial aspect of the lower leg proximal to the ankle in the direction of internal rotation when testing Normal or Good strengths. No resistance is applied when testing Fair strength.

Poor

Client Position: Starting—client is supine with testing hip in internal rotation and knee extension.

Motion—client moves the testing extremity into maximal hip external rotation.

Therapist Position: Stabilize the medial aspect of the thigh. No resistance is applied in the gravity-eliminated position.

Hip: *internal rotation*

The hip internal rotators include the following muscles: gluteus medius, gluteus minimus, and tensor fascia latae.

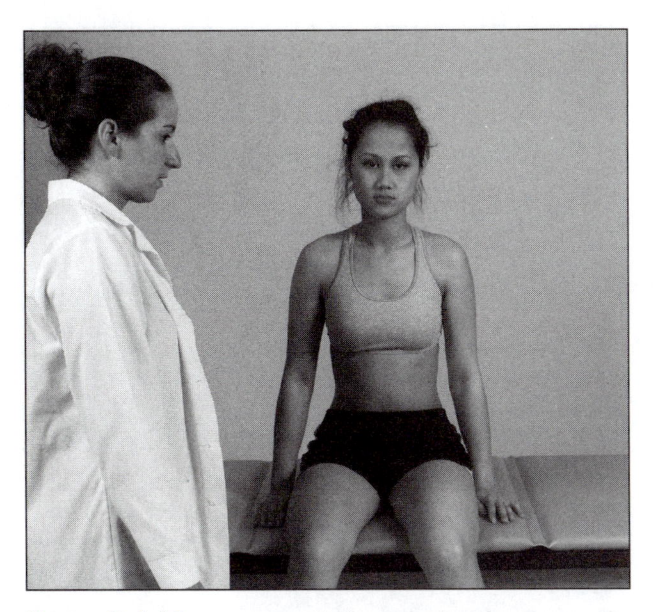

Figure 2-6-11 Start position for hip internal rotation.

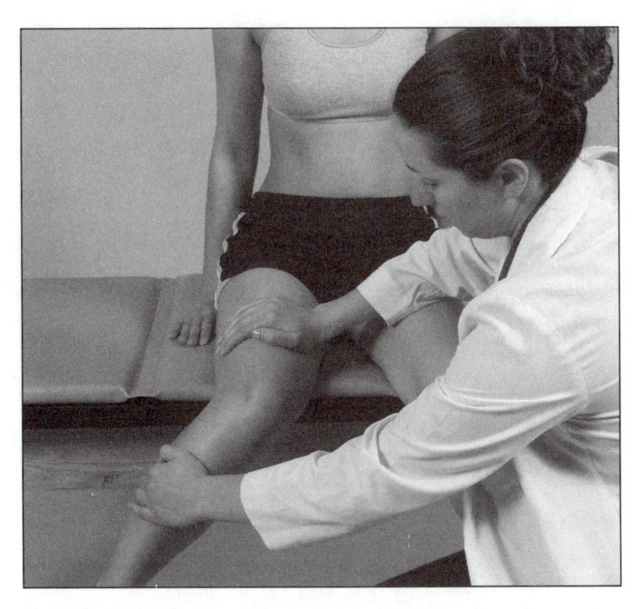

Figure 2-6-12 End position for hip internal rotation.

Normal, Good, Fair

Client Position: Starting—client is sitting with testing hip in 90 degrees of flexion, knees flexed at edge of testing surface. The midpoint of patella is aligned with the ASIS (Figure 2-6-11).

Motion—client moves the testing extremity in the direction of hip internal rotation (Figure 2-6-12).

Therapist Position: Stabilize at the medial aspect of the distal thigh. Resistance is applied over the lateral aspect of the lower leg proximal to the ankle in the direction of external rotation when testing Normal or Good strengths. No resistance is applied when testing Fair strength.

Poor

Client Position: Starting—client is supine with testing hip in external rotation and knee extension.

Motion—client moves the testing extremity into maximal hip internal rotation.

Therapist Position: Stabilize the lateral aspect of the thigh. No resistance is applied in the gravity-eliminated position.

Knee: *flexion*

Knee flexion includes the following muscles: medial hamstrings—semitendinosus and semimembranosus; lateral hamstrings—biceps femoris.

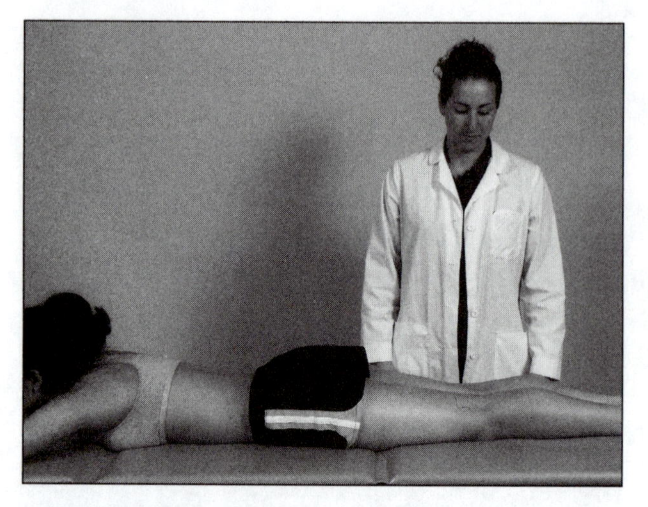

Figure 2-6-13 Start position for knee flexion.

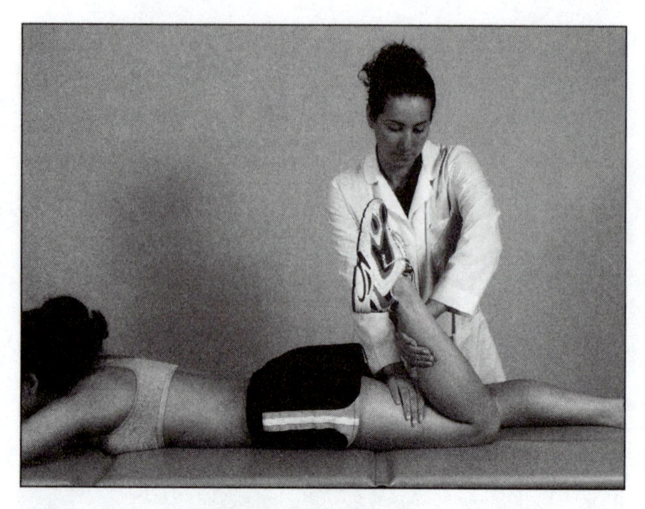

Figure 2-6-14 End position for knee flexion.

Normal, Good, Fair

Client Position: Starting—client is prone. The testing knee is extended and the foot is over edge of testing surface (Figure 2-6-13).

Motion—client moves the testing extremity in the direction of knee flexion (Figure 2-6-14).

Therapist Position: Stabilize the testing thigh. Resistance is applied proximal to the ankle on the posterior aspect of the leg in the direction of knee extension when testing Normal or Good strengths. No resistance is applied when testing Fair strength.

Poor

Client Position: Starting—client is lying on non-test side. The testing hip and knee are extended.

Motion—client moves the testing extremity in the direction of knee flexion.

Therapist Position: Stabilize the thigh. Therapist supports the testing extremity to eliminate gravity without assisting the motion. No resistance is applied in the gravity-eliminated position.

Knee: *extension*

Knee extension includes the following muscles: rectus femoris, vastus intermedius, vastus lateralis, and vastus medialis.

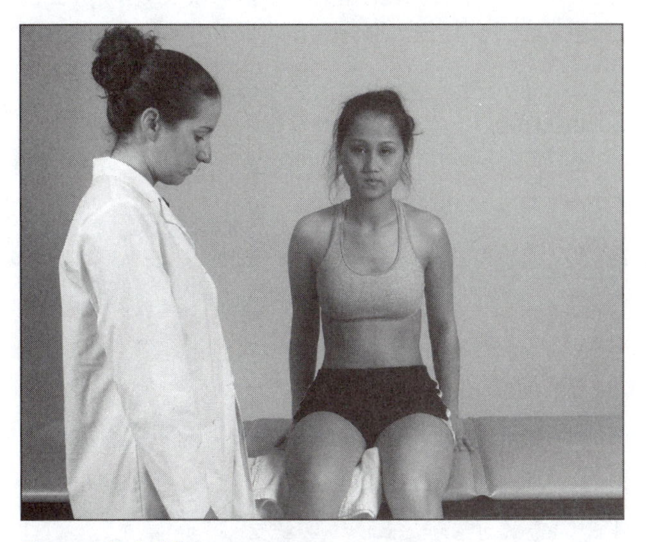

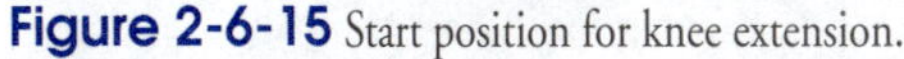

Figure 2-6-15 Start position for knee extension.

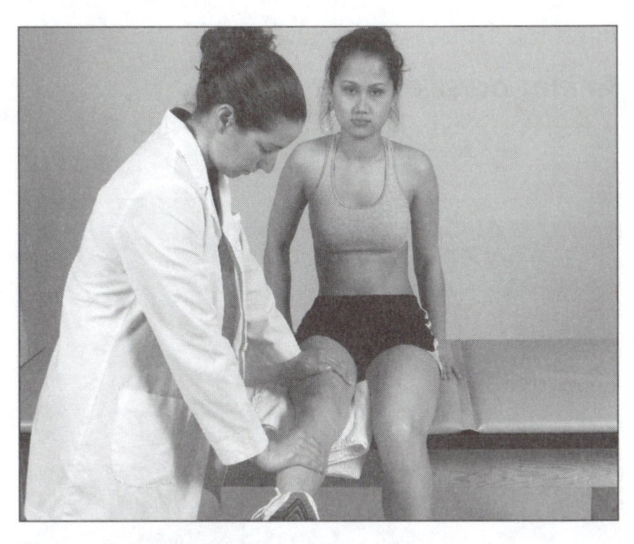

Figure 2-6-16 End position for knee extension.

Normal, Good, Fair

Client Position: Starting—client is sitting with a pad supported under the distal thigh. The testing knee is flexed and lower leg and feet are over edge of testing surface (Figure 2-6-15).

Motion—client moves the testing extremity into knee extension (Figure 2-6-16).

Therapist Position: Stabilize the testing thigh. Resistance is applied on the anterior surface of the distal lower extremity in the direction of knee flexion when testing Normal or Good strengths. No resistance is applied when testing Fair strength.

Poor

Client Position: Starting—client is lying on non-test side. The testing hip is extended and the knee is flexed.

Motion—client moves the testing extremity in the direction of knee extension.

Therapist Position: Stabilize the thigh. Therapist supports the testing extremity to eliminate gravity without assisting the motion. No resistance is applied in the gravity-eliminated position.

SECTION 2-7: Gross Manual Muscle Testing of the Ankle and Foot

Listed after each action in this section are the muscles which act to produce that movement. If deficits are noted during gross manual muscle testing, and isolated manual muscle testing is appropriate, the procedures for the isolated manual muscle testing of these muscles are found in Section 3-7 of this manual.

Ankle: *dorsiflexion*

Ankle dorsiflexion includes the following muscle: tibialis anterior.

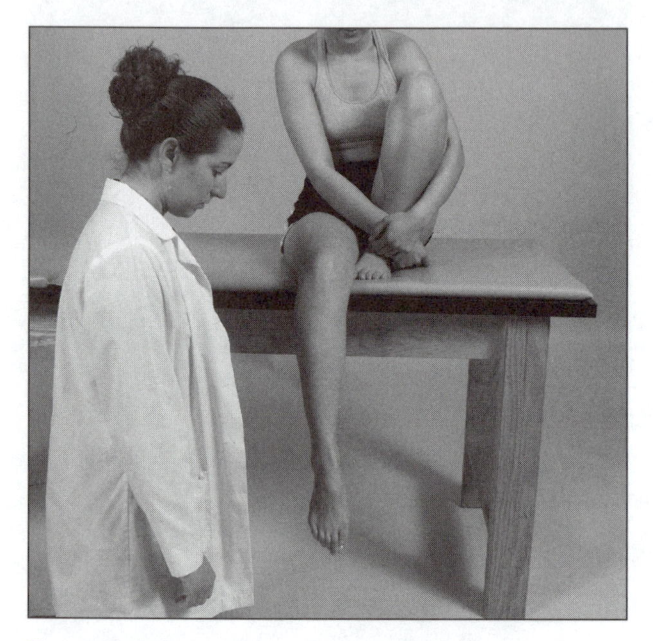

Figure 2-7-1 Start position for ankle dorsiflexion.

Normal, Good, Fair

Client Position: Starting—client is sitting with lower leg and feet over edge of testing surface. The ankle is in plantar flexion and foot is in neutral (Figure 2-7-1).

Motion—client moves the testing extremity into dorsiflexion and with toes relaxed (Figure 2-7-2).

Therapist Position: Stabilize the lower leg proximal to the ankle. Resistance is applied on the medial side and dorsal aspect of the forefoot in the direction of plantar flexion when testing Normal or Good strengths. No resistance is applied when testing Fair strength.

Poor

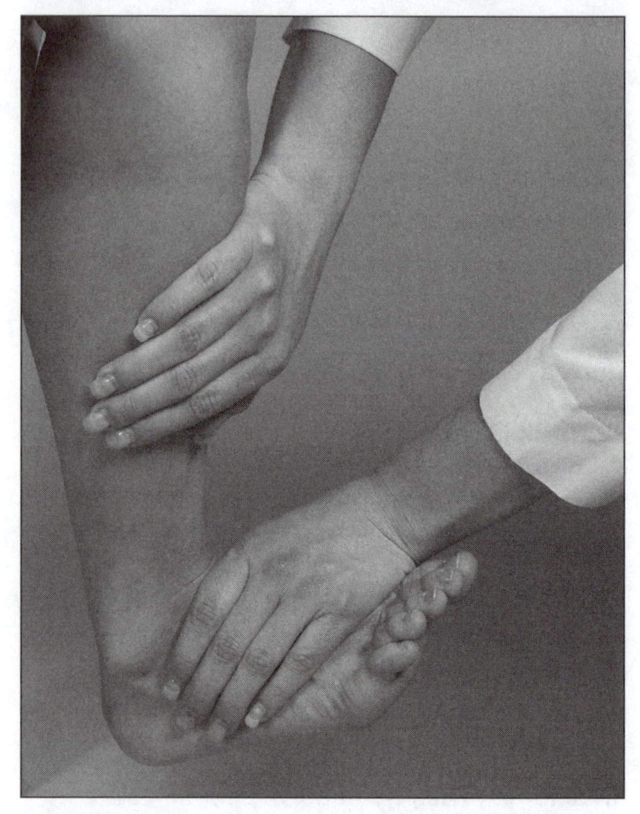

Figure 2-7-2 End position for ankle dorsiflexion.

Client Position: Starting—client is lying on test side. The testing hip is extended, the knee is flexed, the ankle is in plantar flexion.

Motion—client moves the testing extremity into ankle dorsiflexion.

Therapist Position: Stabilize the lower leg proximal to the ankle. Therapist supports the testing extremity to eliminate gravity without assisting the motion. No resistance is applied in the gravity-eliminated position.

Ankle: *plantar flexion*

Ankle plantar flexion includes the following muscles: gastrocnemius, soleus, flexor hallucis longus, flexor digitorum longus, and tibialis posterior.

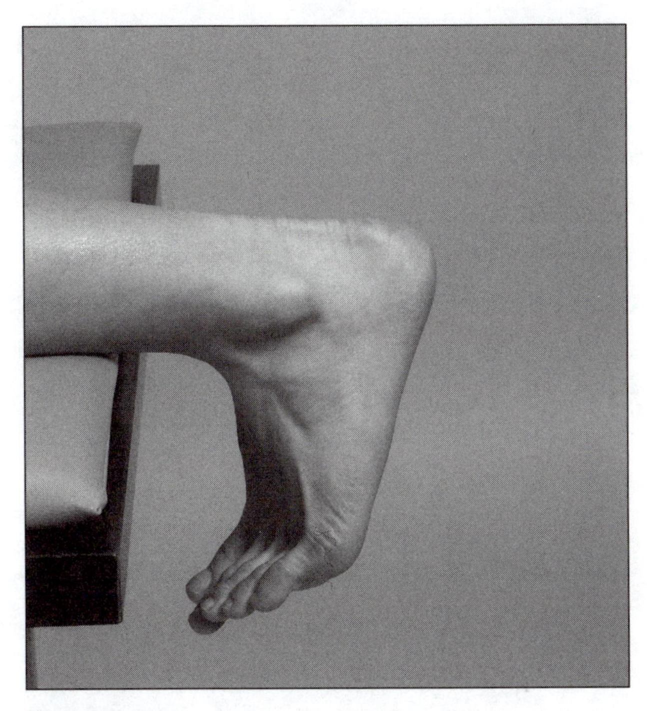

Figure 2-7-3 Start position for ankle plantar flexion.

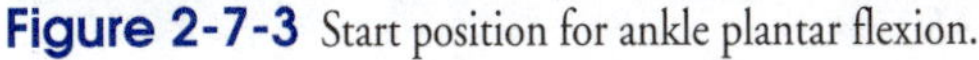

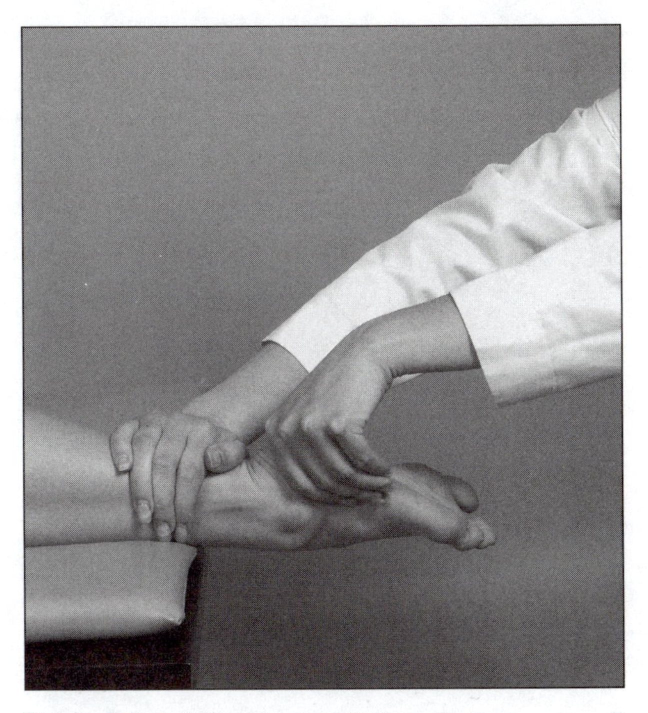

Figure 2-7-4 End position for ankle plantar flexion.

Normal, Good, Fair

Client Position: Starting—client is prone with knee extended and feet are over edge of testing surface. The ankle is in dorsiflexion (Figure 2-7-3).

Motion—client moves the testing extremity into plantar flexion with toes relaxed (Figure 2-7-4).

Therapist Position: Stabilize the lower leg proximal to the ankle. Resistance is applied on the posterior aspect of the calcaneus in the direction of dorsiflexion when testing Normal or Good strengths. No resistance is applied when testing Fair strength.

Poor

Client Position: Starting—client is lying on test side. The nontest knee is flexed. The testing knee is extended and the ankle is in dorsiflexion.

Motion—client moves the testing extremity into ankle plantar flexion.

Therapist Position: Stabilize the lower leg proximal to the ankle. Therapist supports the testing extremity to eliminate gravity without assisting the motion. No resistance is applied in the gravity-eliminated position.

Some references recommend testing ankle plantar flexion by completing heel raises in standing. This test is not included in this manual because of the variability of grading in the literature.

Foot: *inversion*

Foot inversion includes the following muscles: tibialis posterior, extensor hallucis longus, and tibialis anterior.

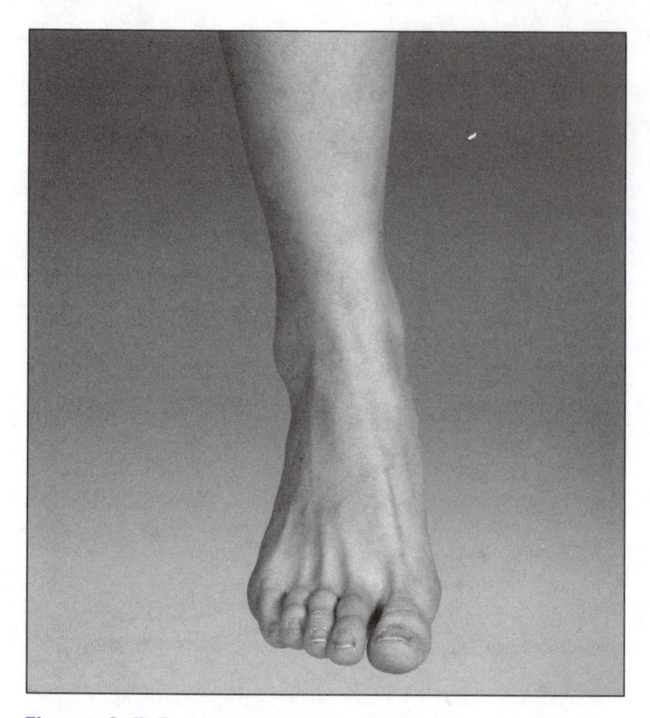

Figure 2-7-5 Start position for foot inversion.

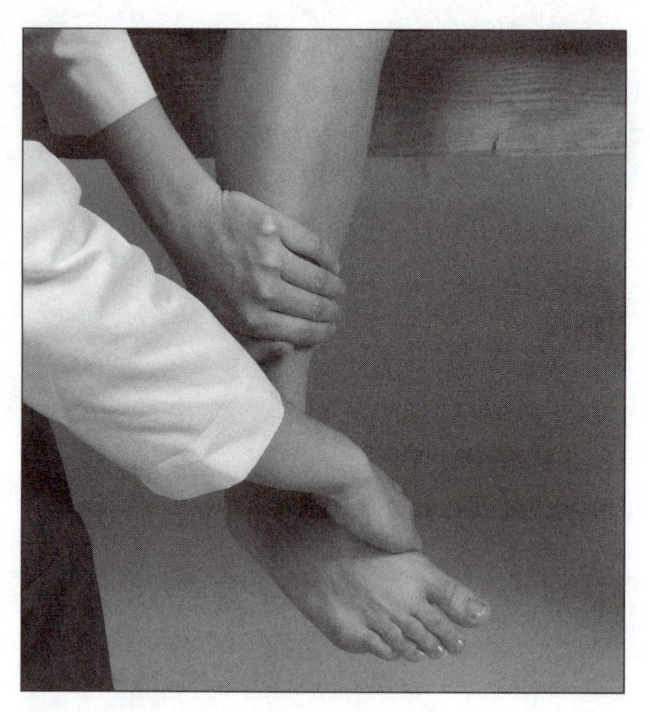

Figure 2-7-6 End position for foot inversion.

Normal, Good, Fair

Client Position: Starting—client is sitting with lower leg and foot over edge of testing surface. The foot and ankle are in neutral (Figure 2-7-5).

Motion—client moves the testing extremity into inversion with toes relaxed (Figure 2-7-6).

Therapist Position: Stabilize the lower leg proximal to the ankle. Resistance is applied on the medial border of the forefoot in the direction of foot eversion when testing Normal or Good strengths. No resistance is applied when testing Fair strength.

Poor

Client Position: Starting—client is supine. The testing knee is extended and the foot and ankle are in neutral.

Motion—client moves the testing extremity into foot inversion.

Therapist Position: Stabilize the lower leg proximal to the ankle. No resistance is applied in the gravity-eliminated position.

Foot: *eversion*

Foot eversion includes the following muscles: peroneus longus, peroneus brevis, and extensor digitorum longus.

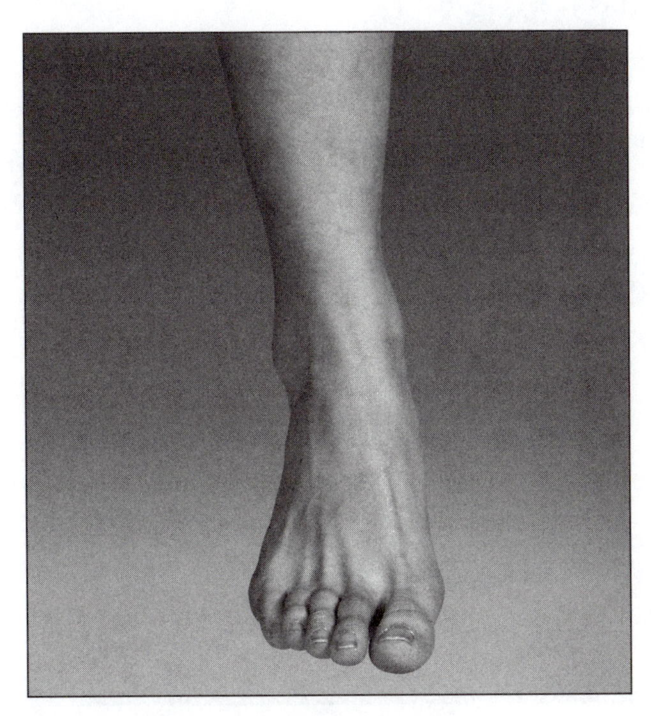

Figure 2-7-7 Start position for foot eversion.

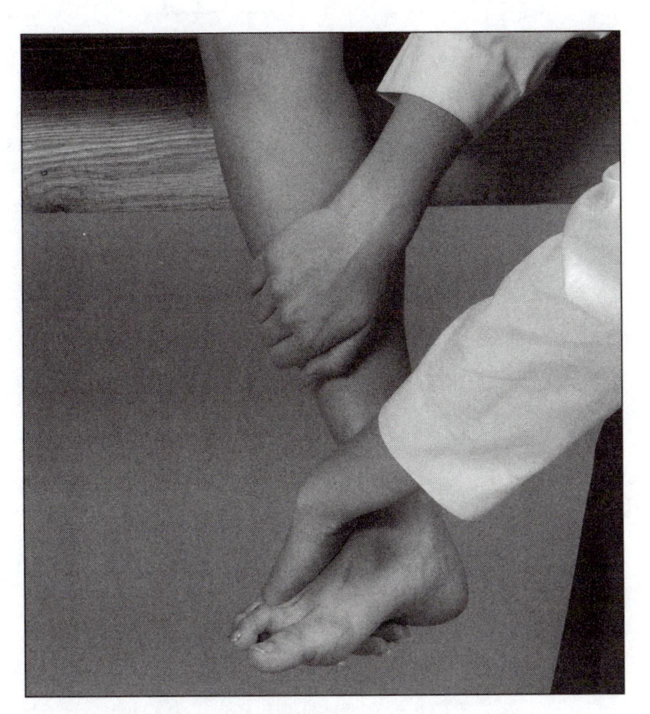

Figure 2-7-8 End position for foot eversion.

Normal, Good, Fair

Client Position: Starting—client is sitting with lower leg and foot over edge of testing surface. The ankle and foot are in neutral (Figure 2-7-7).

Motion—client moves the testing extremity into foot eversion (Figure 2-7-8).

Therapist Position: Stabilize the lower leg. Resistance is applied on the lateral border of the foot in the direction of foot inversion when testing Normal or Good strengths. No resistance is applied when testing Fair strength.

Poor

Client Position: Starting—client is supine with the testing knee extended and the heel resting over the edge of testing surface. The foot and ankle are in neutral.

Motion—client moves the testing extremity into foot eversion.

Therapist Position: Stabilize the lower leg proximal to the ankle. No resistance is applied in the gravity-eliminated position.

In gross manual muscle testing of the toes, gravity is not a consideration. Therefore, the muscle grade of "poor" is not assessed.

Toes: *MTP flexion*

MTP Flexion of the toes includes the following muscles: great toe—flexor hallucis brevis and toes #2–5—lumbricales.

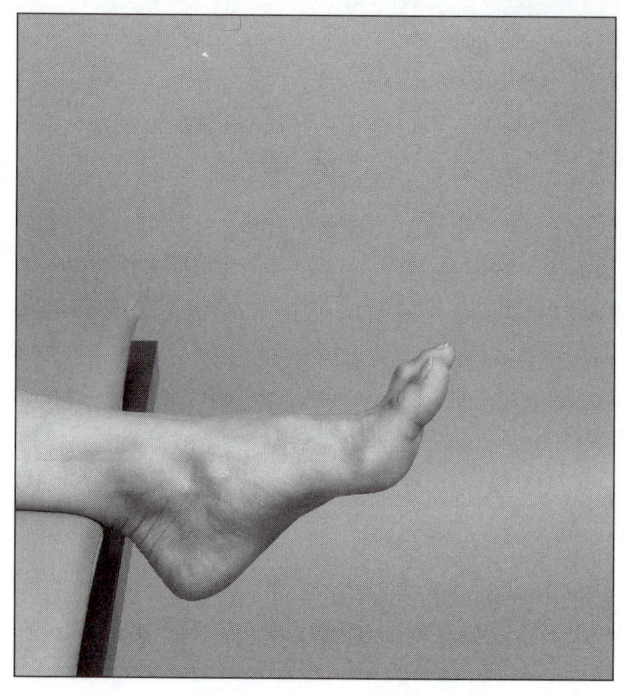

Figure 2-7-9 Start position for toe MTP flexion.

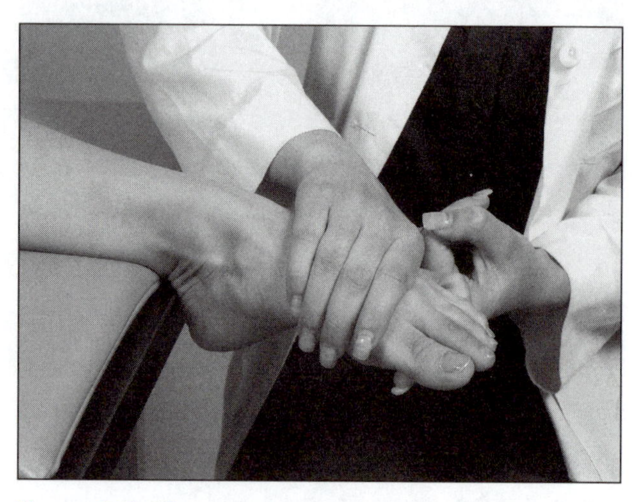

Figure 2-7-10 End position for toe MTP flexion.

Normal, Good, Fair

Client Position: Starting—client is supine. The testing knee is extended and lower leg and feet are resting in neutral on the testing surface (Figure 2-7-9).

Motion—client moves the testing extremity into MTP flexion of each toe (Figure 2-7-10).

Therapist Position: Stabilize the metatarsals and maintain IP joint extension. Resistance is applied on the plantar surface of the proximal phalanges of all toes in the direction of MTP extension when testing Normal or Good strengths. No resistance is applied when testing Fair strength.

Toes: *IP flexion*

IP flexion of the toes includes the following muscles: great toe—flexor hallucis longus; toes #2–5—flexor digitorum longus and flexor digitorum brevis.

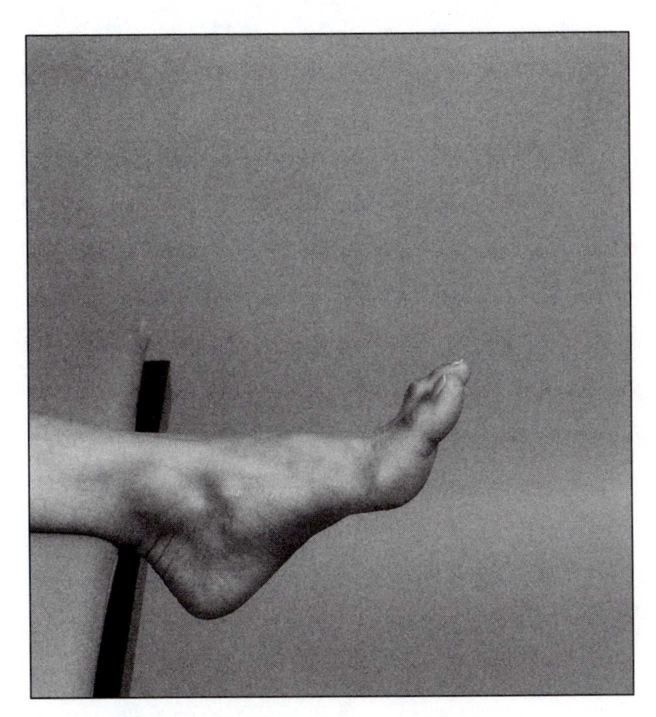

Figure 2-7-11 Start position for toe IP flexion.

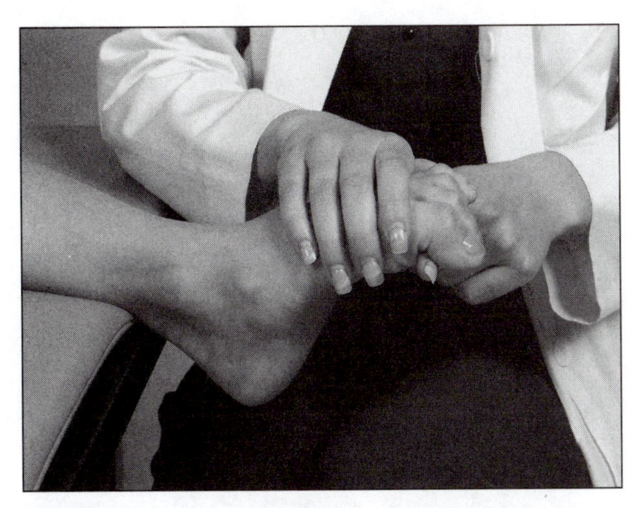

Figure 2-7-12 End position for toe IP flexion.

Normal, Good, Fair

Client Position: Starting—client is supine. The testing knee is extended and lower leg and feet are resting in neutral on the testing surface (Figure 2-7-11).

Motion—client moves the testing extremity into IP flexion of each toe (Figure 2-7-12).

Therapist Position: Stabilize the MTP joint of each toe tested. Resistance is applied on the plantar surface of the distal phalanx of the great toe and the distal and middle phalanges of toes #2–5 individually in the direction of IP extension when testing Normal or Good strengths. No resistance is applied when testing Fair strength.

Toes: *MTP abduction*

MTP abduction includes the following muscles: great toe—abductor hallucis; toes #2–5—abductor digiti minimi and dorsal interossei.

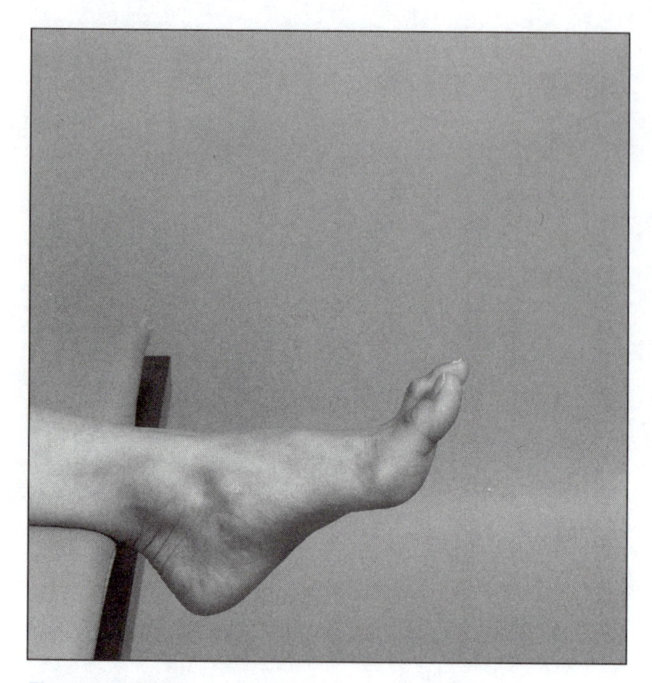

Figure 2-7-13 Start position for toe MTP abduction.

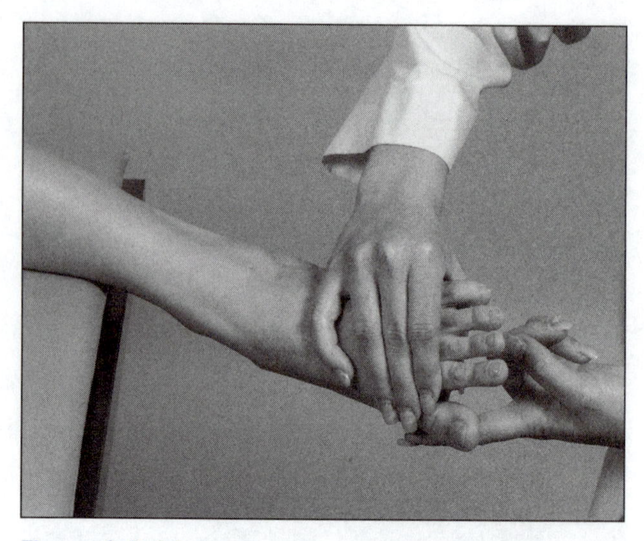

Figure 2-7-14 End position for toe MTP abduction.

Normal, Good, Fair

Client Position: Starting—client is supine. The testing knee is extended and lower leg and feet are resting in neutral on the testing surface. The toes are in adduction (Figure 2-7-13).

Motion—client moves the great toe into abduction (Figure 2-7-14).

Therapist Position: Stabilize the first metatarsal. Resistance is applied on the medial aspect of the proximal phalanx of the great toe in the direction of adduction when testing Normal or Good strengths. No resistance is applied when testing Fair strength.

Gross muscle testing is not performed on toes #2–5. They are only observed functionally.

Toes: *MTP/IP extension*

The extensors of the toes include the following muscles: great toe—extensor hallucis longus, IP of toes #2–5—extensor digitorum longus, and great toe and #2–4—extensor digitorum brevis.

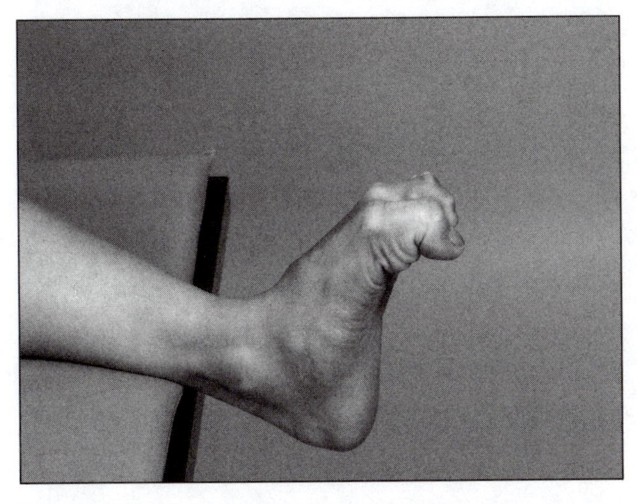

Figure 2-7-15 Start position for toe MTP/IP extension.

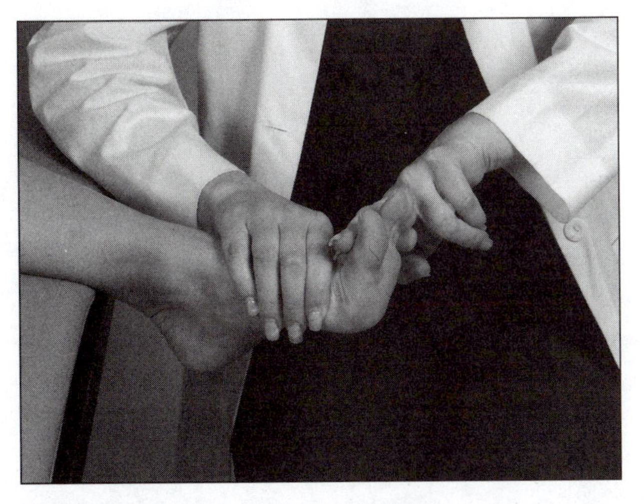

Figure 2-7-16 End position for toe MTP/IP extension.

Normal, Good, Fair

Client Position: Starting—client is supine. The testing knee is extended and lower leg and feet are resting in neutral on the testing surface. The toes are flexed (Figure 2-7-15).

Motion—client moves all toes into MTP extension and into IP extension (Figure 2-7-16). The toes are tested as a group.

Therapist Position: Stabilize the metatarsals of each toe tested. Resistance is applied on the dorsal surface of the distal phalanx of the great toe and the distal surface of toes #2–5 together in the direction of IP flexion when testing Normal or Good strengths. No resistance is applied when testing Fair strength.

chapter 3

Isolated Manual Muscle Testing

SECTION 3-1: Introduction to Isolated Manual Muscle Testing

After completing this chapter, the student should be able to accomplish the following:

- define the terms associated with isolated manual muscle testing
- demonstrate the ability to perform and grade isolated manual muscle testing

As stated in earlier chapters, isolated manual muscle testing is completed as part of the evaluation process of an individual's muscle strength. Before initiating isolated muscle testing, the therapist has completed a functional observation screening of the client, and gross manual muscle testing to identify the muscles that require isolated manual muscle testing. Recall that gross muscle testing tests groups of muscles, such as the hip flexors, while isolated manual muscle testing tests specific muscles. That does not mean that every muscle of the body is tested in isolation. There are certain sets of muscles that are tested together because it is not possible to isolate one from the other. In this chapter such muscles are noted and only one procedure is listed for those muscles.

Chapter two of this manual describes terminology and procedures related to gross manual muscle testing that also apply to isolated manual muscle testing. In review, the client must be positioned in either a gravity-eliminated (movement parallel to the floor) or an against-gravity (movement perpendicular to the floor) position. Once the client is positioned, the therapist must complete passive range of motion (PROM). This is when the therapist moves the client through the complete range of motion to assess the joint integrity/end feel and the muscle tone. Following PROM, the client is asked to demonstrate the motion using active range of motion (AROM). In order to begin the isolated manual muscle testing, the therapist places one hand proximal to the joint on which the testing muscle acts. This is the stabilizing hand. The other hand is generally placed distal to that same joint and applies pressure in the direction opposite to the client's motion. This is the resistance hand. Once the isolated manual muscle test is complete, the therapist grades the muscle strength and tests the contralateral side. The grading of muscles is found in Table 2-1-1.

Please refer to chapter two for specific information regarding precautions and contraindications for isolated manual muscle testing.

SECTION 3-2: Isolated Manual Muscle Testing of the Trunk and Neck

As stated in section 2-2 of this manual (Gross Manual Muscle Testing of the Trunk and Neck), the majority of muscles of the trunk and neck cannot be tested in an isolated manner. Because of this, there is only one muscle listed in this section. All others are tested only in the gross manual muscle testing format.

Trunk: *quadratus lumborum*

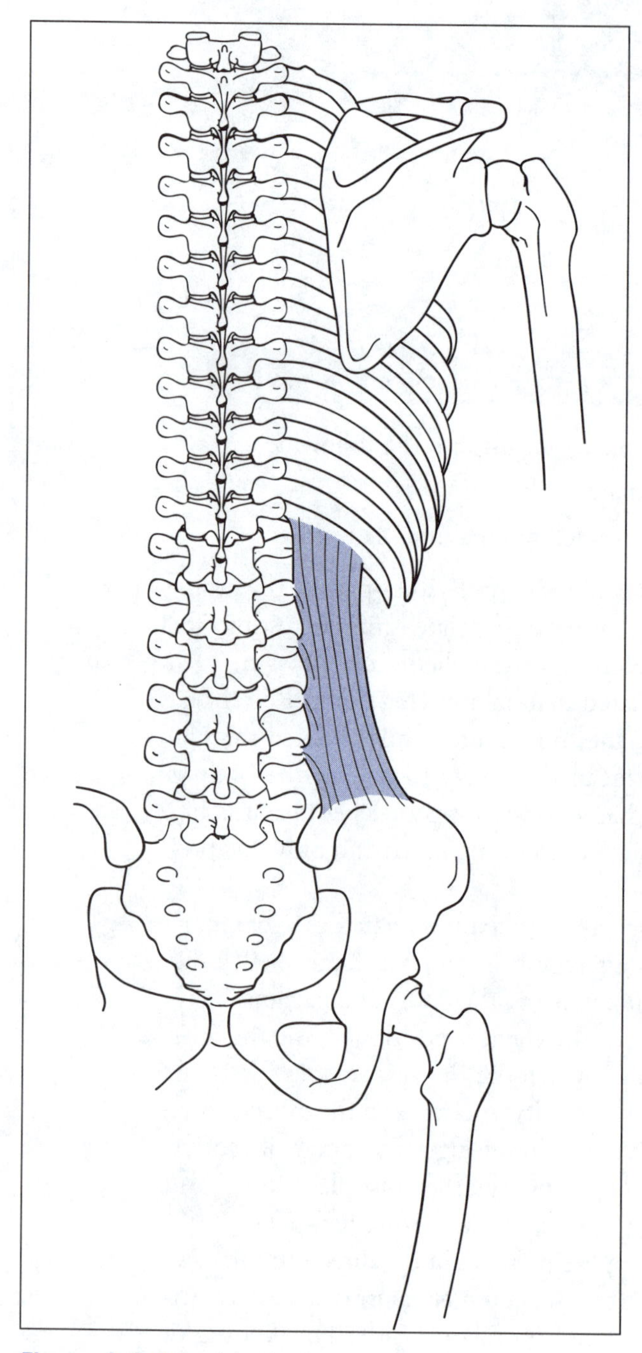

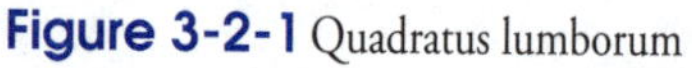

Figure 3-2-1 Quadratus lumborum

Origin: Iliolumbar ligament, iliac crest

Insertion: Inferior border of last rib, transverse processes of upper four lumbar vertebrae

Innervation: T12, L1–4

Action: Pelvic elevation, trunk lateral flexion

The quadratus lumborum is tested in the gravity-eliminated position. This is the most accurate test because when tested in standing (against gravity) other muscles act on the pelvis to a greater extent.

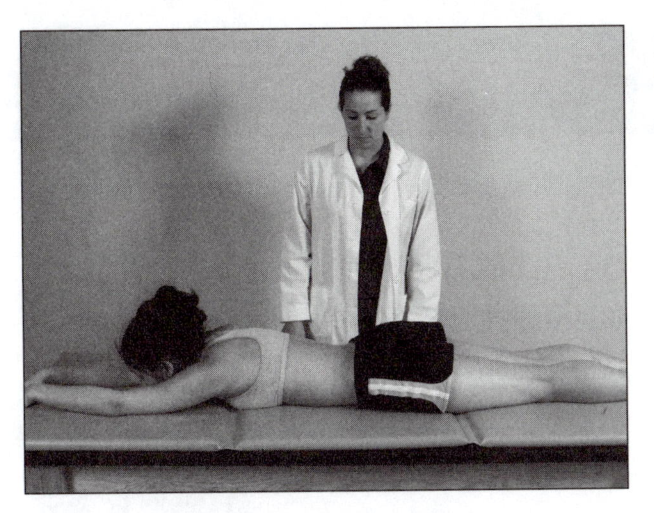

Figure 3-2-2 Start position for quadratus lumborum.

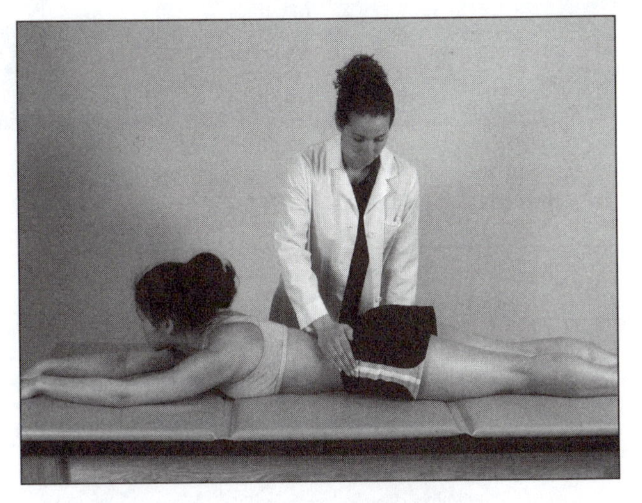

Figure 3-2-3 End position for quadratus lumborum.

Normal, Good, Fair

Client Position: Starting—client is prone with the hip in adduction and the feet off of the plinth (Figure 3-2-2).

Motion—client moves in the direction of pelvic elevation on the test side (Figure 3-2-3).

Therapist Position: Resistance is applied on the iliac crest in the direction of pelvic depression (Figure 3-2-3), or on the femur pulling into pelvic depression (Figure 3-2-3a), when testing Normal or Good strengths. No resistance is applied when testing Fair strength. No manual stabilization is used during this test.

Poor

Client Position: Starting—client is prone with the hip in adduction and the feet off the plinth.

Motion—client moves in the direction of pelvic elevation on the test side.

Therapist Position: No manual stabilization or resistance is applied during this test except that the therapist may be required to support the testing extremity against gravity while the client moves the pelvis.

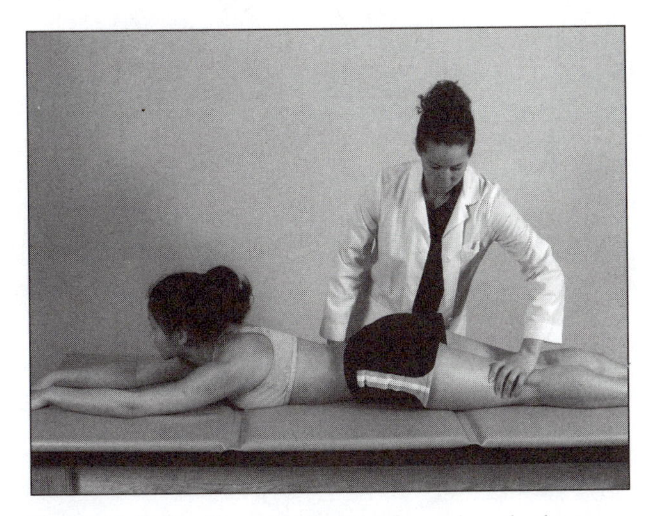

Figure 3-2-3a Alternate end position for quadratus lumborum.

Trace

It is difficult to palpate the quadratus lumborum because it is deeply located; however, at times it can be palpated superior to the ilium crest, lateral to the trunk extensors' muscle mass.

SECTION 3-3: Isolated Manual Muscle Testing of the Scapula and Shoulder Complex

Shoulder: *posterior deltoid*

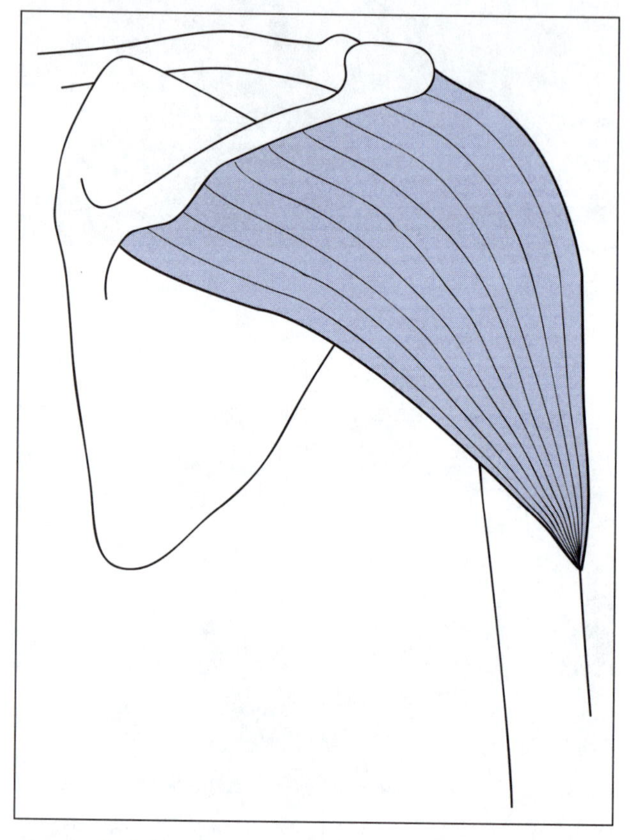

Figure 3-3-1 Posterior deltoid

Origin: Inferior lip, spine of scapula

Insertion: Deltoid tuberosity of the humerus

Innervation: Axillary nerve

Action: Humeral extension, humeral horizontal abduction, and humeral external rotation.

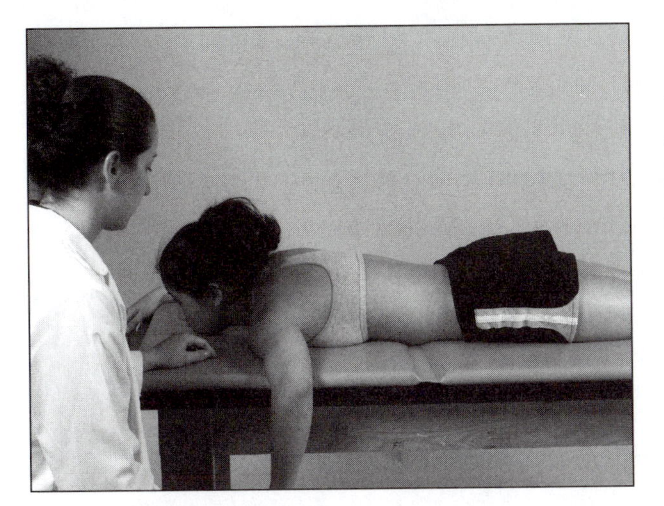

Figure 3-3-2 Start position for posterior deltoid.

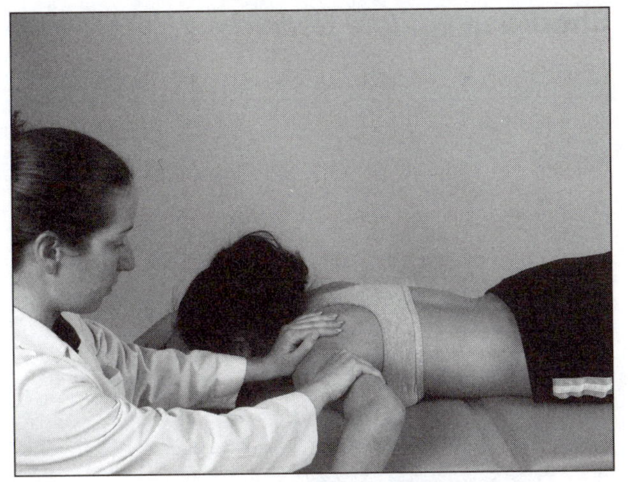

Figure 3-3-3 End position for posterior deltoid.

Normal, Good, Fair

Client Position: Starting—client is prone with the testing extremity in abduction and slight external rotation. Elbow is flexed at 90 degrees (over the edge of the table) (Figure 3-3-2).

Motion—client moves the testing extremity in the direction of humeral horizontal abduction (Figure 3-3-3).

Therapist Position: Stabilize at the scapula to avoid scapular retraction/adduction. Observe elbow for compensation of the triceps (elbow extension). Resistance is applied at the posterior–lateral aspect of the distal humerus in the direction of horizontal adduction when testing Normal or Good strengths. No resistance is applied when testing Fair strength.

Poor

Client Position: Starting—client is sitting with the testing extremity in 90 degrees of humeral flexion and 90 degrees of elbow flexion, supported on a table or by the therapist.

Motion—client moves the testing extremity in the direction of horizontal abduction.

Therapist Position: Stabilize at the scapula to avoid scapular retraction/adduction. Observe elbow for compensation of the triceps (elbow extension). Support the testing extremity to eliminate gravity; however, do not assist the motion. No resistance is applied in the gravity-eliminated position.

Trace

The posterior deltoid can be palpated on the dorsal/proximal one-third of the humerus.

Shoulder: *middle deltoid*

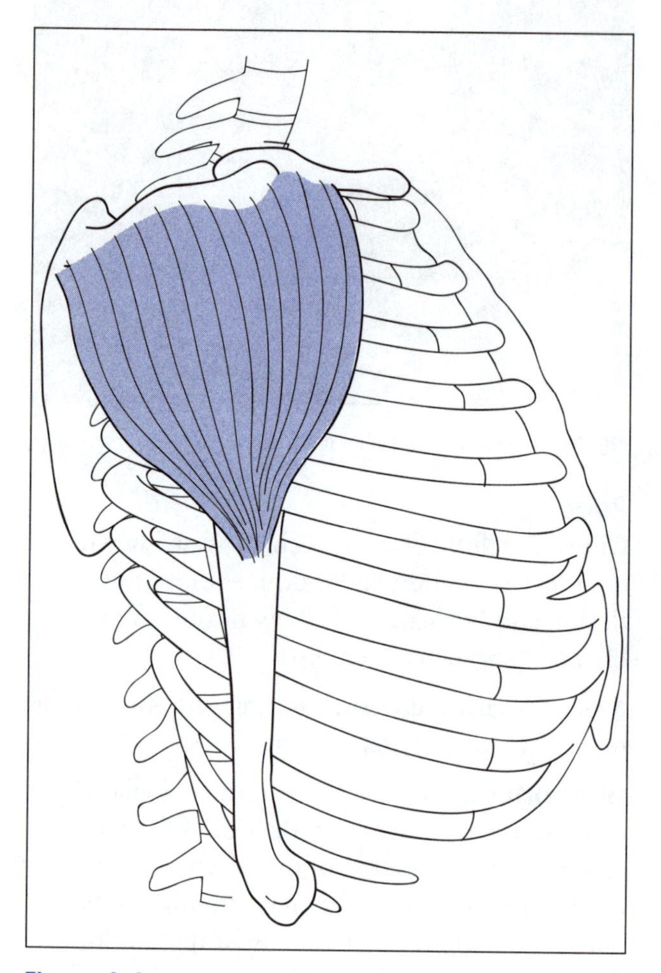

Figure 3-3-4 Middle deltoid

Origin: Acromion process

Insertion: Deltoid tuberosity of the humerus

Innervation: Axillary nerve

Action: Humeral abduction

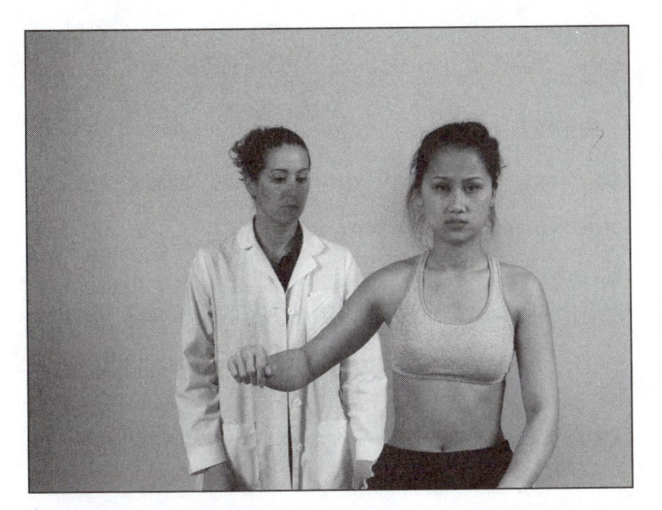

Figure 3-3-5 Start position for middle deltoid.

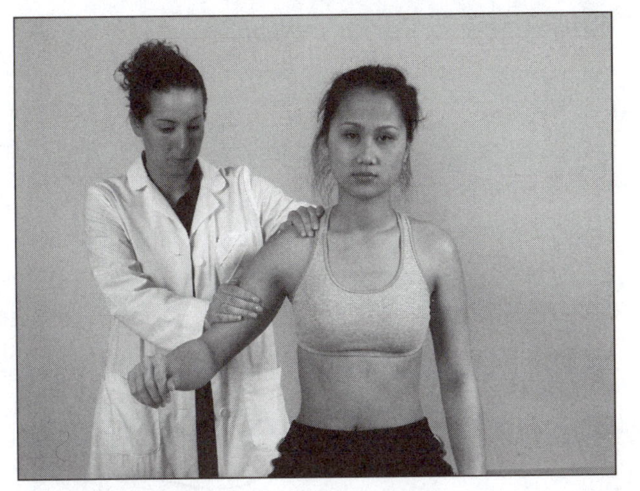

Figure 3-3-6 End position for middle deltoid.

Normal, Good, Fair

Client Position: Starting—client is sitting or standing with the testing extremity between zero and 45 degrees of humeral abduction and the elbow is flexed to 90 degrees (Figure 3-3-5).

Motion—client moves the testing extremity in the direction of humeral abduction (Figure 3-3-6).

Therapist Position: Stabilize at the shoulder to avoid compensation of scapular elevation. Resistance is applied at the distal humerus in the direction of adduction when testing Normal or Good strengths. No resistance is applied when testing Fair strength.

Poor

Client Position: Starting—client is supine with the testing extremity in humeral adduction.

Motion—client moves the testing extremity in the direction of humeral abduction.

Therapist Position: Stabilize at the shoulder to avoid compensation of scapular elevation. No resistance is applied when testing in the gravity-eliminated position.

Trace

The middle deltoid can be palpated below the acromion process on the lateral/proximal one-third of the humerus.

Shoulder: *anterior deltoid*

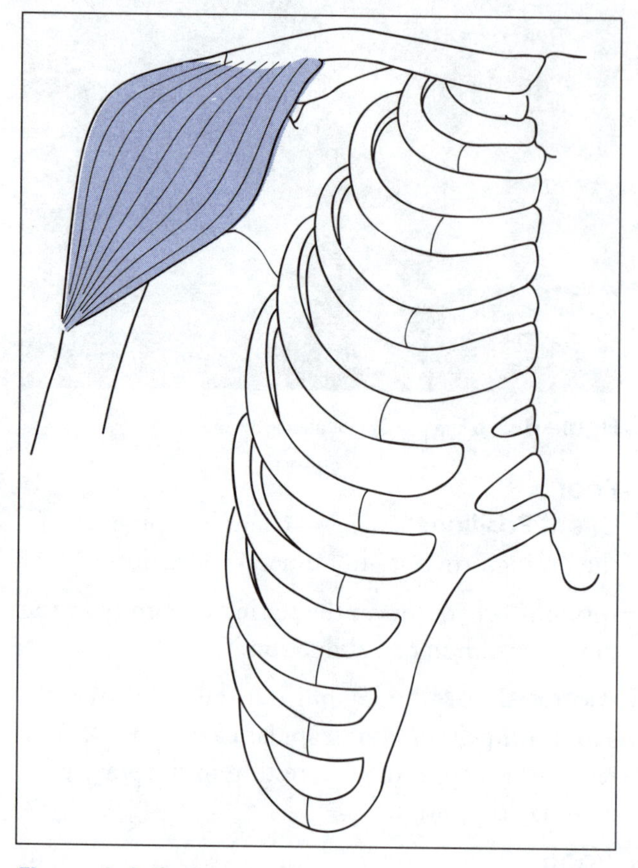

Figure 3-3-7 Anterior deltoid

Origin: Lateral 1/3 of clavicle

Insertion: Deltoid tuberosity of the humerus

Innervation: Axillary nerve

Action: Humeral flexion, humeral horizontal adduction, and humeral internal rotation

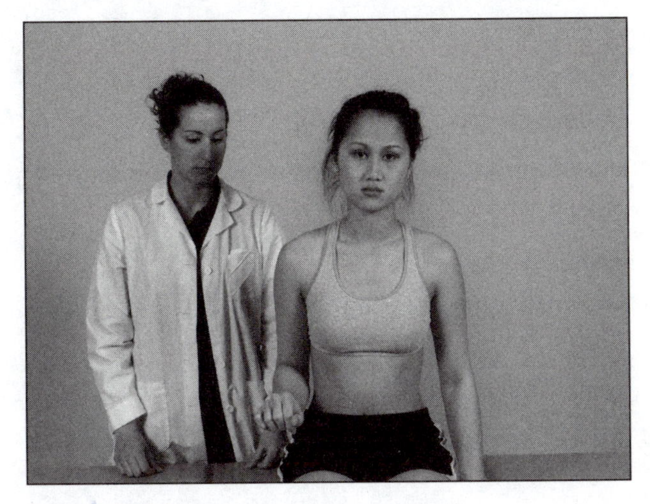

Figure 3-3-8 Start position for anterior deltoid.

Normal, Good, Fair

Client Position: Starting—client is sitting or standing with the testing extremity at the side with slight elbow flexion and forearm pronation (Figure 3-3-8).

Motion—client moves the testing extremity in the direction of humeral flexion (Figure 3-3-9).

Therapist Position: Stabilize at the shoulder to avoid compensation of humeral rotation or horizontal movement. Resistance is applied at the proximal humerus in the direction of humeral extension when testing Normal or Good strengths. No resistance is applied when testing Fair strength.

Poor

Client Position: Starting—client is lying on the uninvolved side and the testing extremity is at the side with slight elbow flexion, and forearm pronation, supported on a table or by the therapist.

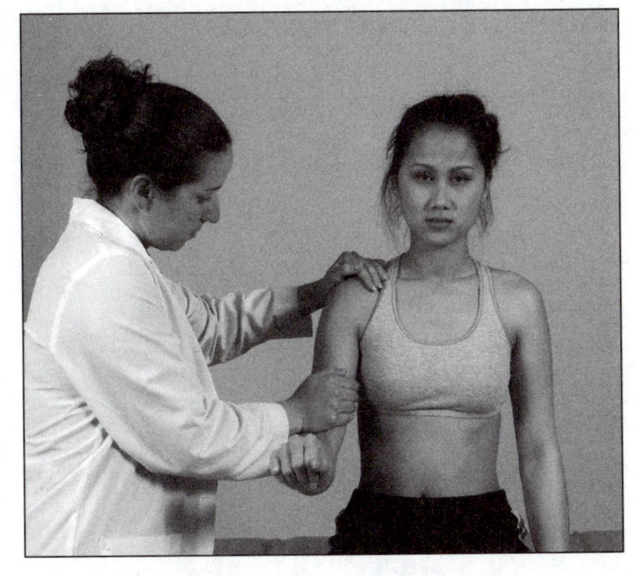

Figure 3-3-9 End position for anterior deltoid.

Motion—client moves the testing extremity in the direction of humeral flexion.

Therapist Position: Stabilize at the shoulder to avoid compensation of humeral rotation or horizontal movement. Support the testing extremity to eliminate gravity; however, do not assist the motion. No resistance is applied when testing in the gravity-eliminated position.

Trace

Anterior deltoid is palpated by locating the acromion process and bringing the therapist's fingers 2 to 3 inches anteriorly along the client's shoulder.

Shoulder: *coracobrachialis*

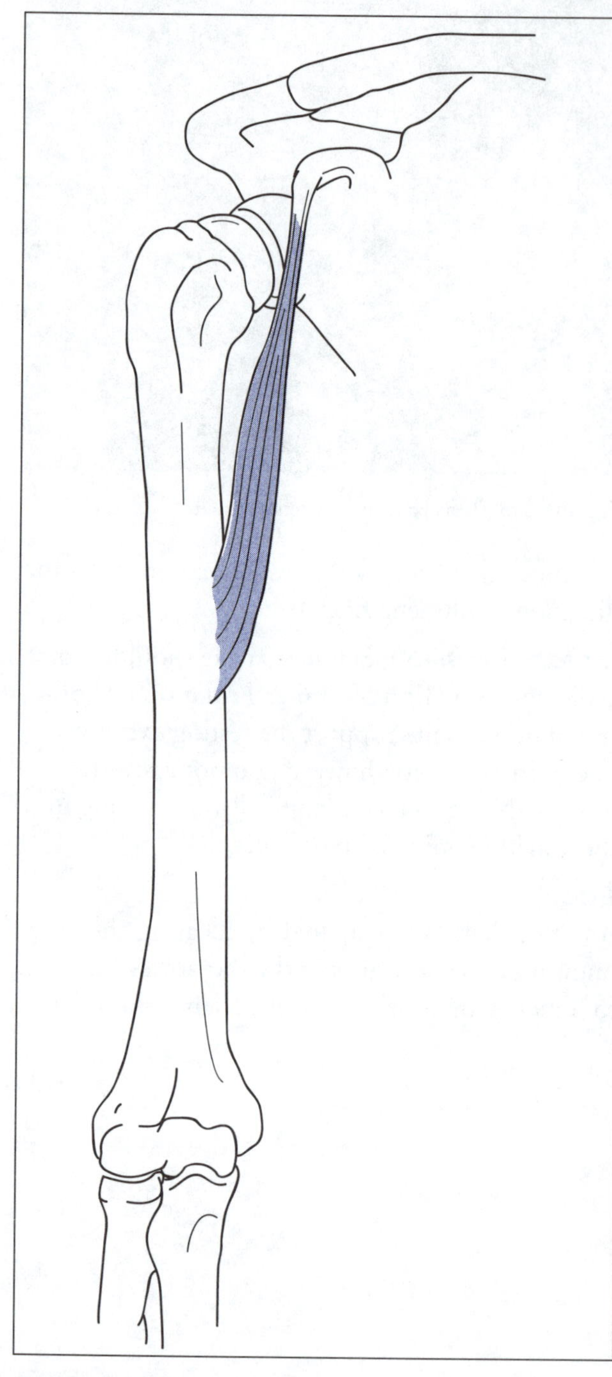

Figure 3-3-10 Coracobrachialis

Origin: Coracoid process of scapula

Insertion: Opposite deltoid tuberosity on the medial aspect of the mid-humerus

Innervation: Musculocutaneous nerve

Action: Humeral flexion

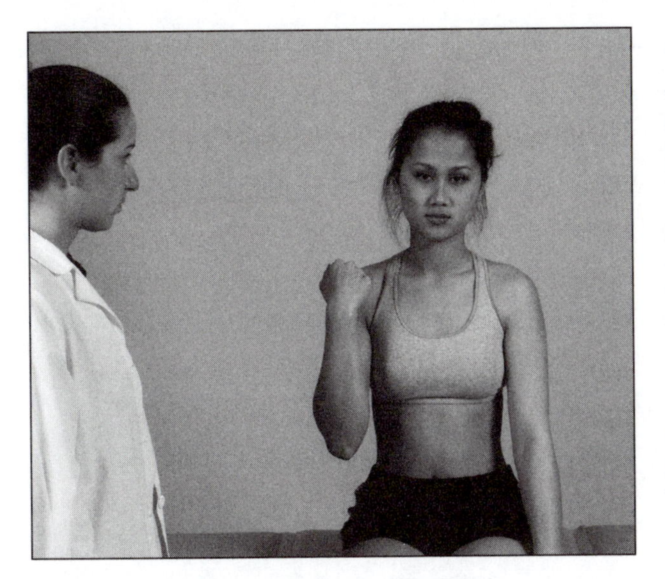

Figure 3-3-11 Start position for coracobrachialis.

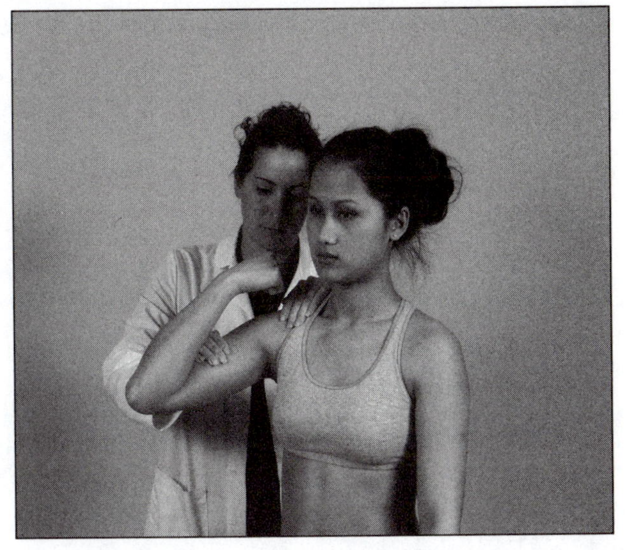

Figure 3-3-12 End position for coracobrachialis.

Normal, Good, Fair

Client Position: Starting—client is sitting or standing with the testing extremity at the side with slight humeral external rotation, full elbow flexion, and forearm supination (Figure 3-3-11).

Motion—client moves the testing extremity in the direction of humeral flexion while keeping the elbow flexed (Figure 3-3-12).

Therapist Position: Stabilize at the shoulder to avoid compensation. Resistance is applied at the proximal humerus in the direction of humeral extension and slight humeral internal rotation when testing Normal or Good strengths. No resistance is applied when testing Fair strength.

Poor

Client Position: Starting—client is lying on the unaffected side with the testing extremity at the side with slight humeral external rotation, full elbow flexion, and forearm supination.

Motion—client moves the testing extremity in the direction of humeral flexion while keeping the elbow flexed.

Therapist Position: Stabilize at the shoulder to avoid compensation. No resistance is applied when testing in the gravity-eliminated position.

Trace

Muscle is too deep to be palpated.

Shoulder: *pectoralis major (clavicular head)*

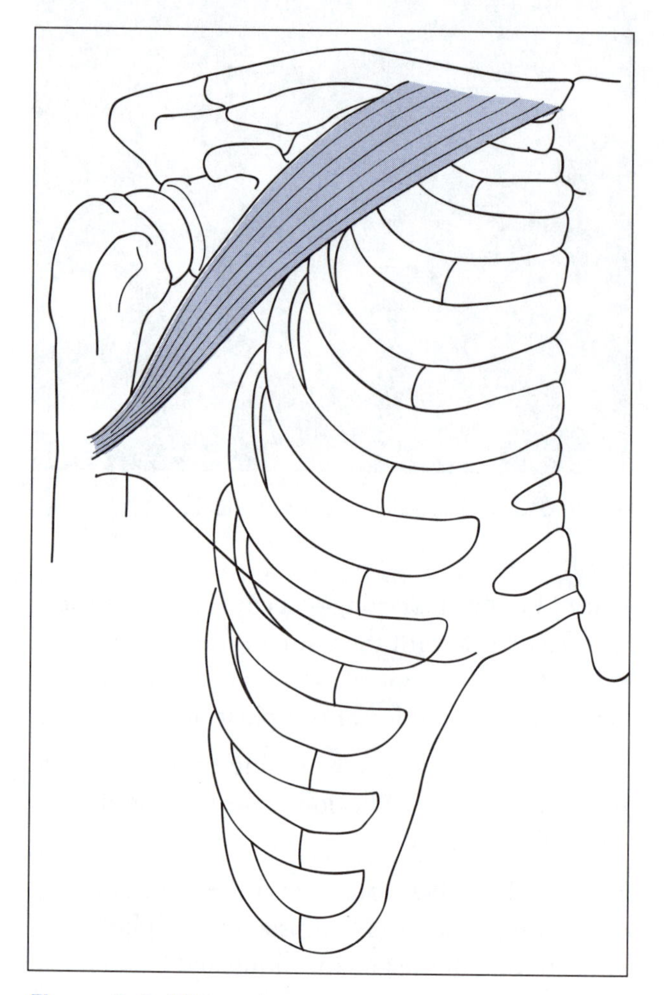

Figure 3-3-13 Pectoralis major (clavicular head)

Origin: Medial 2/3 of the clavicle

Insertion: Crest of greater tubercle of humerus

Innervation: Medial pectoral nerve

Action: Humeral flexion, humeral horizontal adduction, humeral adduction

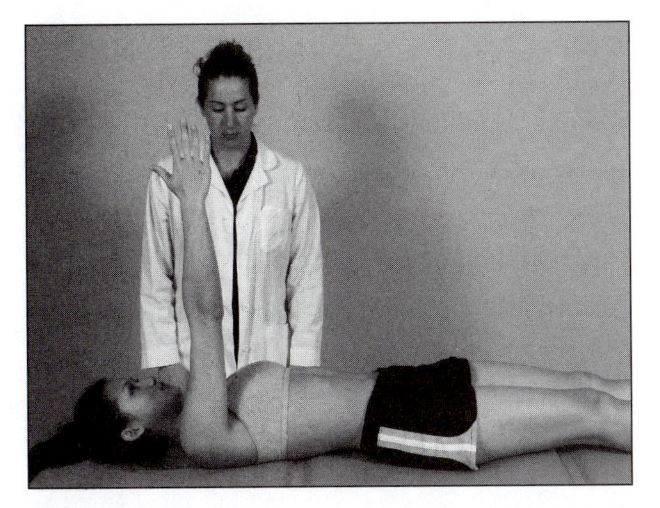

Figure 3-3-14 Start position for pectoralis major (clavicular head).

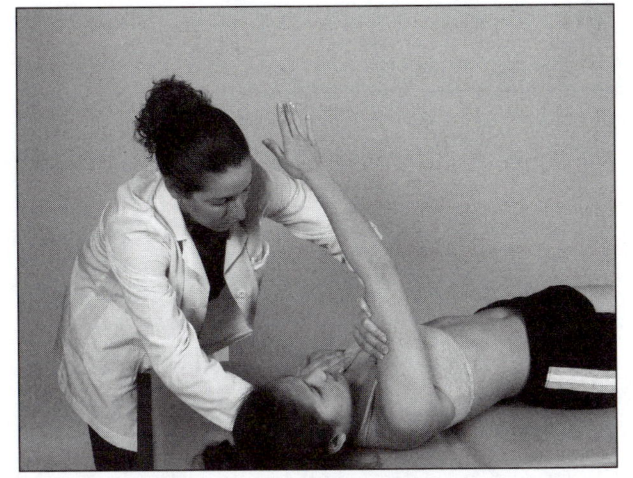

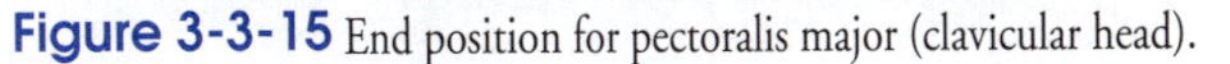

Figure 3-3-15 End position for pectoralis major (clavicular head).

Normal, Good, Fair

Client Position: Starting—client is supine with the testing extremity positioned in 90 degrees of humeral flexion, slight humeral internal rotation, and complete elbow extension (Figure 3-3-14).

Motion—client moves the testing extremity in the direction of the horizontal adduction (Figure 3-3-15).

Therapist Position: Stabilize at the contralateral shoulder to avoid compensation. Resistance is applied at the proximal humerus in the direction of horizontal abduction when testing Normal or Good strengths. No resistance is applied when testing Fair strength.

Poor

Client Position: Starting—client is sitting with the testing extremity positioned in 90 degrees of humeral flexion, slight humeral internal rotation, and complete elbow extension, supported by the therapist.

Motion—client moves the testing extremity in the direction of humeral horizontal adduction.

Therapist Position: Stabilize at the contralateral shoulder to avoid compensation. Support the testing extremity to eliminate gravity; however, do not assist the motion. No resistance is applied when testing in the gravity-eliminated position.

Trace

Pectoralis major (clavicular) can be palpated below the middle of the clavicle.

Shoulder: *pectoralis major (sternal head)*

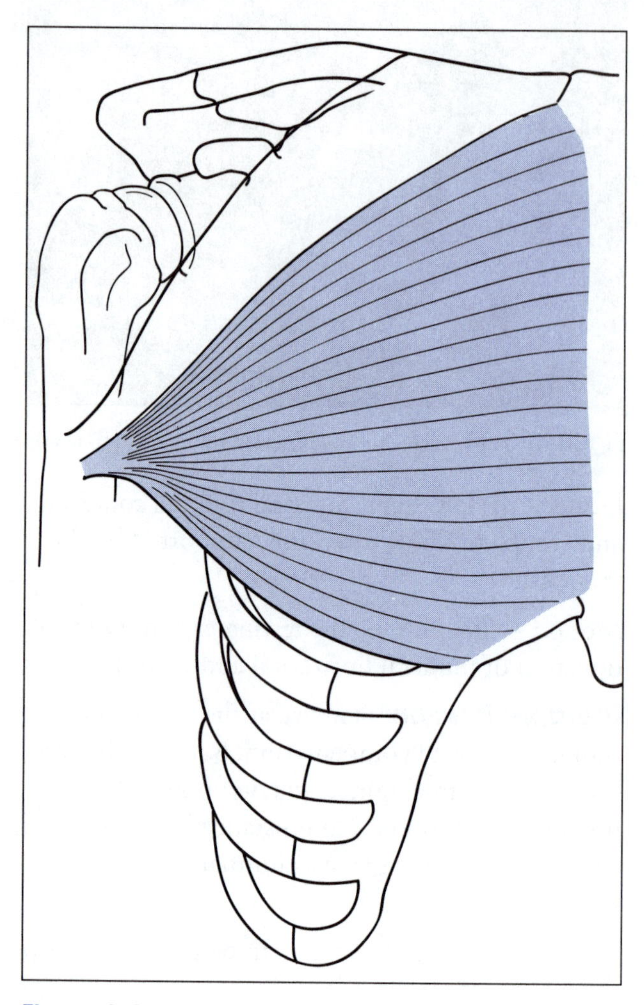

Figure 3-3-16 Pectoralis major (sternal head)

Origin: Sternum, costal cartilage ribs 1–6

Insertion: Crest of greater tubercle of the humerus

Innervation: Lateral pectoral nerve

Action: Humeral horizontal adduction, humeral extension

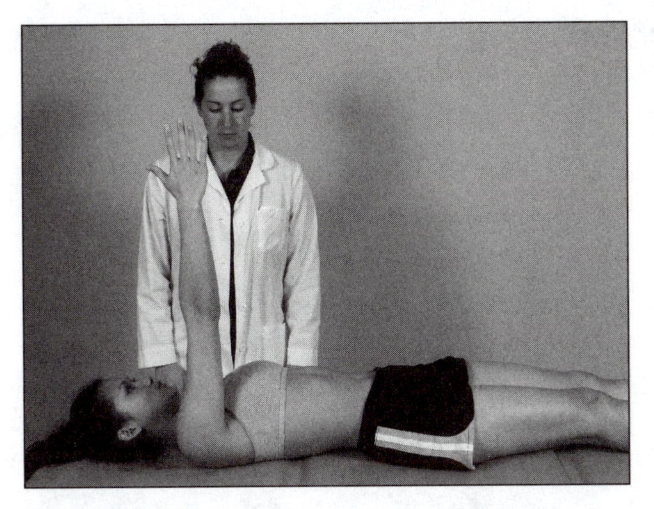

Figure 3-3-17 Start position for pectoralis major (sternal head).

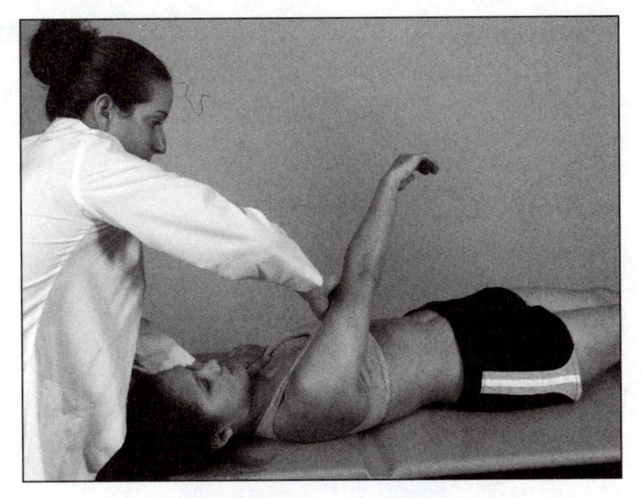

Figure 3-3-18 End position for pectoralis major (sternal head).

Normal, Good, Fair

Client Position: Starting—client is supine with the testing extremity in 90 degrees of humeral flexion, slight humeral internal rotation, and complete elbow extension (Figure 3-3-17).

Motion—client moves the testing extremity in the direction of humeral horizontal adduction, but in a diagonal pattern toward the opposite iliac crest (Figure 3-3-18).

Therapist Position: Stabilize at the opposite iliac crest to avoid trunk rotation. Resistance is applied at the proximal humerus in a diagonal pattern of humeral horizontal abduction when testing Normal or Good strengths. No resistance is applied when testing Fair strength.

Poor

Client Position: Starting—client is sitting with the testing extremity in 90 degrees humeral flexion, slight humeral internal rotation, and complete elbow flexion, supported by the therapist.

Motion—client moves the testing extremity in the direction of humeral horizontal adduction, but in a diagonal pattern toward the opposite iliac crest.

Therapist Position: Stabilize at the opposite iliac crest to avoid compensation of trunk rotation. Support the testing extremity to eliminate gravity; however, do not assist the motion. No resistance is applied when testing in the gravity-eliminated position.

Trace

The pectoralis major (sternal end) is palpated on the anterior aspect of the axilla.

Shoulder: *latissimus dorsi*, and *teres major* (tested together)

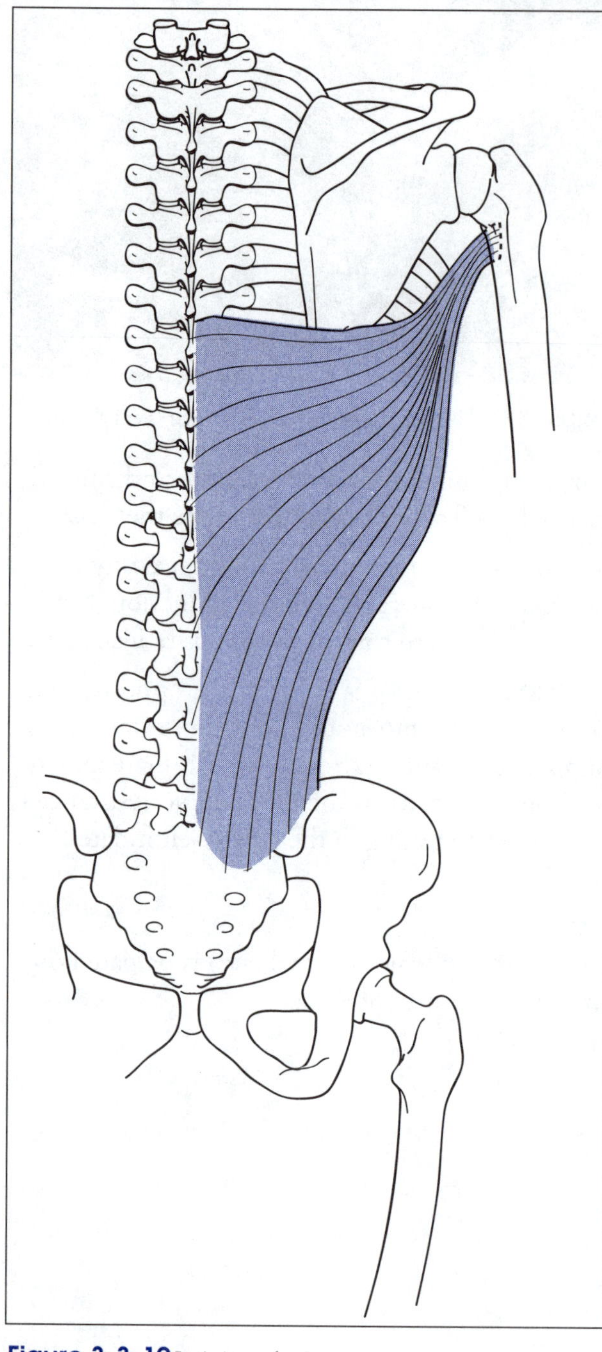

Figure 3-3-19 Latissimus dorsi

Latissimus dorsi

Origin: Spinous process of last 6 thoracic vertebrae, all lumbar and all sacral vertebrae, posterior iliac crest, posterior last 3 ribs, inferior angle of the scapula

Insertion: Bottom of intertubercular groove of humerus

Innervation: Thoracodorsal nerves

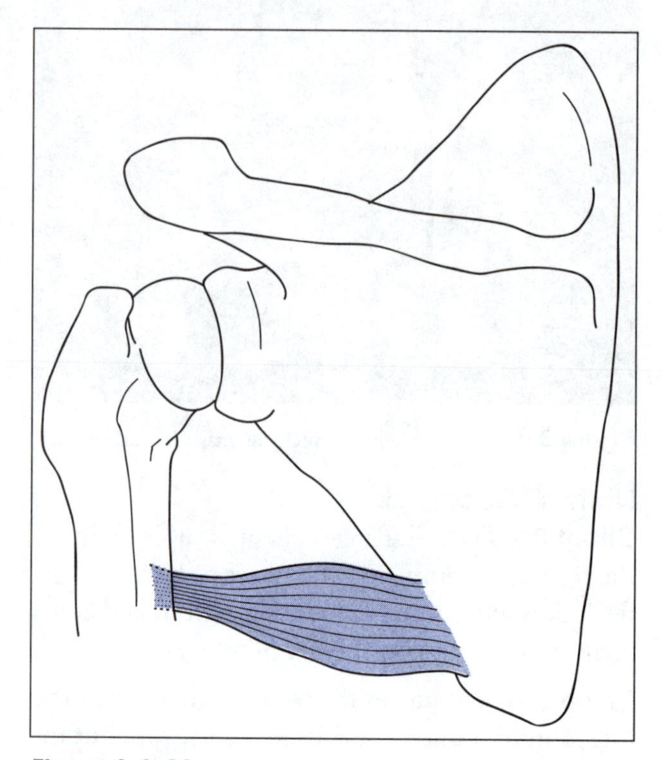

Figure 3-3-20 Teres major

Action: Humeral extension, humeral adduction, humeral internal rotation, and scapular depression

Teres major

Origin: Dorsal surface of the inferior angle of the scapula

Insertion: Below the lesser tuberosity of the humerus, posterior to the latissimus dorsi insertion

Innervation: Inferior subscapular nerve

Action: Humeral extension, humeral internal rotation, and humeral adduction

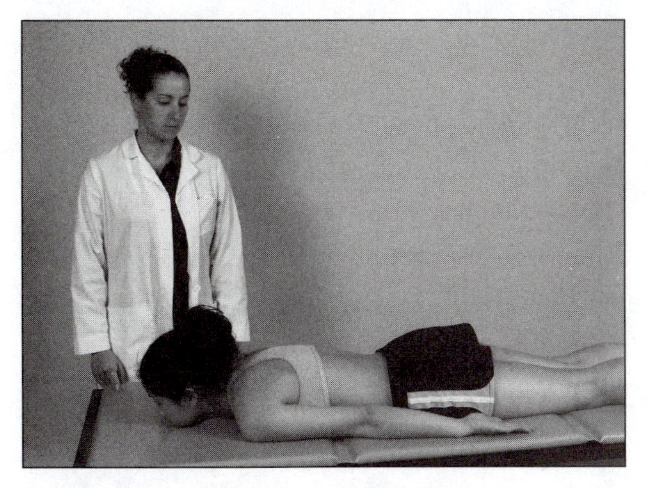

Figure 3-3-21 Start position for latissimus dorsi and teres major.

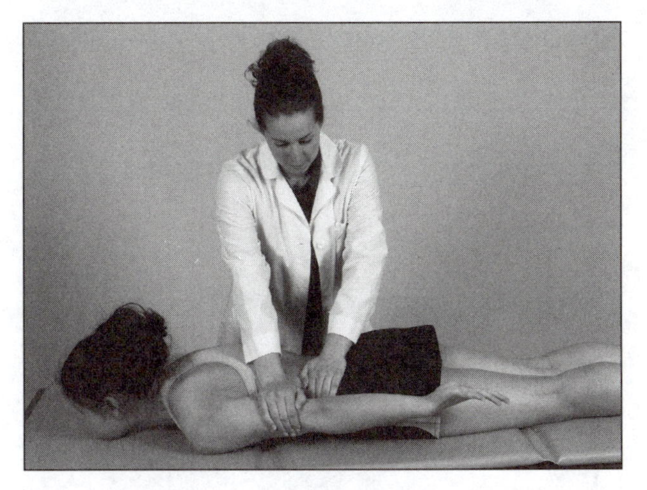

Figure 3-3-22 End position for latissimus dorsi and teres major.

Normal, Good, Fair

Client Position: Starting—client is prone with the testing extremity at side in humeral internal rotation (Figure 3-3-21).

Motion—client moves the testing extremity in the direction of humeral extension and humeral adduction while also depressing the scapula. (Reach toward feet while maintaining extension.) (Figure 3-3-22).

Therapist Position: Stabilize at the lateral pelvis to avoid the compensation of trunk rotation. Resistance is applied on the distal humerus in the direction of humeral flexion and humeral abduction when testing Normal or Good strengths. No resistance is applied when testing Fair strength.

Poor

Client Position: Starting—client is prone with the testing extremity in humeral extension, humeral internal rotation, and humeral adduction.

Motion—client moves the testing extremity in the direction of humeral extension and humeral adduction while also depressing the scapula. (Reach toward feet while maintaining extension.) A grade of poor is given when the client moves through partial range only.

Therapist Position: Stabilize at the lateral trunk to avoid the compensation of rotation. No resistance is applied when testing in the gravity-eliminated position.

Trace

The latissimus dorsi is palpated on the lower border of the scapula below the teres major fibers. The teres major is palpated along the lower border of the scapula.

Shoulder: *subscapularis*

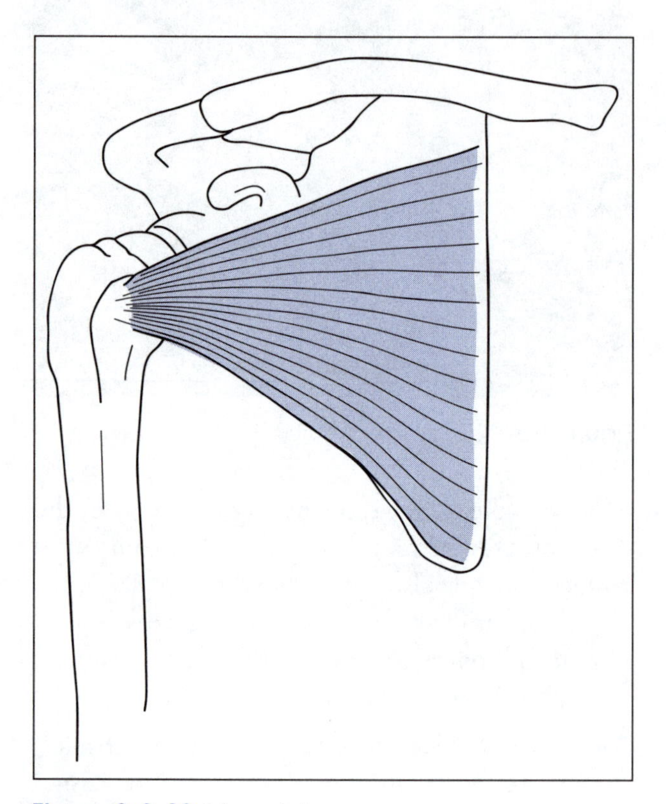

Figure 3-3-23 Subscapularis

Origin: Subscapular fossa of scapula

Insertion: Lesser tubercle of humerus, capsule of shoulder joint

Innervation: Superior upper and inferior lower subscapular nerves

Action: Humeral internal rotation, one of the muscles of the rotator cuff

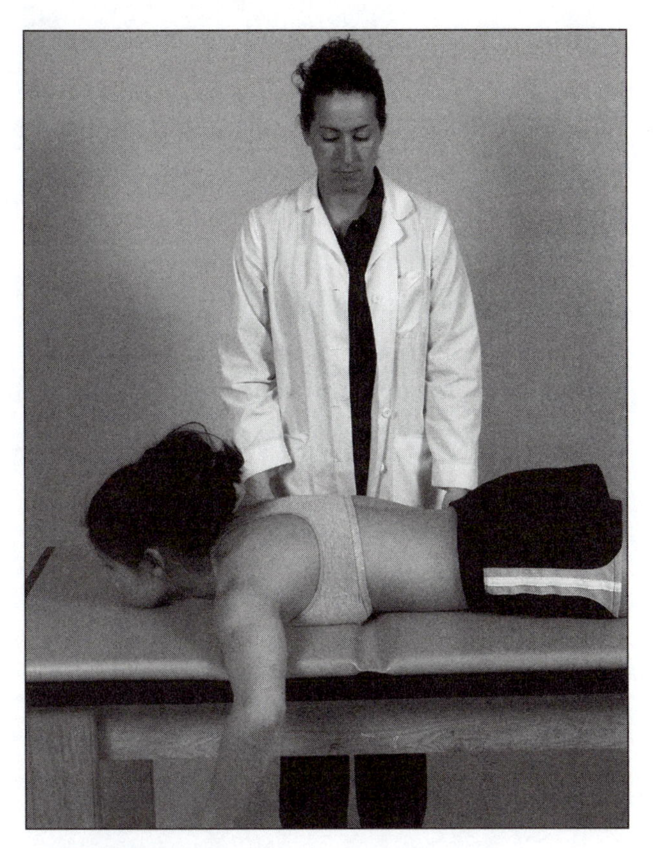

Figure 3-3-24 Start position for subscapularis.

Normal, Good, Fair

Client Position: Starting—client is prone with the testing extremity in 90 degrees of humeral abduction and 90 degrees of elbow flexion (fingers pointed toward the floor) (Figure 3-3-24).

Motion—client moves the testing extremity in the direction of humeral internal rotation (Figure 3-3-25).

Therapist Position: Stabilize under the humerus to avoid compensation. Resistance is applied at the forearm in the direction of humeral external rotation when testing Normal or Good strengths. No resistance is applied when testing Fair strength.

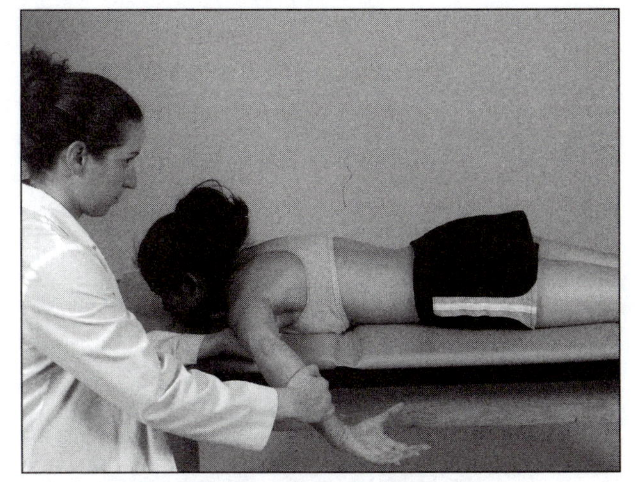

Figure 3-3-25 End position for subscapularis.

Poor

Client Position: Starting—client is prone with the entire humerus off the table (fingers point toward the floor).

Motion—client moves the testing extremity in the direction of humeral internal rotation (LUE = clockwise, RUE = counter-clockwise).

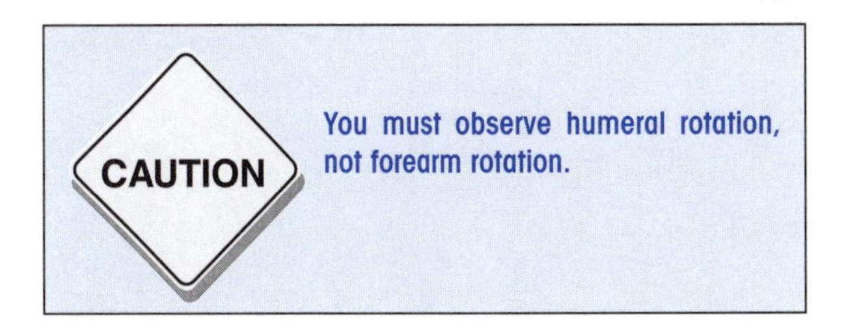

Therapist Position: Stabilize at the scapula to avoid compensation. No resistance is applied when testing in the gravity-eliminated position.

Trace

The subscapularis is palpated deep in the axilla, near the insertion.

Alternate Position

Client Position: Starting—client is sitting with the testing extremity in humeral adduction, and elbow flexion to 90 degrees.

Motion—client moves the testing extremity in the direction of humeral internal rotation (hand moves toward the body).

Shoulder: *infraspinatus* (tested with *teres minor*)

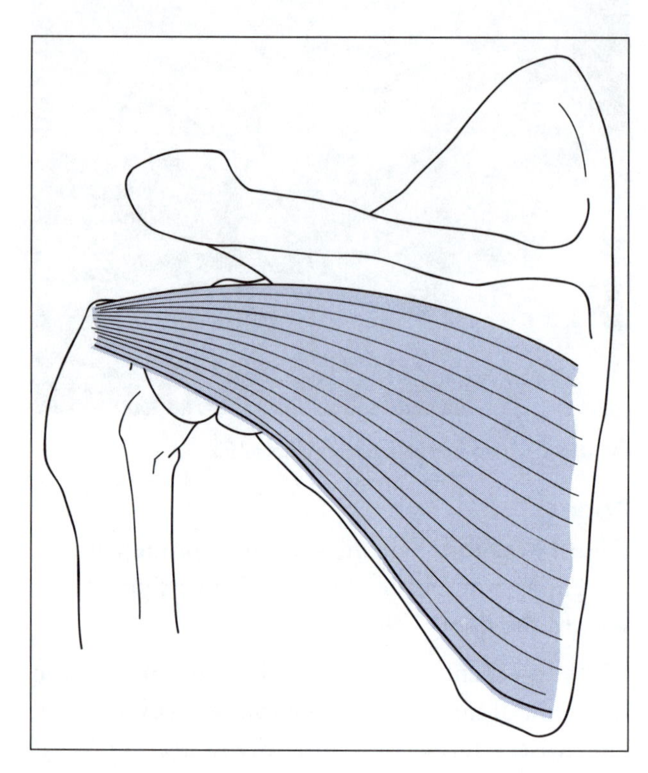

Figure 3-3-26 Infraspinatus

Origin: Medial 2/3 of infraspinatus fossa of the scapula

Insertion: Greater tubercle of humerus, capsule of the shoulder joint

Innervation: Suprascapular nerve

Action: Humeral external rotation and humeral horizontal abduction, one of the muscles of the rotator cuff

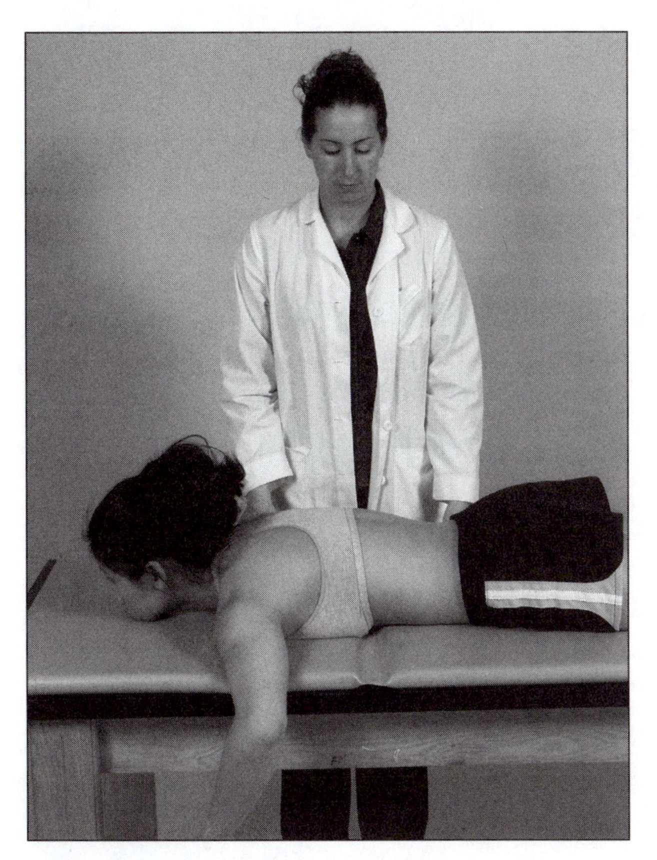

Figure 3-3-27 Start position for infraspinatus.

Normal, Good, Fair

Client Position: Starting—client is prone with the testing extremity in 90 degrees of humeral abduction and 90 degrees of elbow flexion (fingers point toward the floor) (Figure 3-3-27).

Motion—client moves the testing extremity in the direction of humeral external rotation (Figure 3-3-28).

Therapist Position: Stabilize under the humerus to avoid compensation. Resistance is applied at the forearm in the direction of humeral internal rotation when testing Normal or Good strengths. No resistance is applied when testing Fair strength.

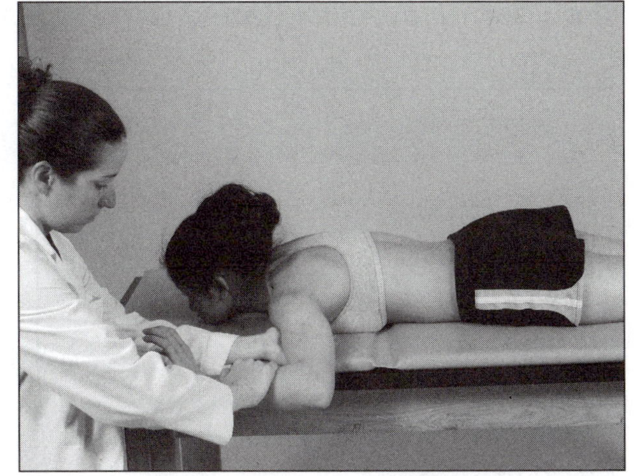

Figure 3-3-28 End position for infraspinatus.

Poor

Client Position: Starting—client is prone with the entire extremity off the table (fingers point toward the floor).

Motion—client moves the testing extremity in the direction of humeral external rotation (LUE = counter-clockwise, RUE = clockwise).

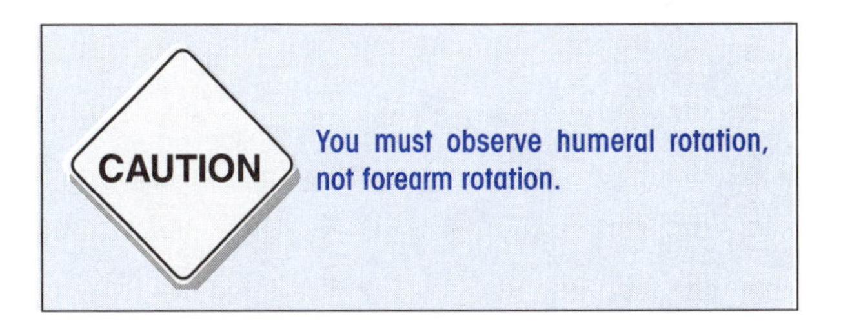

You must observe humeral rotation, not forearm rotation.

Therapist Position: Stabilize at the scapula to avoid compensation. No resistance is applied when testing in the gravity-eliminated position.

Trace

The infraspinatus is palpated below the spine of the scapula.

Alternate Position

Client Position: Starting—client is sitting with the testing extremity in humeral adduction, and elbow flexion to 90 degrees.

Motion—client moves the testing extremity in the direction of humeral external rotation (hand moves away from the body).

Shoulder: *teres minor* (tested with *infraspinatus*)

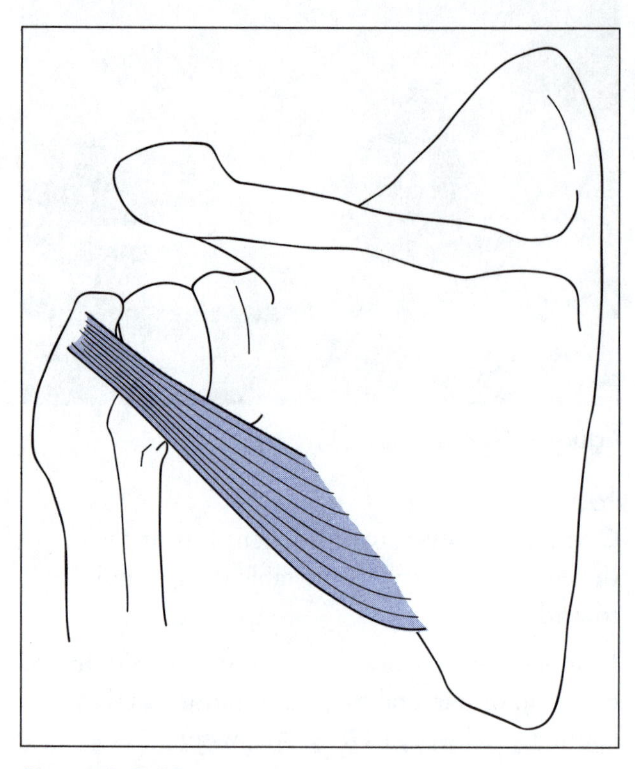

Figure 3-3-29 Teres minor

Origin: Upper 2/3 of the lateral, dorsal border of the scapula

Insertion: Greater tubercle of humerus and capsule of the shoulder joint

Innervation: Axillary nerve

Action: Humeral external rotation and humeral horizontal abduction, one of the muscles of the rotator cuff

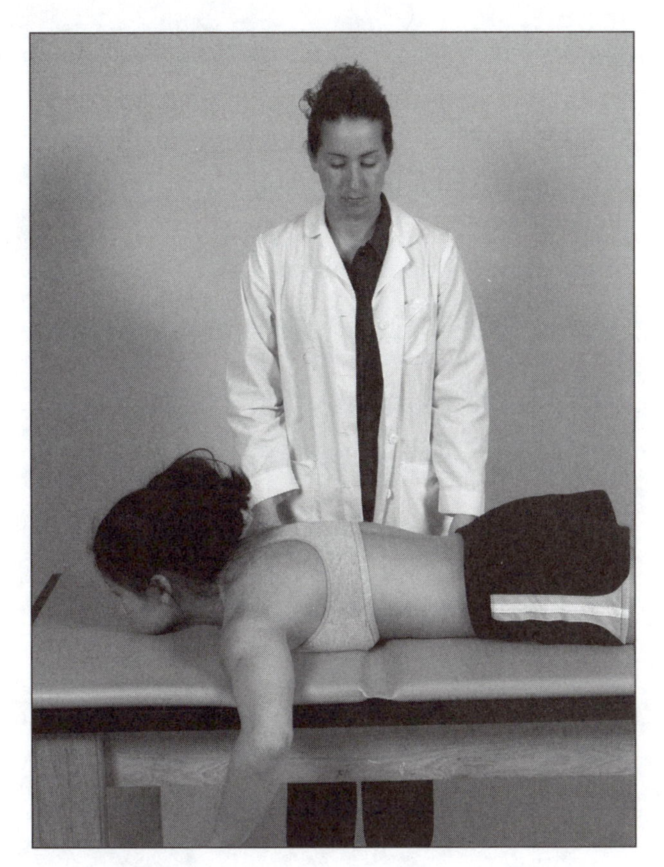

Figure 3-3-30 Start position for teres minor.

Normal, Good, Fair

Client Position: Starting—client is prone with the testing extremity in 90 degrees of humeral abduction and 90 degrees of elbow flexion (fingers point toward the floor) (Figure 3-3-30).

Motion—client moves the testing extremity in the direction of humeral external rotation (Figure 3-3-31).

Therapist Position: Stabilize under the humerus to avoid compensation. Resistance is applied at the forearm in the direction of humeral internal rotation when testing Normal or Good strengths.

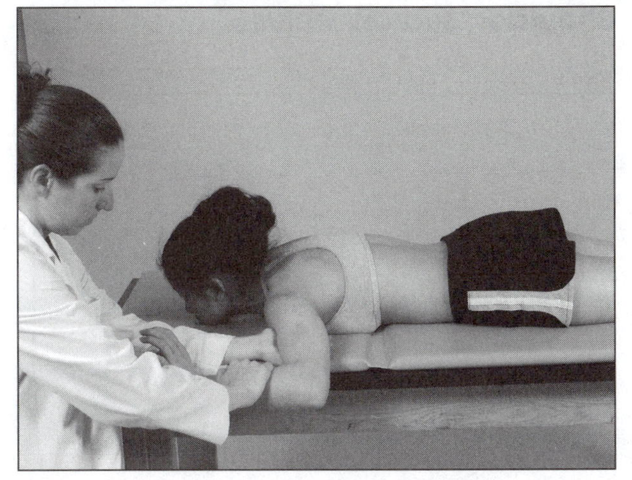

Figure 3-3-31 End position for teres minor.

No resistance is applied when testing Fair strength.

Poor

Client Position: Starting—client is prone with the entire extremity off the table (fingers point toward the floor).

Motion—client moves the testing extremity in the direction of humeral external rotation (LUE = counter-clockwise, RUE = clockwise).

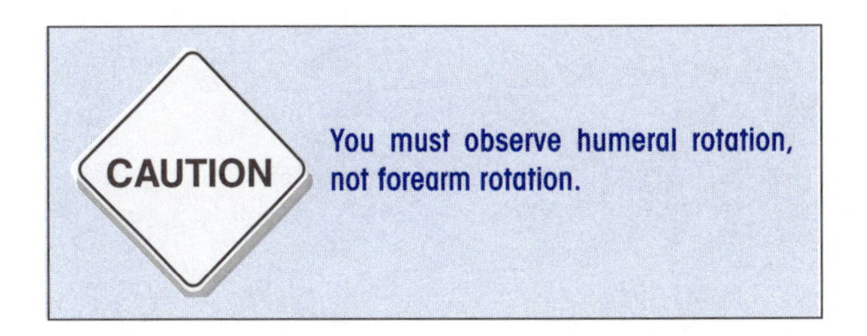

You must observe humeral rotation, not forearm rotation.

Therapist Position: Stabilize at the scapula to avoid compensation. No resistance is applied when testing in the gravity-eliminated position.

Trace

The teres minor is not palpatable.

Alternate Position

Client Position: Starting—client is sitting with the testing extremity in humeral adduction, and elbow flexion to 90 degrees.

Motion—client moves the testing extremity in the direction of humeral external rotation (hand moves away from the body).

Shoulder: *supraspinatus*

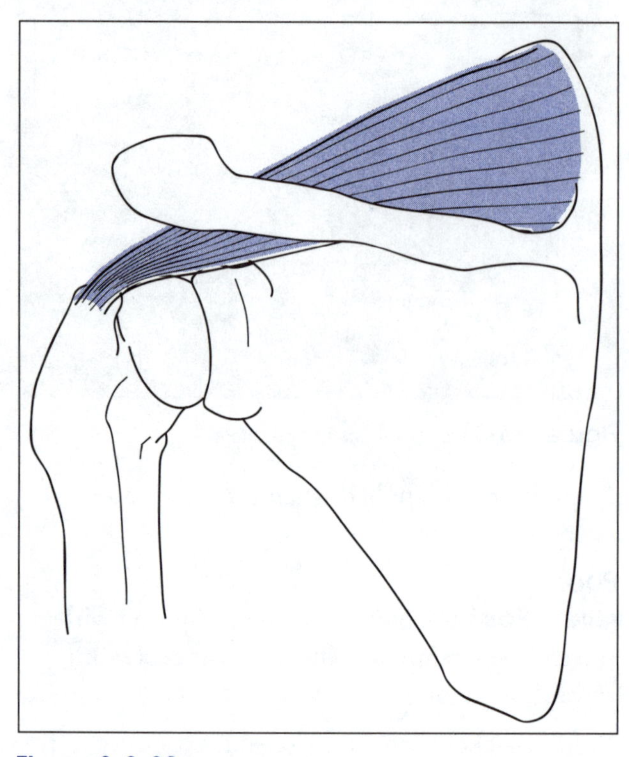

Figure 3-3-32 Supraspinatus

Origin: Medial 2/3 of the supraspinous fossa

Insertion: Greater tubercle of the humerus and shoulder joint capsule

Innervation: Suprascapular nerve

Action: Humeral abduction; one of the muscles of the rotator cuff

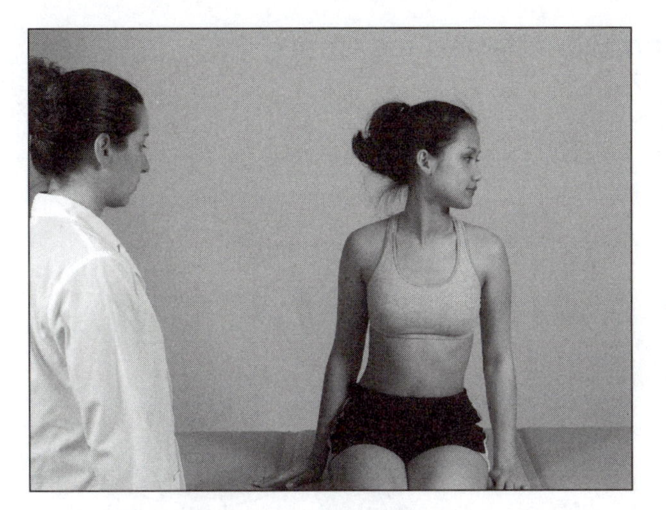

Figure 3-3-33 Start position for supraspinatus.

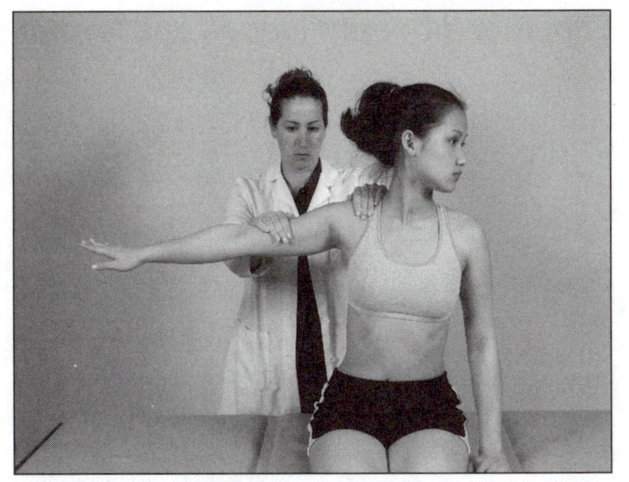

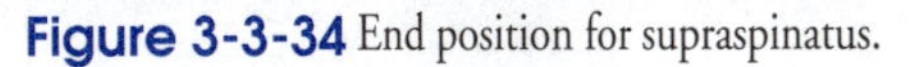

Figure 3-3-34 End position for supraspinatus.

Normal, Good, Fair

Client Position: Starting—client is sitting or standing with the testing extremity in 90 degrees of humeral abduction and the head rotated to the contralateral side (Figure 3-3-33).

Motion—client moves the testing extremity in the direction of humeral abduction (Figure 3-3-34).

Therapist Position: Stabilize at the shoulder to avoid compensation. Resistance is applied at the humerus in the direction of humeral adduction when testing Normal or Good strengths. No resistance is applied when testing Fair strength.

Poor

Client Position: Client is prone or supine with the testing extremity in humeral adduction and the head rotated to the contralateral side.

Motion—client moves the testing extremity in the direction of humeral abduction.

Therapist Position: Stabilize at the shoulder to avoid compensation. No resistance is applied when testing in the gravity-eliminated position.

Trace

The supraspinatus is too deep to palpate.

Shoulder: *trapezius (upper)* and *levator scapulae* (tested together)

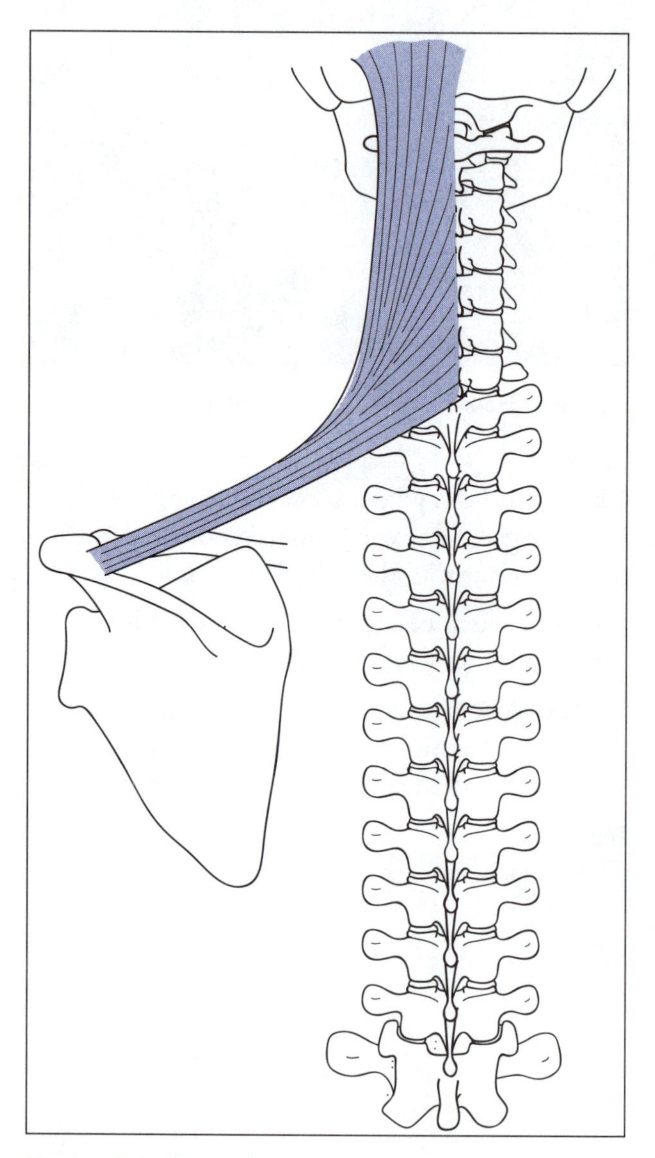

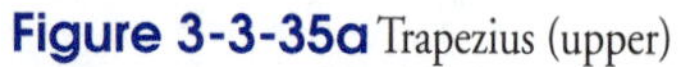

Figure 3-3-35a Trapezius (upper)

Upper trapezius

Origin: Occipital protruberance, medial 1/3 of nuchal line of occipital bone, ligamentum nuchae, and spinous process of C1–C7

Insertion: Lateral 1/3 of clavicle and acromion process

Innervation: Spinal accessory nerve

Action: Scapular elevation, scapular upward rotation

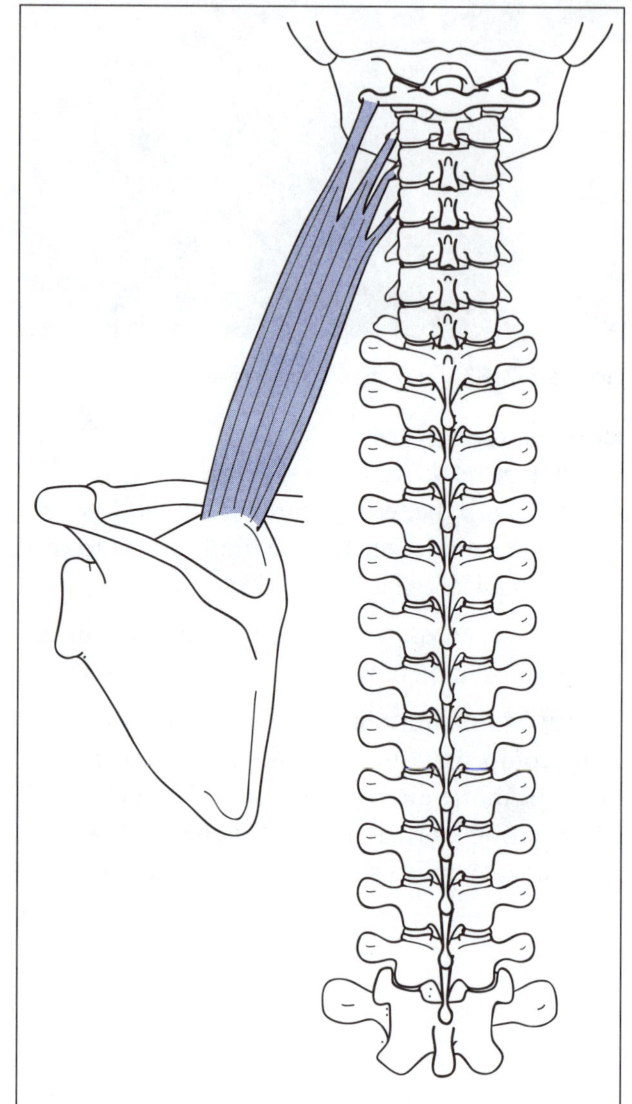

Figure 3-3-35b Levator scapulae

Levator scapulae

Origin: Transverse process of C1–C4

Insertion: Superior angle of the scapula

Innervation: Dorsal scapular nerve

Action: Scapular elevation

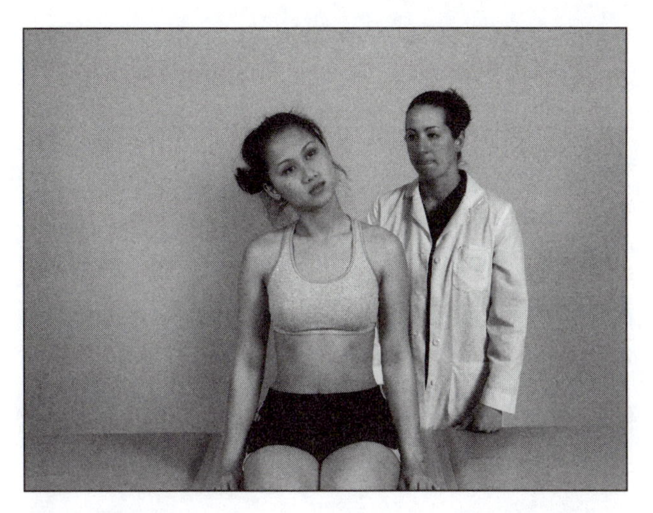

Figure 3-3-36 Start position for trapezius (upper) and levator scapulae.

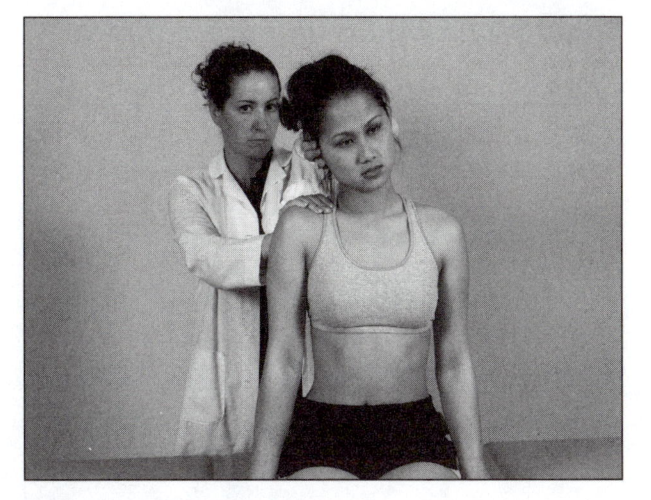

Figure 3-3-37 End position for trapezius (upper) and levator scapulae.

Normal, Good, Fair

Client Position: Starting—client is sitting with the testing extremity at the side. The head is tilted toward the testing side and rotated away from the testing side (Figure 3-3-36).

Motion—client moves the scapula being tested in the direction of scapular elevation (Figure 3-3-37).

Therapist Position: Stabilize at the lateral head. Resistance is applied at the shoulder/scapula in the direction of scapular depression when testing Normal or Good strengths. No resistance is applied when testing Fair strength.

Poor

Client Position: Starting—client is supine or prone with the testing extremity at the side. The head is tilted toward the testing side and rotated away from the testing side.

Motion—client moves the scapula being tested in the direction of scapular elevation.

Therapist Position: Stabilize at the lateral head. No resistance is applied when testing in the gravity-eliminated position.

Trace

The upper trapezius can be palpated next to C7, and above the lateral 1/3 of the clavicle.

Shoulder/scapula: *trapezius (middle)*

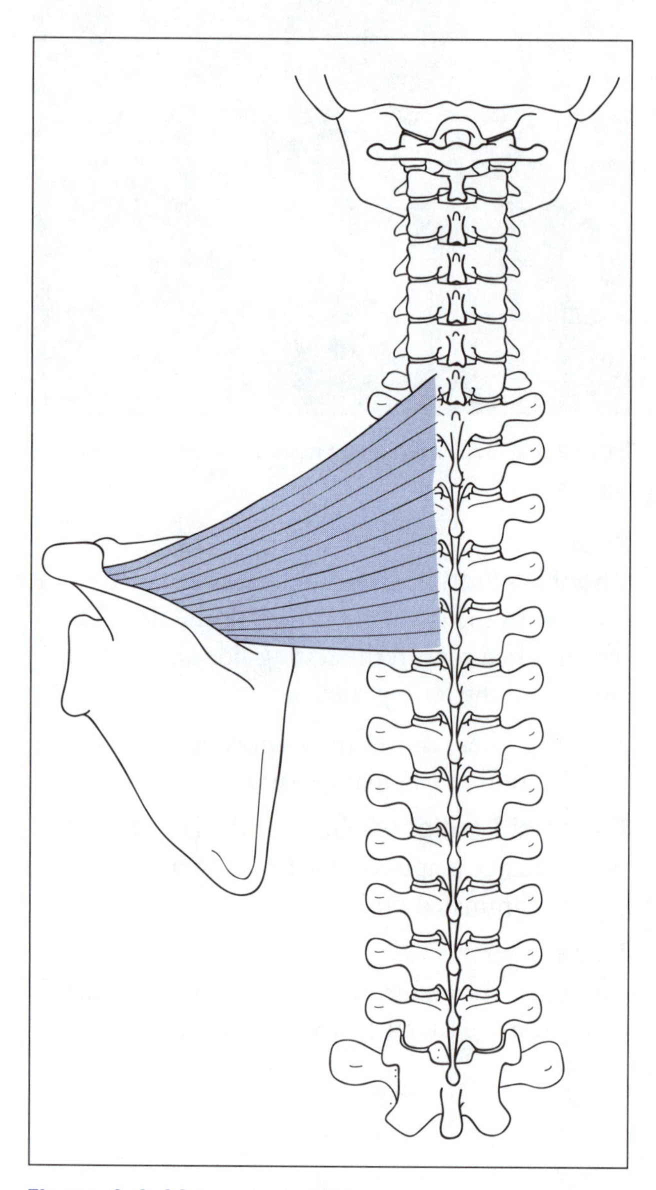

Figure 3-3-38 Trapezius (middle)

Origin: Inferior aspect of the ligamentum nuchae and C7–T5

Insertion: Medial margin of the acromion process, superior spine of the scapula

Innervation: Spinal accessory nerve

Action: Scapular adduction

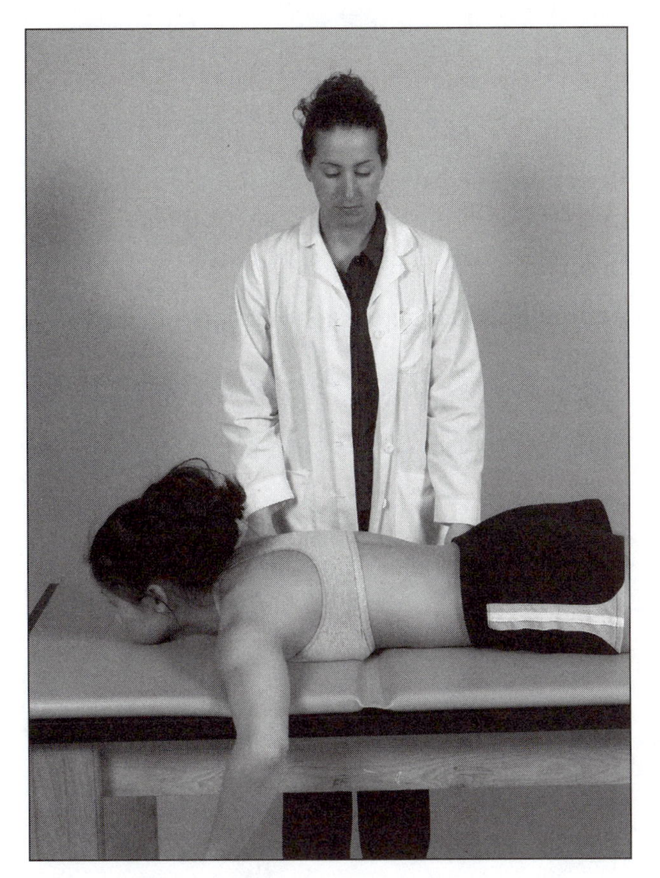

Figure 3-3-39 Start position for trapezius (middle).

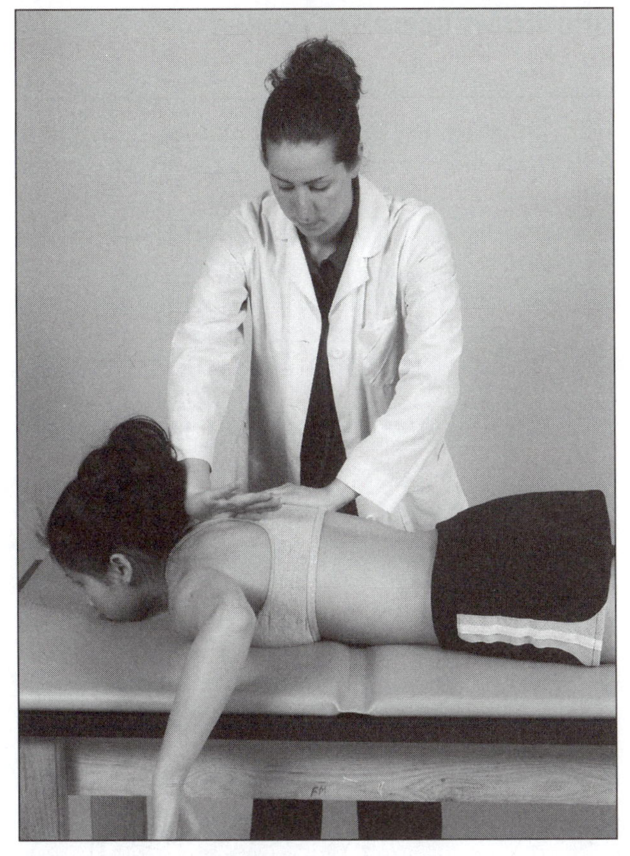

Figure 3-3-40 End position for trapezius (middle).

Normal, Good, Fair

Client Position: Starting—client is prone with the testing extremity at 90 degrees of humeral abduction and 90 degrees of elbow flexion (fingers point toward floor) (Figure 3-3-39).

Motion—client moves the scapula being tested in the direction of scapular abduction. Humerus will follow in the direction of horizontal abduction; however, testing should isolate this motion from scapular adduction (Figure 3-3-40).

Therapist Position: Stabilize at the thorax to avoid compensation. Resistance is applied along the medial border of the scapula in the direction of scapular abduction when testing Normal or Good strengths. No resistance is applied when testing Fair strength.

It is difficult to isolate the middle trapezius from the humeral horizontal abductors.

Poor

Client Position: Starting—client is sitting with the testing extremity in 90 degrees of humeral abduction and 90 degrees of elbow flexion, supported on a table or by the therapist.

Motion—client moves the scapula being tested in the direction of scapular adduction.

Therapist Position: Stabilize at the thorax to avoid compensation. Support the testing extremity to eliminate gravity; however, do not assist the motion. No resistance is applied when testing in the gravity-eliminated position.

Trace

The middle trapezius is palpated above the spine of the scapula.

Shoulder: *trapezius (lower)*

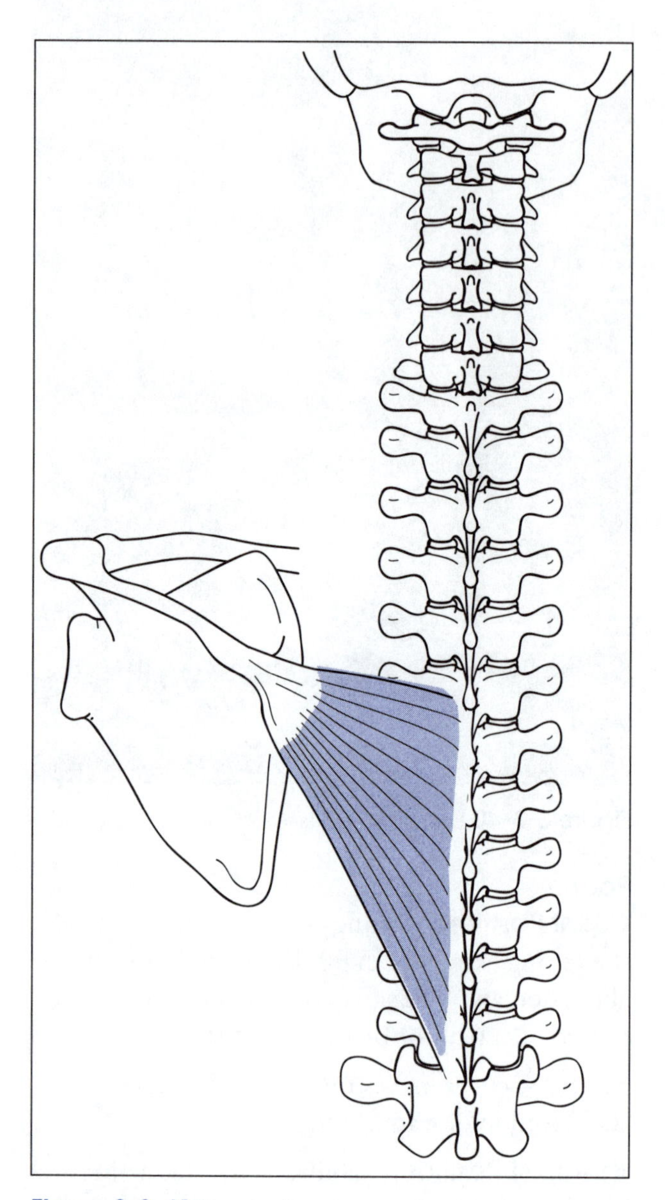

Figure 3-3-41 Trapezius (lower)

Origin: T6–T12

Insertion: Medial spine of the scapula and tubercle at the apex of the spine of the scapula

Innervation: Spinal accessory nerve

Action: Scapular depression, scapular upward rotation

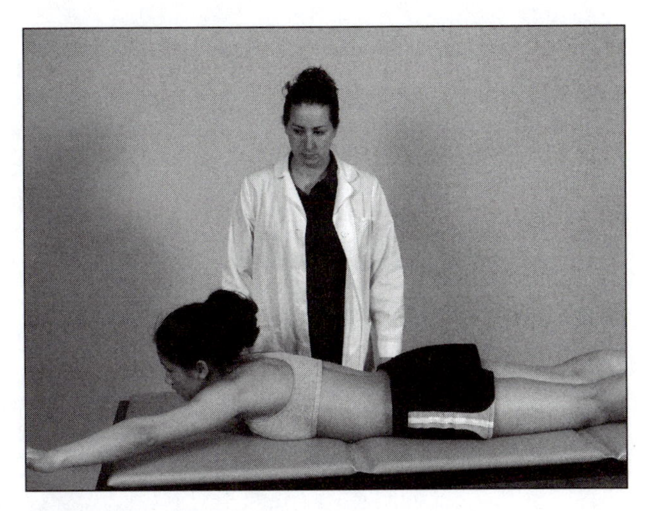

Figure 3-3-42 Start position for trapezius (lower).

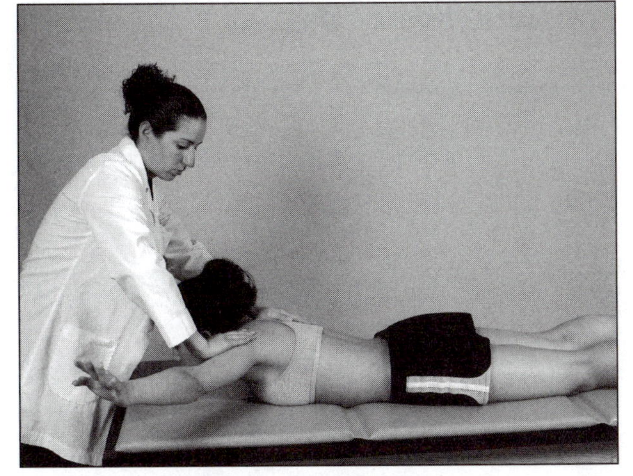

Figure 3-3-43 End position for trapezius (lower).

Normal, Good, Fair

Client Position: Starting—client is prone with the testing extremity at approximately 140 degrees of humeral abduction (Figure 3-3-42).

Motion—client raises the testing extremity toward the ceiling and depresses the scapula (Figure 3-3-43).

Therapist Position: Stabilize at the thorax. Resistance is applied at the distal humerus in a downward motion when testing Normal or Good strengths. No resistance is applied when testing Fair strength.

Poor

Client Position: Client is prone with the testing extremity at approximately 140 degrees of humeral abduction.

Motion—client raises the testing extremity toward the ceiling and depresses the scapula.

Therapist Position: Stabilize at the thorax and stabilize the extremity against gravity without assisting the motion. No resistance is applied when testing in the gravity-eliminated position.

Trace

The lower trapezius is palpated along T6–T12 and at the medial spine of the scapula.

Scapula: *rhomboids*

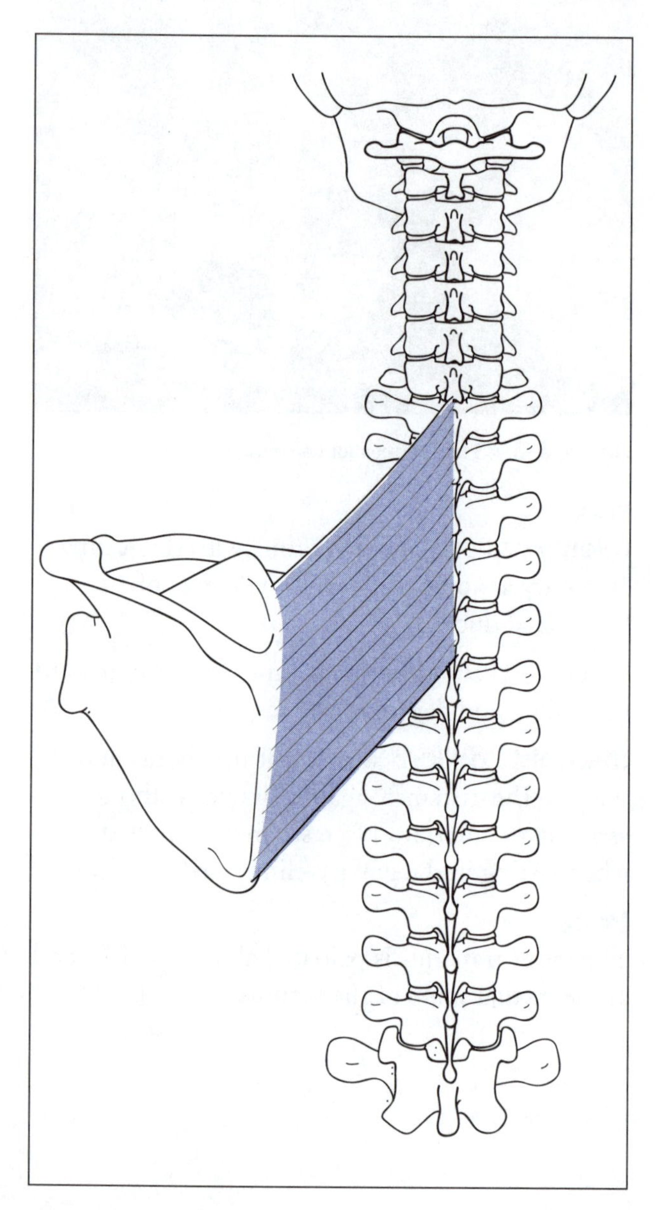

Figure 3-3-44 Rhomboids

Origin: Spinous process C7–T5, ligamentum nuchae

Insertion: Entire medial border of the scapula

Innervation: Dorsal scapular nerve

Action: Scapular adduction and scapular downward rotation

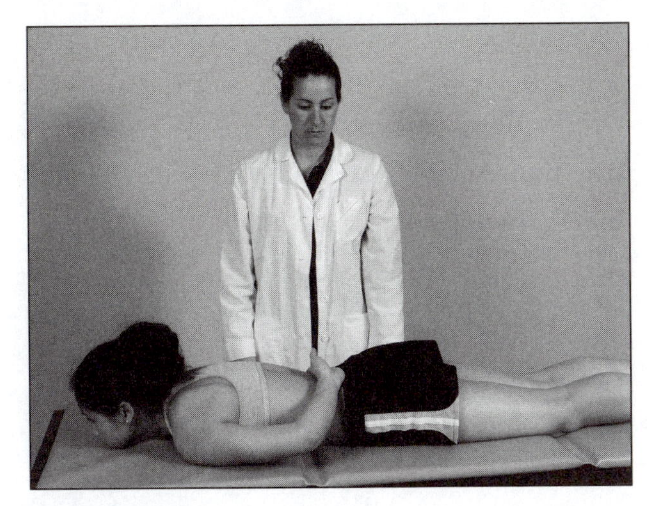

Figure 3-3-45 Start position for rhomboids.

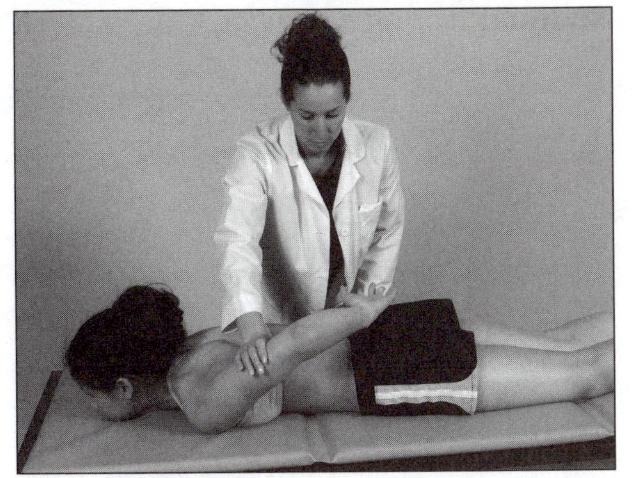

Figure 3-3-46 End position for rhomboids.

Normal, Good, Fair

Client Position: Starting—client is prone with the testing extremity hand placed behind the back (internal rotation, adduction of humerus) (Figure 3-3-45).

Motion—client moves the testing extremity away from the back (toward the ceiling) (Figure 3-3-46).

Therapist Position: Stabilization is usually not required. Resistance is applied at the distal humerus in the direction of humeral abduction and humeral external rotation when testing Normal or Good strengths. No resistance is applied when testing Fair strength.

Poor

Client Position: Starting—client is sitting with the testing extremity hand placed behind the back (internal rotation, adduction of humerus).

Motion—client moves the testing extremity away from the back.

Therapist Position: Stabilization is usually not required. No resistance is applied when testing in the gravity-eliminated position.

Trace

The rhomboids can be palpated medial to the vertebral border of the scapula.

Scapula: *serratus anterior*

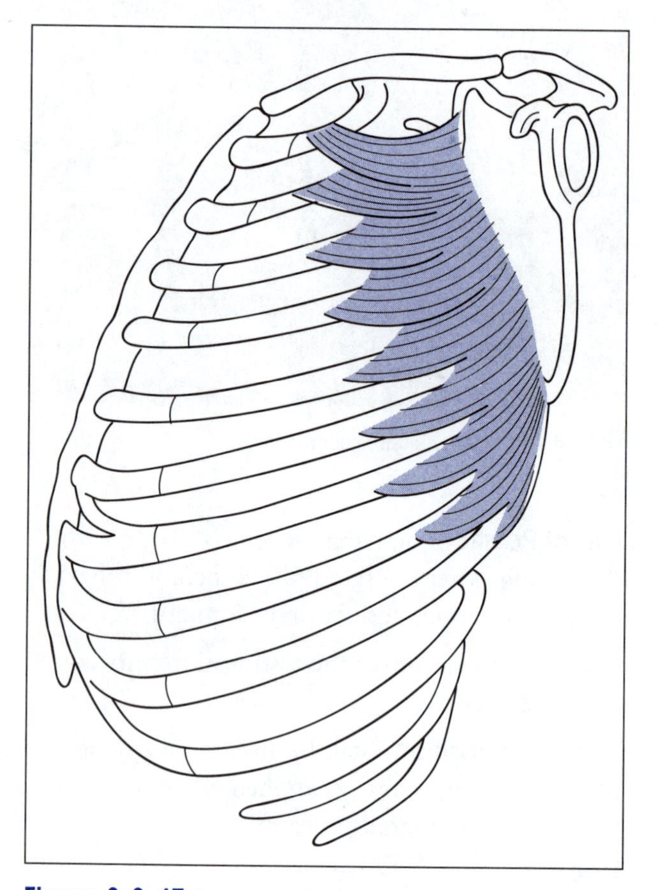

Figure 3-3-47 Serratus anterior

Origin: Ribs 1 through 9

Insertion: Anterior, medial border of the scapula

Innervation: Long thoracic nerve

Action: Scapular abduction

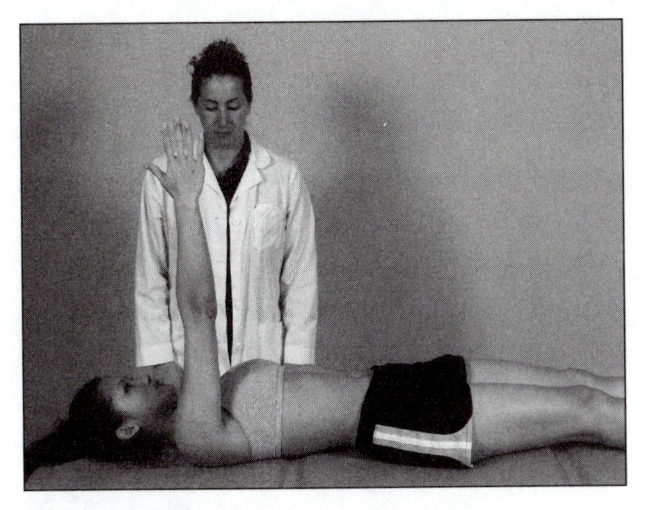

Figure 3-3-48 Start position for serratus anterior.

Normal, Good, Fair

Client Position: Starting—client is supine with testing extremity in 90 degrees of humeral flexion and elbow extension (Figure 3-3-48).

Motion—client moves the testing extremity in the direction of scapular abduction (reaches toward the ceiling) (Figure 3-3-49).

Therapist Position: Stabilize at the trunk to avoid trunk rotation. Resistance is applied at the proximal humerus in the direction of scapular adduction when testing Normal or Good strengths. No resistance is applied when testing Fair strength.

Poor

Client Position: Starting—client is sitting with the testing extremity in 90 degrees of humeral flexion and elbow extension, supported on a table or by the therapist.

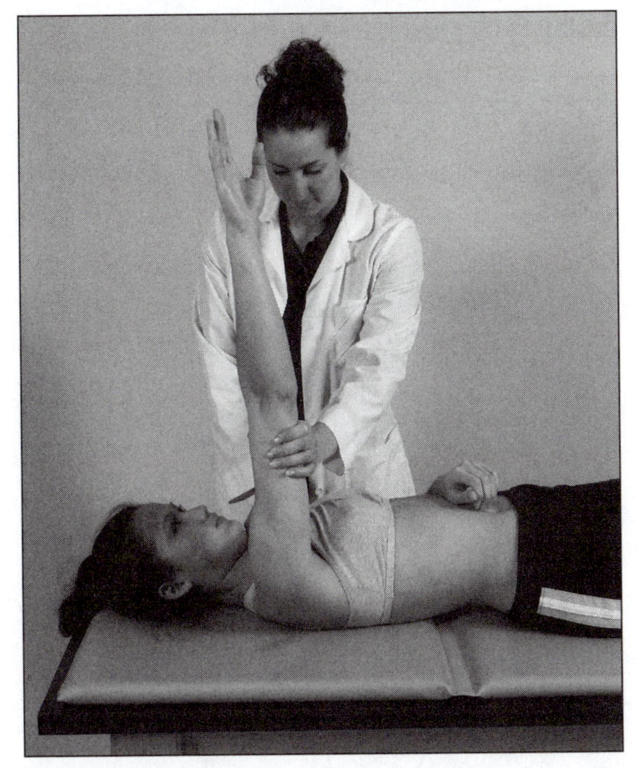

Figure 3-3-49 End position for serratus anterior.

Motion—client moves the testing extremity in the direction of scapular abduction.

Therapist Position: Stabilize at the trunk to avoid trunk rotation. Support the testing extremity to eliminate gravity; however, do not assist the motion. No resistance is applied in the gravity-eliminated position.

Trace

The serratus anterior can be palpated at the anterior–lateral border of the scapula when the testing extremity is positioned as stated above.

Scapula: *pectoralis minor*

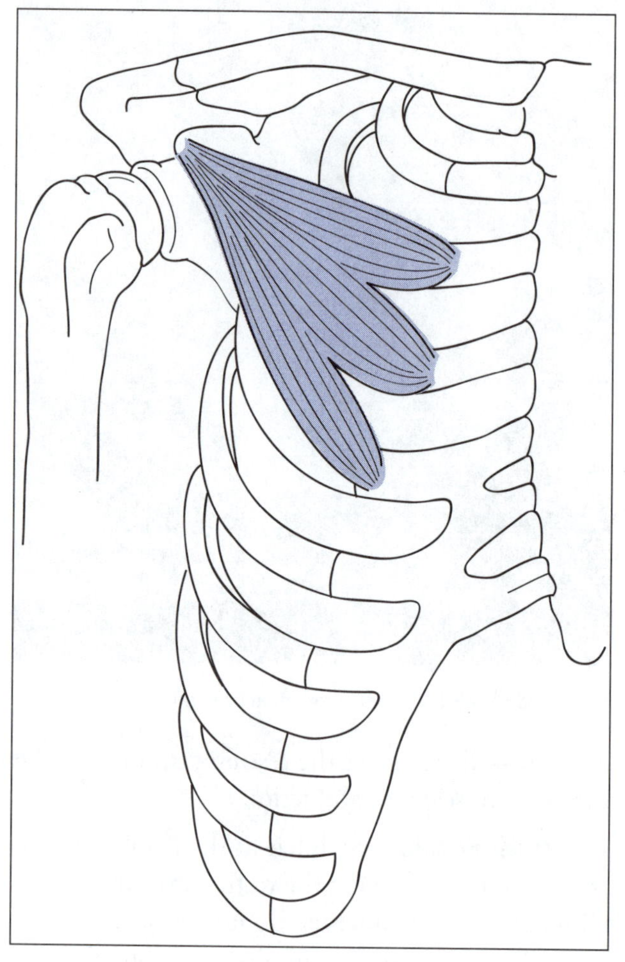

Figure 3-3-50 Pectoralis minor

Origin: Ribs 3, 4, and 5

Insertion: Coracoid process of the scapula, superior surface

Innervation: Medial and lateral pectoral nerves

Action: Scapular abduction, scapular downward rotation

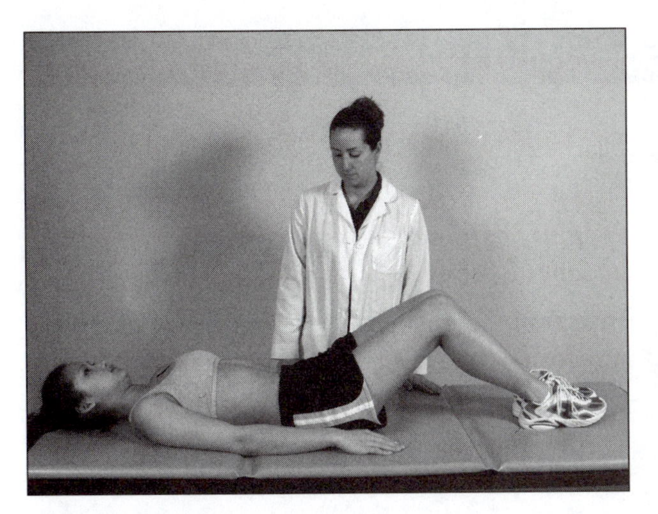

Figure 3-3-51 Start position for pectoralis minor.

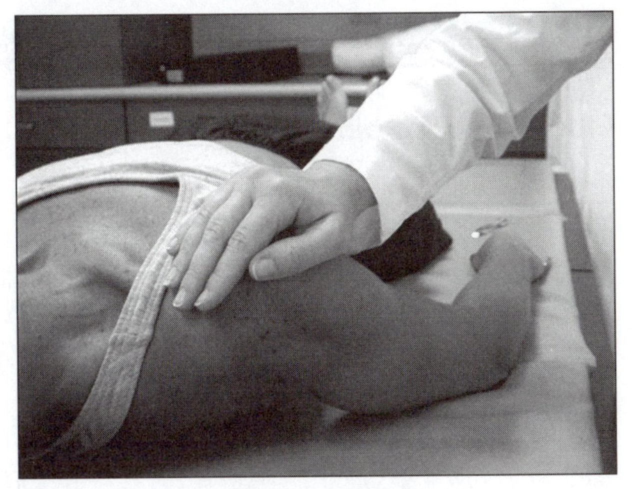

Figure 3-3-52 End position for pectoralis minor.

Normal, Good, Fair

Client Position: Starting—client is supine with testing extremity at side and raised slightly off the table (Figure 3-3-51).

Motion—client moves the testing extremity in the direction of scapular abduction (brings shoulder toward the ceiling) (Figure 3-3-52).

Therapist Position: Stabilize at the trunk to avoid trunk rotation. Resistance is applied at the anterior aspect of the shoulder in the direction of scapular adduction when testing Normal and Good strengths. No resistance is applied when testing Fair strength.

Poor

Client Position: Starting—client is sitting with testing extremity at the side.

Motion—client moves the testing extremity in the direction of scapular abduction.

Therapist Position: Stabilize at the trunk to avoid trunk rotation. No resistance is applied in the gravity-eliminated position.

Trace

The pectoralis minor is too difficult to palpate because it lies under the pectoralis major.

SECTION 3-4: Isolated Manual Muscle Testing of the Elbow and Forearm

Elbow flexion: *biceps brachii*

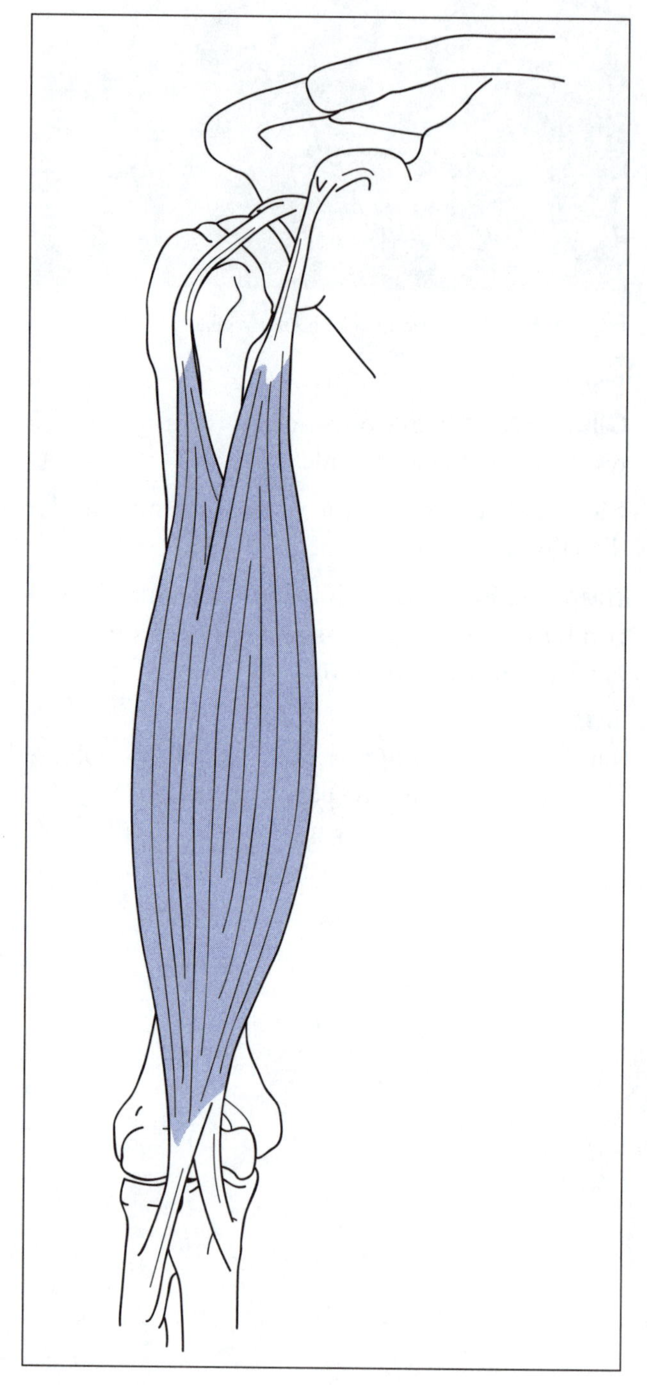

Figure 3-4-1 Biceps brachii

Origin: Short head—scapular coracoid process; long head—scapular supraglenoid process

Insertion: Short head—posterior aspect of radial tuberosity; long head—bicipital aponeurosis

Innervation: Musculocutaneous nerve

Action: Elbow flexion, forearm supination

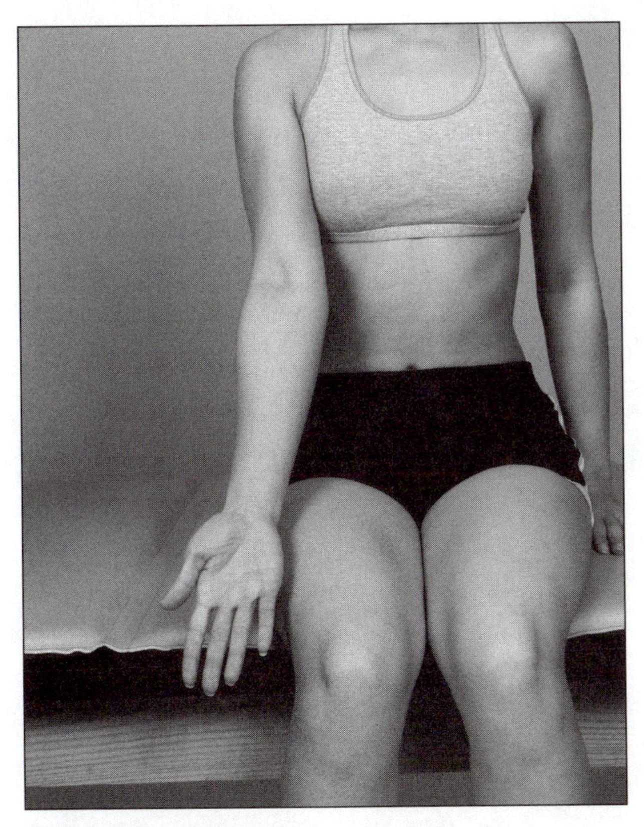

Figure 3-4-2 Start position for biceps brachii.

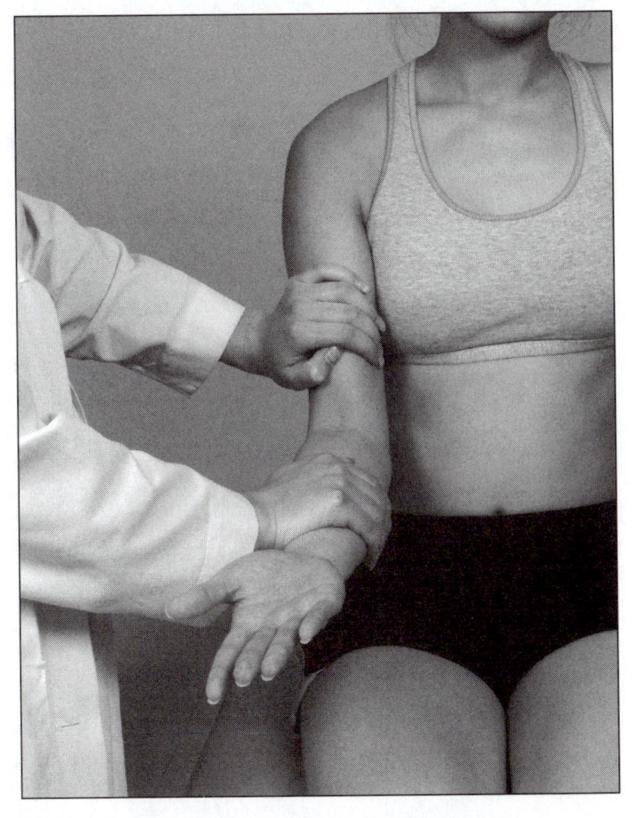

Figure 3-4-3 End position for biceps brachii.

Normal, Good, Fair

Client Position: Client is sitting with the testing extremity in humeral adduction, elbow extension, and forearm supination (Figure 3-4-2).

Motion—client moves the testing extremity in the direction of elbow flexion (Figure 3-4-3).

Therapist Position: Stabilize at the humerus to avoid compensation. Resistance is applied at the forearm in the direction of elbow extension when testing Normal or Good strengths. No resistance is applied when testing Fair strength.

Poor

Client Position: Starting—client is sitting with the testing extremity in 90 degrees of humeral flexion or abduction, elbow extension, and forearm in supination, supported on a table or by the therapist.

Motion—client moves the testing extremity in the direction of elbow flexion.

Therapist Position: Stabilize at the humerus to avoid compensation. Support the testing extremity to eliminate gravity; however, do not assist the motion. No resistance is applied when testing in the gravity-eliminated position.

Trace

The biceps brachii is palpated on the volar aspect of the distal/medial humerus when the forearm is in supination.

Elbow flexion: *brachialis*

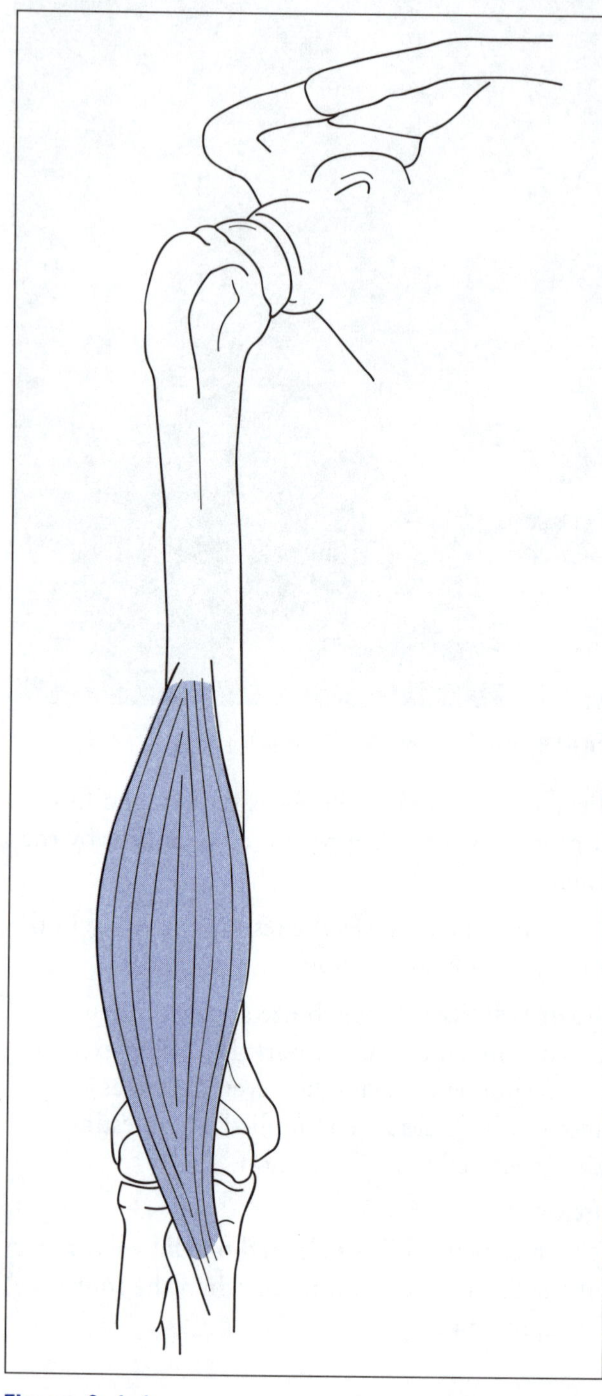

Figure 3-4-4 Brachialis

Origin: Distal 1/2 of the anterior aspect of the humerus and medial/lateral intermuscular septa

Insertion: Tuberosity and coronoid process of the ulna

Innervation: Musculocutaneous and radial nerves

Action: Elbow flexion

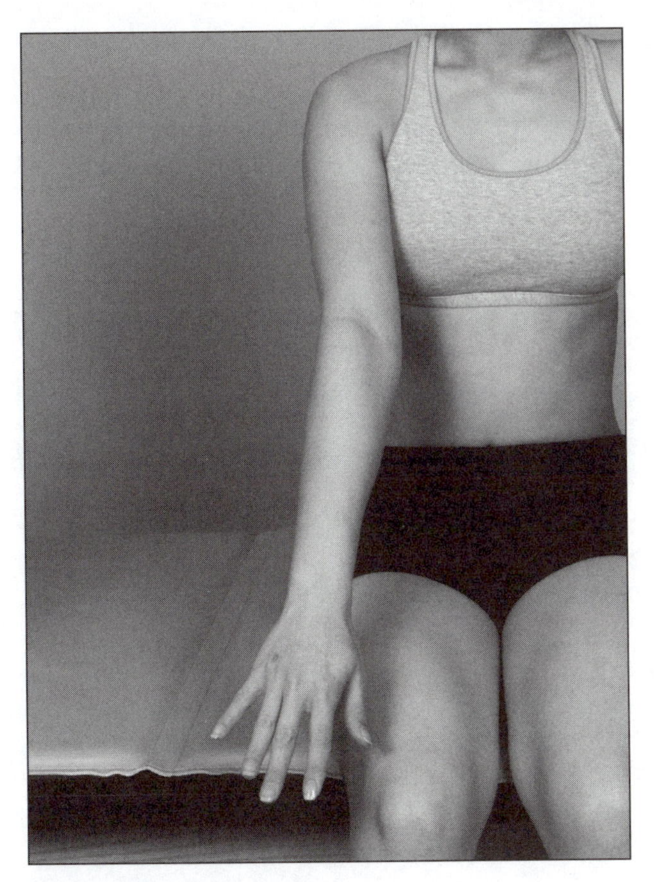

Figure 3-4-5 Start position for brachialis.

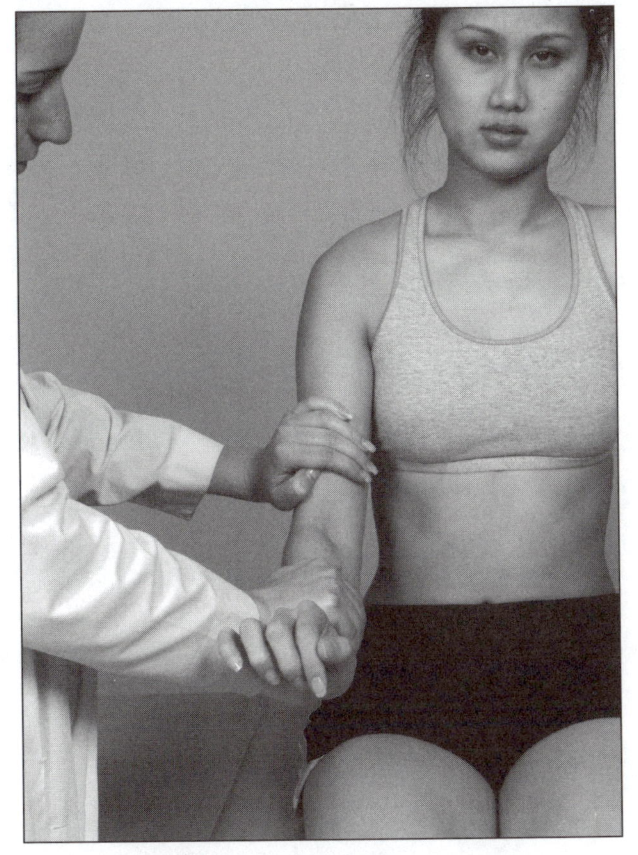

Figure 3-4-6 End position for brachialis.

Normal, Good, Fair

Client Position: Starting—client is sitting with the testing extremity in humeral adduction, elbow extension, and forearm pronation (Figure 3-4-5).

Motion—client moves the testing extremity in the direction of elbow flexion, while remaining in forearm pronation (Figure 3-4-6).

Therapist Position: Stabilize at the humerus to avoid compensation. Resistance is applied at the mid-forearm, in the direction of elbow extension when testing Normal or Good strengths. No resistance is applied when testing Fair strength.

Poor

Client Position: Starting—client is sitting with the testing extremity in 90 degrees of humeral flexion or abduction, elbow extension, and forearm pronation, supported on a table or by the therapist.

Motion—client moves the testing extremity in the direction of elbow flexion while remaining in forearm pronation.

Therapist Position: Stabilize at the humerus to avoid compensation. Support the testing extremity to eliminate gravity; however, do not assist the motion. No resistance is applied when testing in the gravity-eliminated position.

Trace

The brachialis is palpated medial to the biceps brachii tendon when the forearm is in pronation.

Elbow flexion: *brachioradialis*

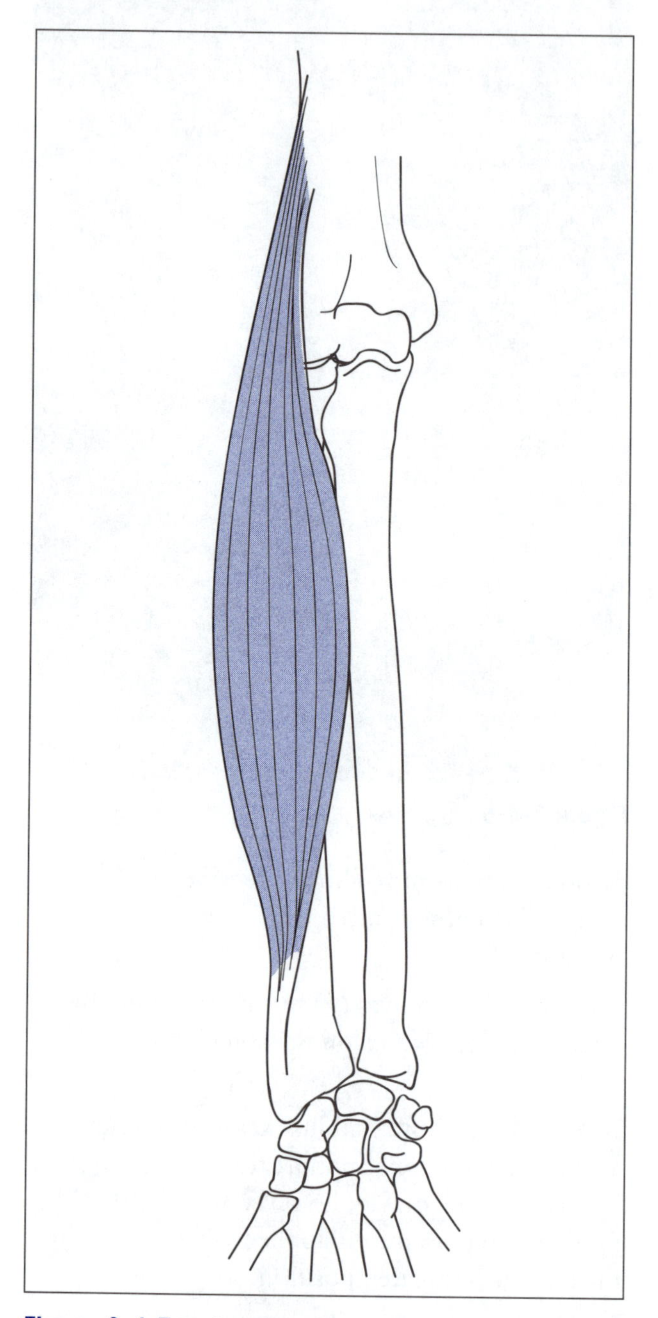

Figure 3-4-7 Brachioradialis

Origin: Proximal, lateral supracondylar ridge of humerus

Insertion: Lateral side of radial styloid process

Innervation: Radial nerve

Action: Elbow flexion

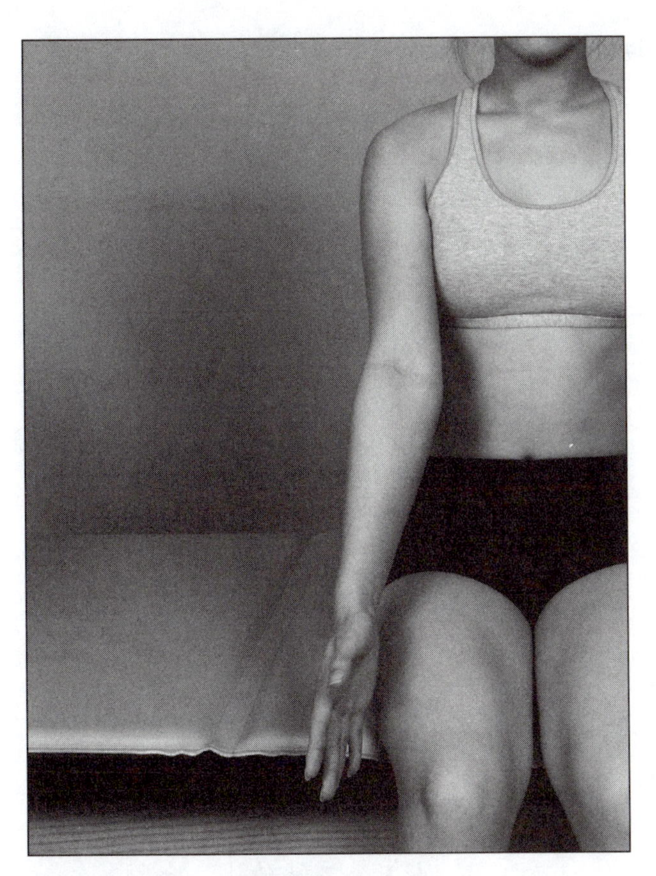

Figure 3-4-8 Start position for brachioradialis.

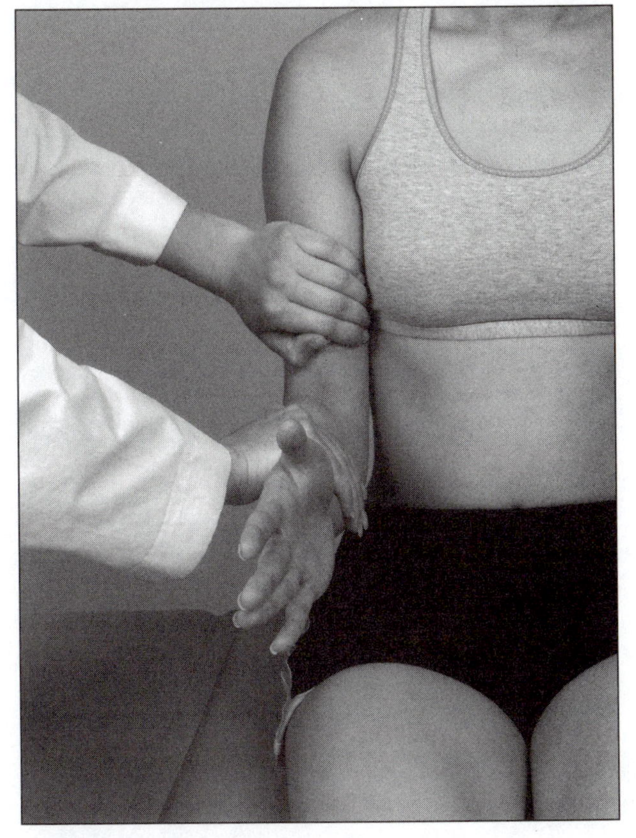

Figure 3-4-9 End position for brachioradialis.

Normal, Good, Fair

Client Position: Starting—client is sitting with the testing extremity in humeral adduction, elbow extension, and the forearm in neutral (Figure 3-4-8).

Motion—client moves the testing extremity in the direction of elbow flexion, while forearm remains in neutral (Figure 3-4-9).

Therapist Position: Stabilize at the humerus to avoid compensation. Resistance is applied at the mid-forearm in the direction of elbow extension when testing Normal or Good strengths. No resistance is applied when testing Fair strength.

Poor

Client Position: Starting—client is sitting with the testing extremity in 90 degrees of humeral flexion or abduction, elbow extension, and forearm in neutral, supported on a table or by the therapist.

Motion—client moves the testing extremity in the direction of elbow flexion while the forearm remains in neutral.

Therapist Position: Stabilize the humerus to avoid compensation. Support the testing extremity to eliminate gravity; however, do not assist the motion. No resistance is applied when testing in the gravity-eliminated position.

Trace

The brachioradialis is palpated at the distal/lateral humerus when the forearm is in neutral.

Elbow extension: *triceps* and *anconeus* (tested together)

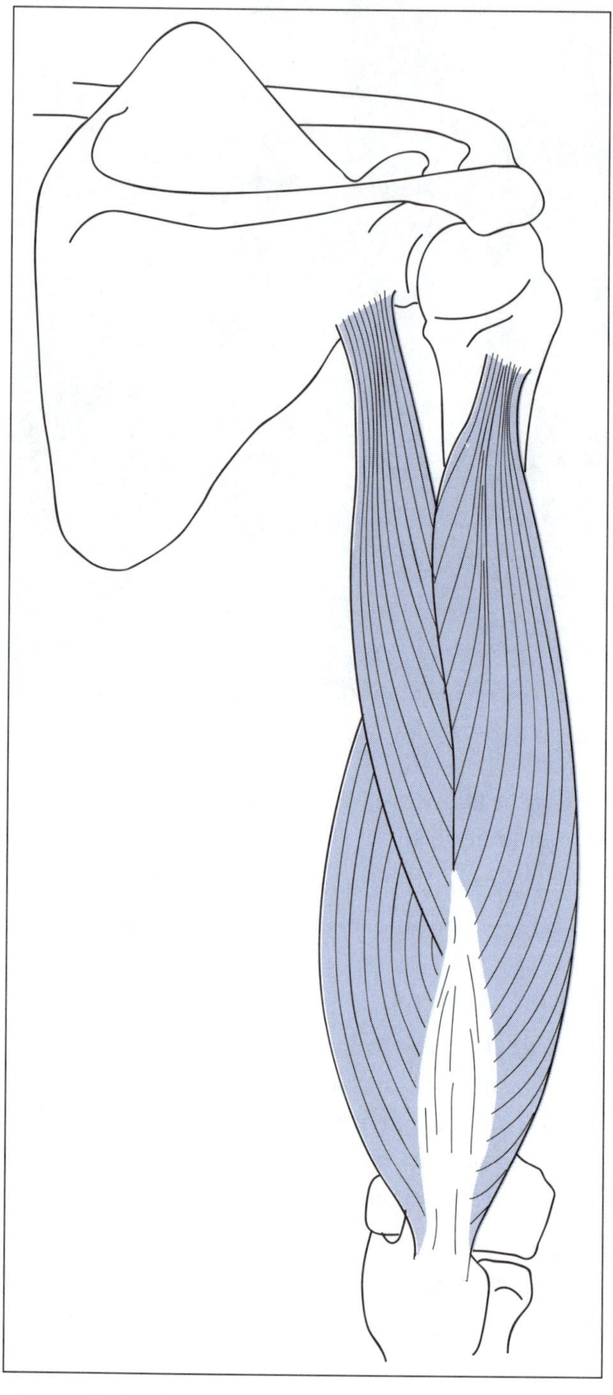

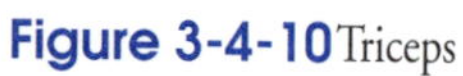

Figure 3-4-10 Triceps

Triceps

Origin: Long head—infraglenoid tubercle of the scapula. Lateral head—posterolateral surface of the humerus between the radial groove and the insertion of teres minor. Medial head—posterior surface of the humerus below the radial groove.

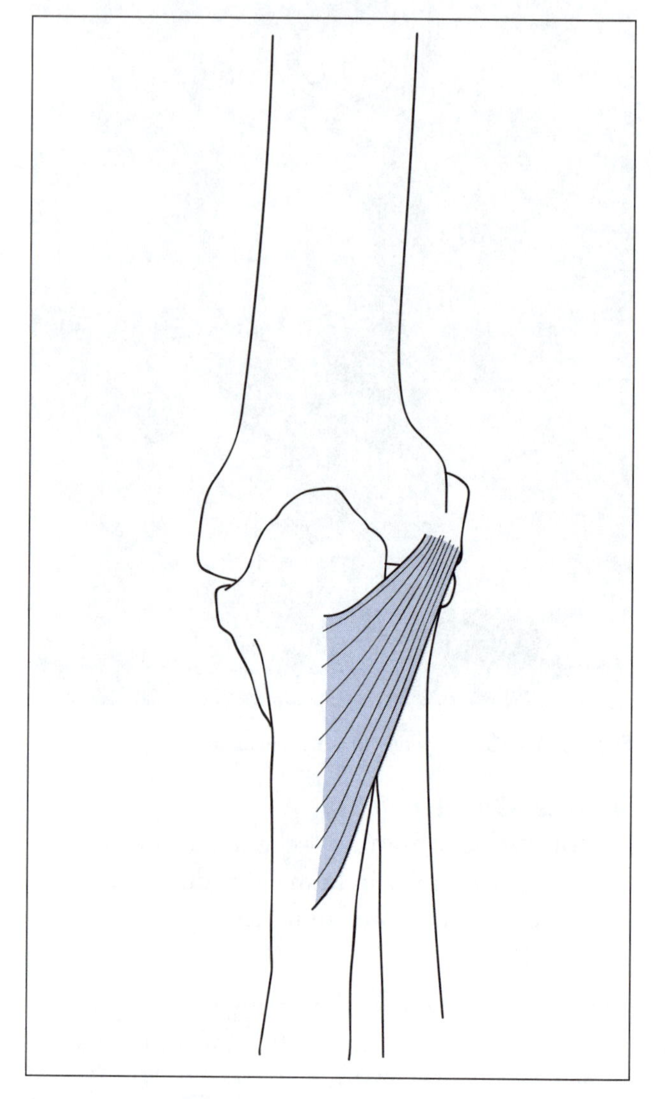

Figure 3-4-11 Anconeus

Insertion: Posterior surface of olecranon process

Innervation: Radial nerve

Action: Elbow extension

Anconeus

Origin: Lateral epicondyle of the humerus

Insertion: Lateral side of olecranon process and upper 1/4 of ulna

Innervation: Radial nerve

Action: Elbow extension

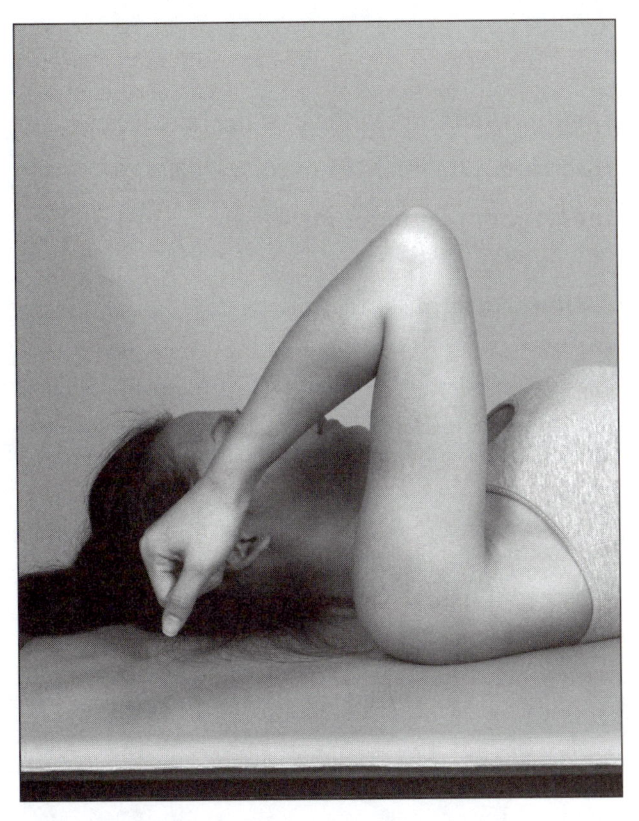

Figure 3-4-12 Start position for triceps and anconeus.

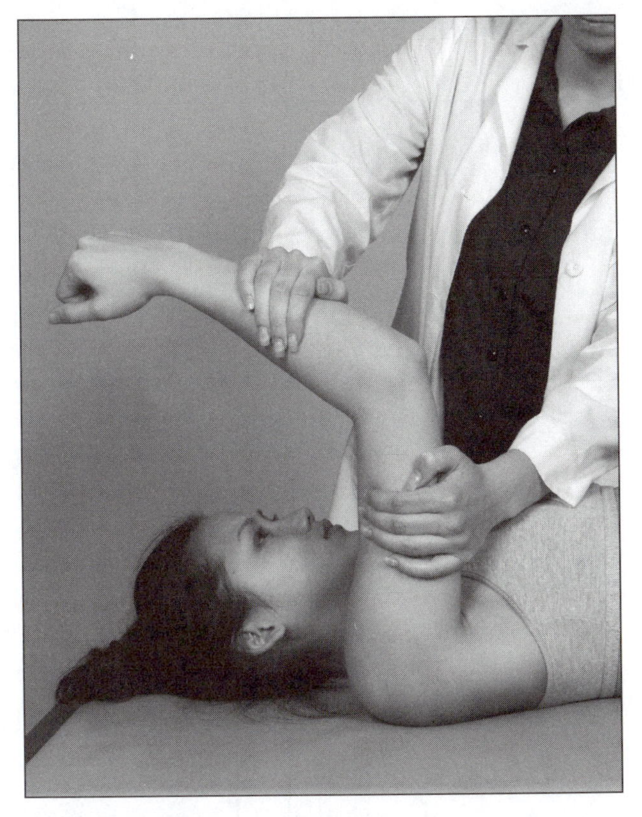

Figure 3-4-13 End position for triceps and anconeus.

Normal, Good, Fair

Client Position: Starting—client is supine with the testing extremity in humeral flexion, elbow flexion, and forearm supination (Figure 3-4-12).

Motion—client moves the testing extremity in the direction of elbow extension (Figure 3-4-13).

Therapist Position: Stabilize at the humerus to avoid compensation. Resistance is applied at the posterior aspect of the forearm in the direction of elbow flexion when testing Normal or Good strengths. No resistance is applied when testing Fair strength.

Poor

Client Position: Starting—client is sitting with the testing extremity in humeral flexion or abduction, elbow flexion, and forearm is neutral, supported on a table or by the therapist.

Motion—client moves the testing extremity in the direction of elbow extension.

Therapist Position: Stabilize at the humerus to avoid compensation. Support the testing extremity to eliminate gravity; however, do not assist the motion. No resistance is applied when testing in the gravity-eliminated position.

Trace

The triceps are palpated at the posterior, mid-humerus. The anconeus is unable to be palpated.

Alternate Position

Standing or sitting with the testing extremity in 180 degrees of humeral flexion, elbow flexion, and forearm supination.

Forearm supination: *supinator*

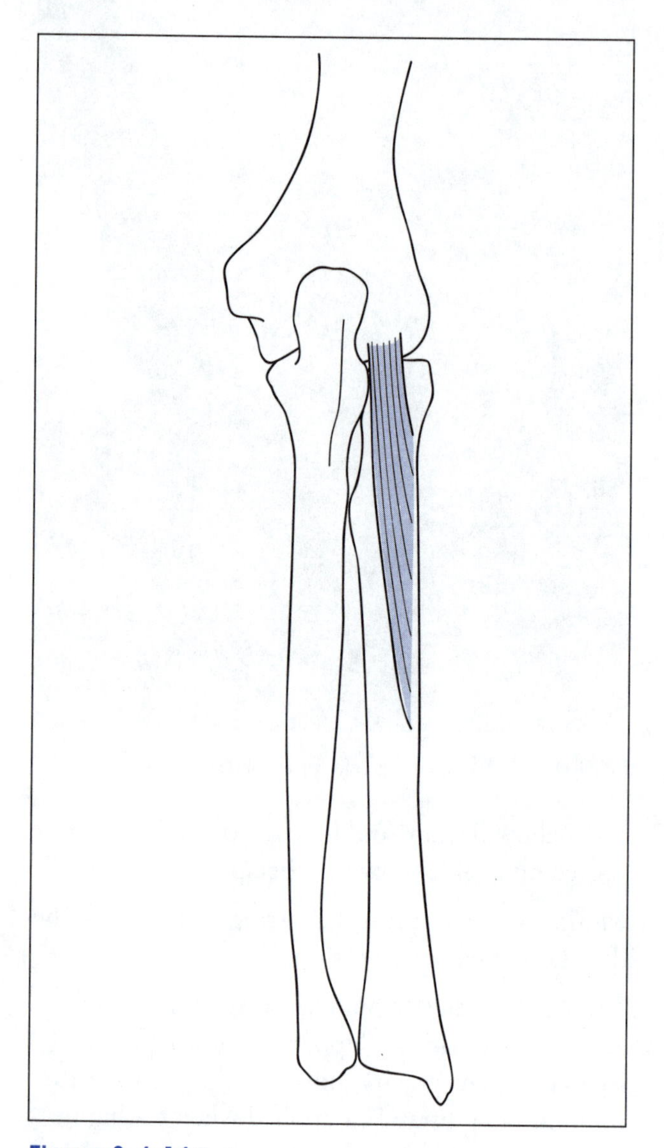

Figure 3-4-14 Supinator

Origin: Lateral epicondyle of the humerus

Insertion: Proximal 1/3 of the radius

Innervation: Posterior interosseus branch of the radial nerve

Action: Forearm supination

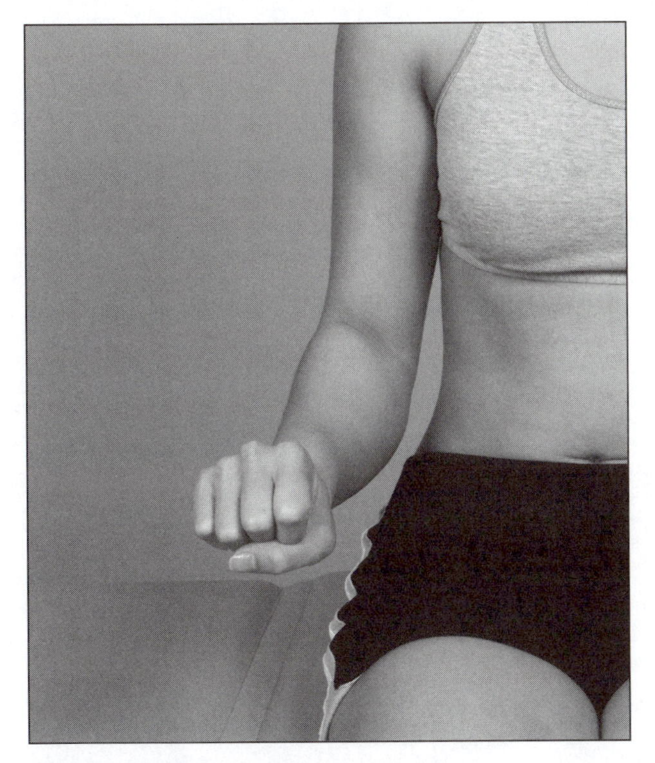

Figure 3-4-15 Start position for the supinator.

Normal, Good, Fair

Client Position: Starting—client is sitting with the testing extremity in adduction, 90 degrees of elbow flexion, and forearm pronation. (Figure 3-4-15).

Motion—client moves the testing extremity in the direction of forearm supination (Figure 3-4-16).

Therapist Position: Stabilize at the distal humerus to avoid compensation. Resistance is applied at the posterior aspect of the distal end of the forearm in the direction of forearm pronation when testing Normal or Good strengths. No resistance is applied when testing Fair strength.

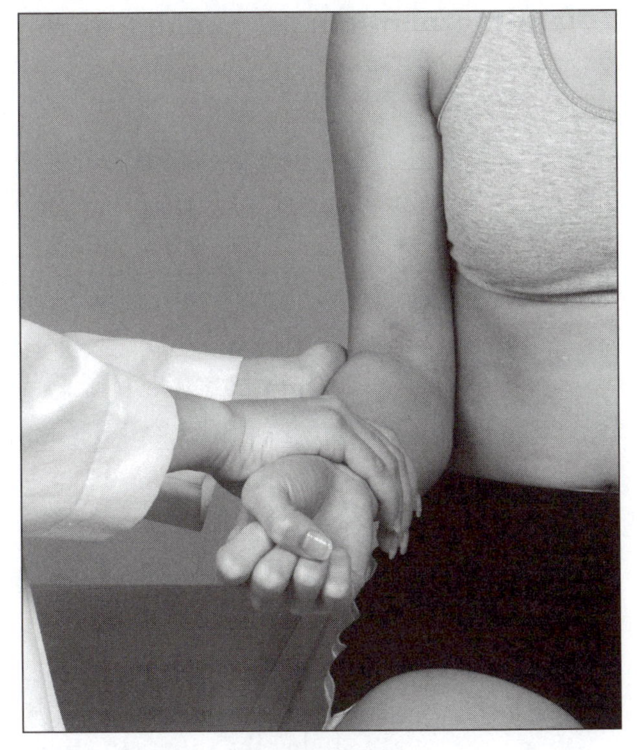

Figure 3-4-16 End position for the supinator.

Poor

Client Position: Starting—client is sitting with the testing extremity in humeral flexion, elbow flexion, and forearm pronation with the elbow supported on the table.

Motion—client moves the testing extremity in the direction of forearm supination.

Therapist Position: Stabilize at the humerus to avoid compensation. No resistance is applied when testing in the gravity-eliminated position.

Trace

The supinator is palpated at the posterior, proximal forearm over the radius.

Forearm pronation: *pronator teres*

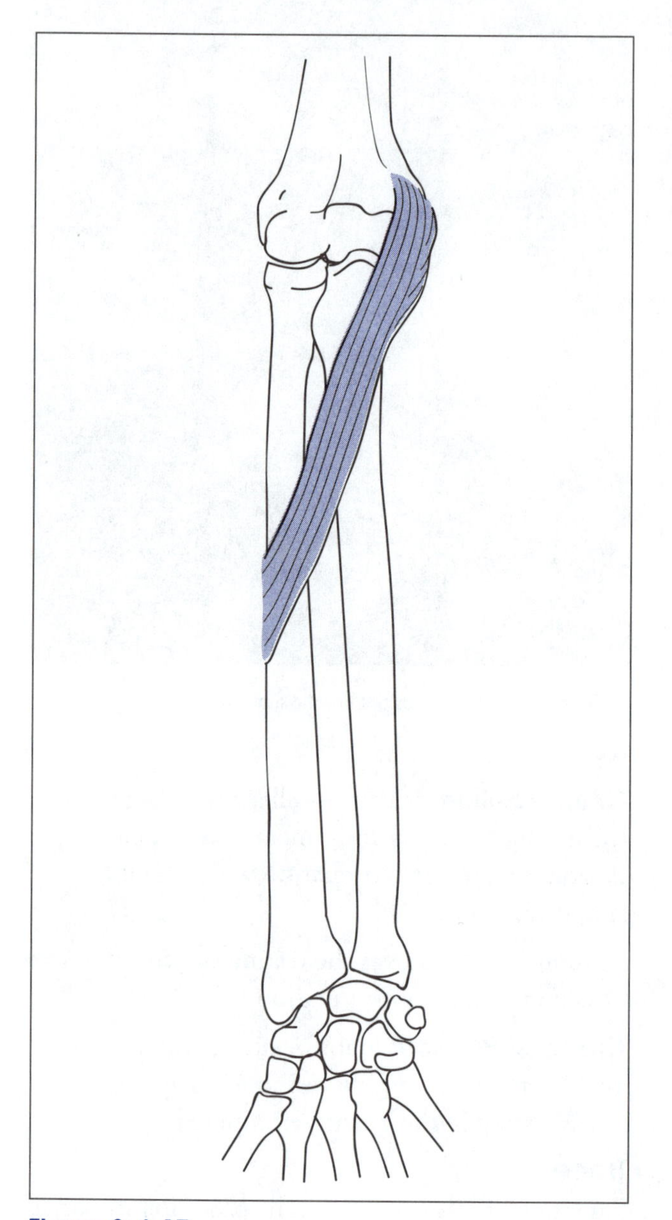

Figure 3-4-17 Pronator teres

Origin: Humeral head—proximal to the medial epicondyle and common flexor tendon. Ulnar head—medial side of coronoid process of ulna.

Insertion: Lateral surface of radial shaft

Innervation: Median nerve

Action: Forearm pronation

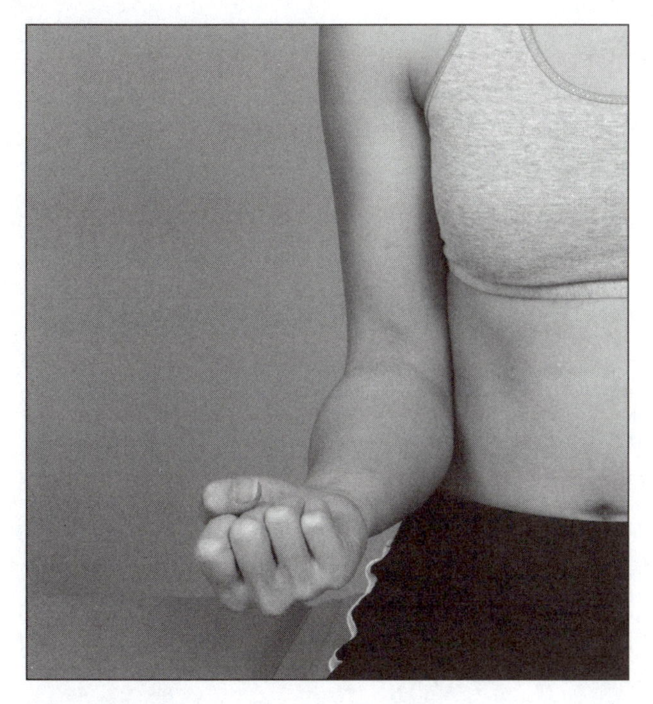

Figure 3-4-18 Start position for the pronator teres.

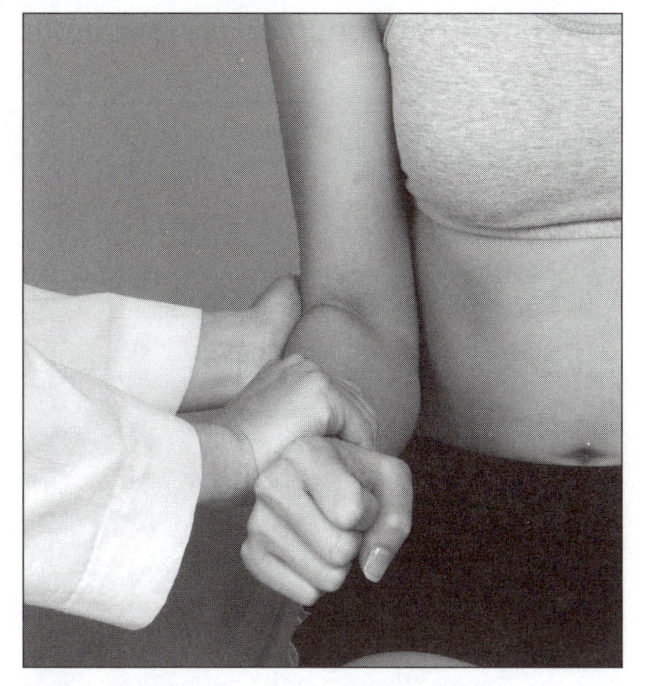

Figure 3-4-19 End position for the pronator teres.

Normal, Good, Fair

Client Position: Starting—client is sitting with the testing extremity in humeral adduction, partial elbow flexion, and forearm supination (Figure 3-4-18).

Motion—client moves the testing extremity in the direction of forearm pronation (Figure 3-4-19).

Therapist Position: Stabilize at the humerus. Resistance is applied at the posterior aspect of the distal end of the forearm in the direction of forearm supination when testing Normal or Good strengths. No resistance is applied when testing Fair strength.

Poor

Client Position: Starting—client is sitting with the testing extremity in 90 degrees of humeral flexion, elbow partially flexed, and forearm in supination with elbow supported on a table.

Motion—client moves the testing extremity in the direction of forearm pronation.

Therapist Position: Stabilize at the humerus. No resistance is applied when testing in the gravity-eliminated position.

Trace

The pronator teres is palpated at the anterior, proximal forearm between the radius and the ulna.

Forearm pronation: *pronator quadratus*

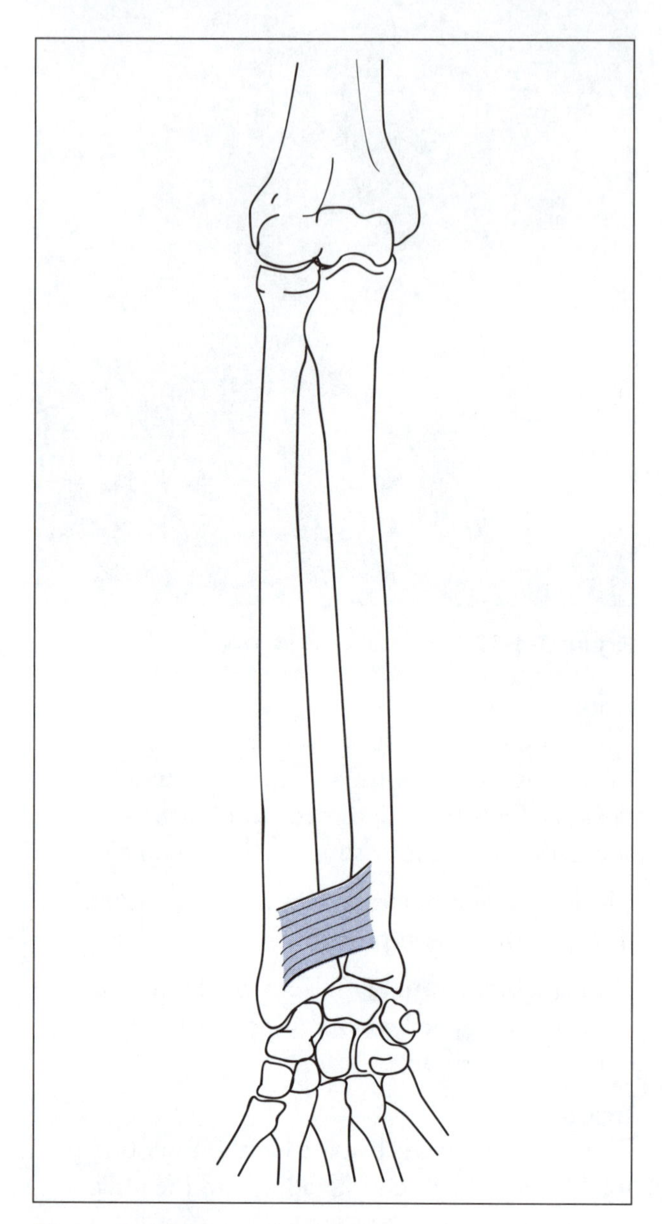

Figure 3-4-20 Pronator quadratus

Origin: Distal 1/4 of the anterior surface of the ulnar shaft

Insertion: Distal 1/4 of the anterior surface of the radial shaft

Innervation: Anterior interosseous branch of the median nerve

Action: Forearm pronation

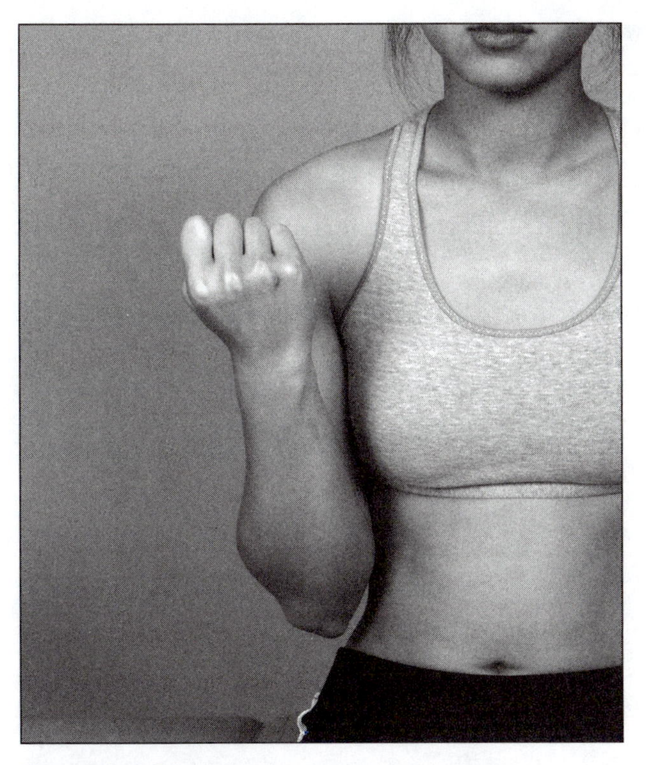

Figure 3-4-21 Start position for the pronator quadratus.

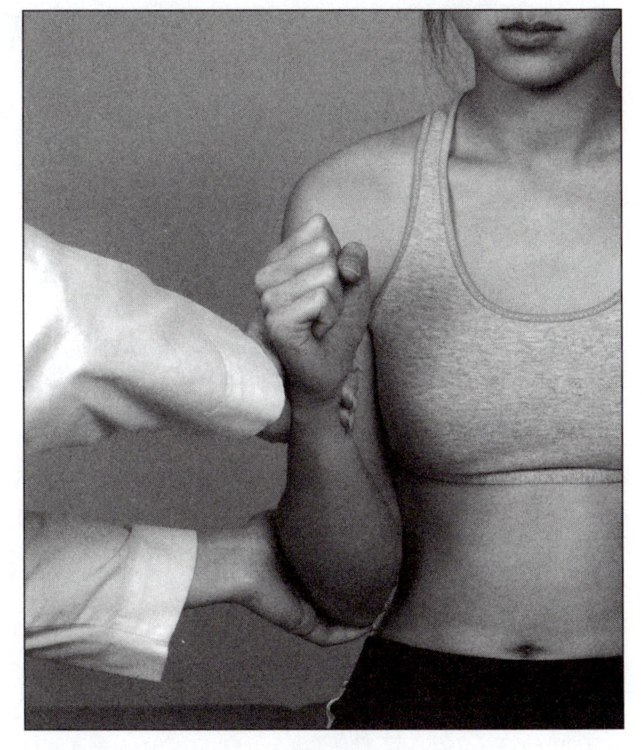

Figure 3-4-22 End position for the pronator quadratus.

Normal, Good, Fair

Client Position: Starting—client is sitting with the testing extremity in humeral adduction, elbow fully flexed, and forearm supinated (Figure 3-4-21).

Motion—client moves the testing extremity in the direction of forearm pronation (Figure 3-4-22).

Therapist Position: Stabilize at the humerus to avoid compensation. Resistance is applied at the posterior aspect of the distal end of the forearm in the direction of forearm supination when testing Normal or Good strengths. No resistance is applied when testing Fair strength.

Poor

Client Position: Starting—client is sitting with the testing extremity in 90 degrees of humeral flexion, elbow fully flexed, and forearm in supination with the elbow supported on the table.

Motion—client moves the testing extremity in the direction of forearm pronation.

Therapist Position: Stabilize at the humerus to avoid compensation. No resistance is applied when testing in the gravity-eliminated position.

Trace

The pronator quadratus is too deep to palpate.

SECTION 3-5: Isolated Manual Muscle Testing of the Wrist and Hand

Wrist: *flexor carpi radialis*

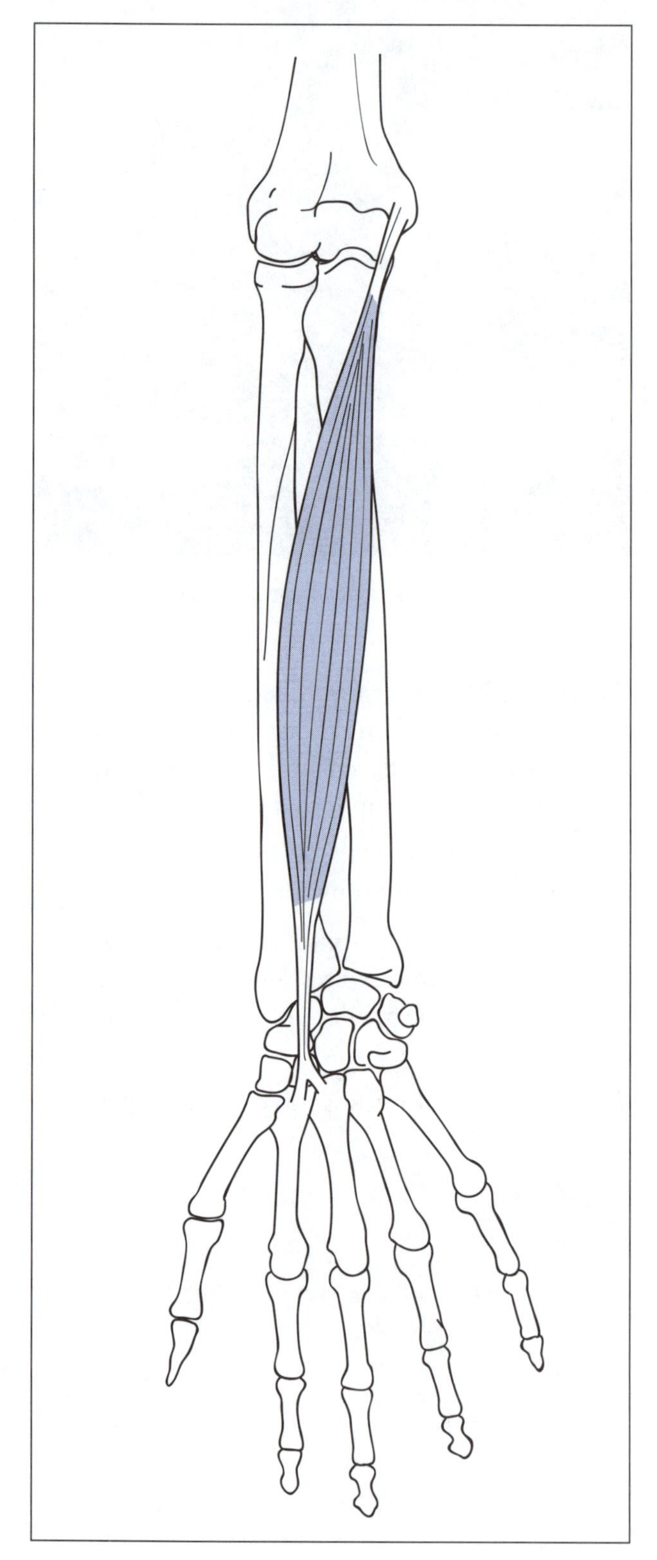

Figure 3-5-1 Flexor carpi radialis

Origin: Medial epicondyle, common extensor tendon

Insertion: Base of the second metacarpal

Innervation: Median nerve

Action: Wrist flexion, wrist radial deviation

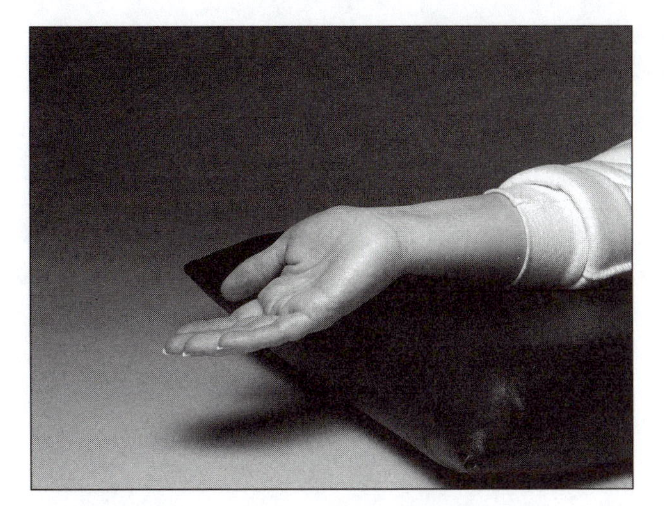

Figure 3-5-2 Start position for flexor carpi radialis.

Normal, Good, Fair

Client Position: Starting—client is sitting with the testing extremity on a table with the forearm in supination, and the wrist over the edge of the table in slight extension (Figure 3-5-2).

Motion—client moves the testing extremity in the directions of both wrist flexion and wrist radial deviation (Figure 3-5-3).

Therapist Position: Stabilize at the distal forearm to avoid compensation. Resistance is applied at the second metacarpal in the directions of both extension and ulnar deviation when testing Normal or Good strengths. No resistance is applied when testing Fair strength.

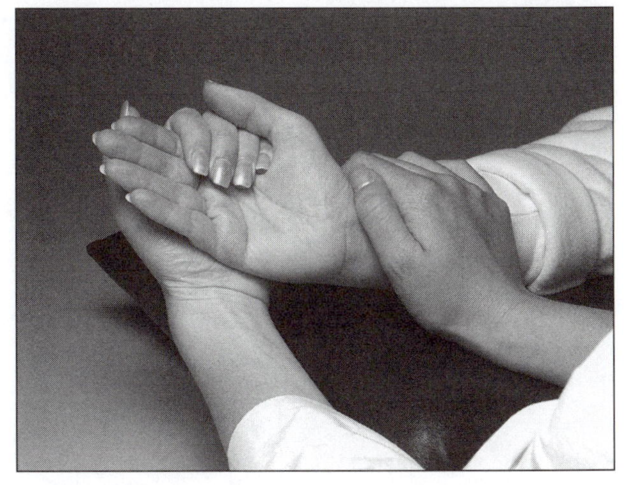

Figure 3-5-3 End position for flexor carpi radialis.

Poor

Client Position: Starting—client is sitting with the testing extremity on a table with the wrist in neutral and the forearm in supination.

Motion—client moves the testing extremity in the directions of both wrist flexion and wrist radial deviation.

Therapist Position: Stabilize at the distal forearm to avoid compensation. No resistance is applied when testing in the gravity-eliminated position.

Trace

The flexor carpi radialis is palpated on the anterior surface of the forearm in line with the second metacarpal, just lateral to the palmaris longus.

Wrist: *flexor carpi ulnaris*

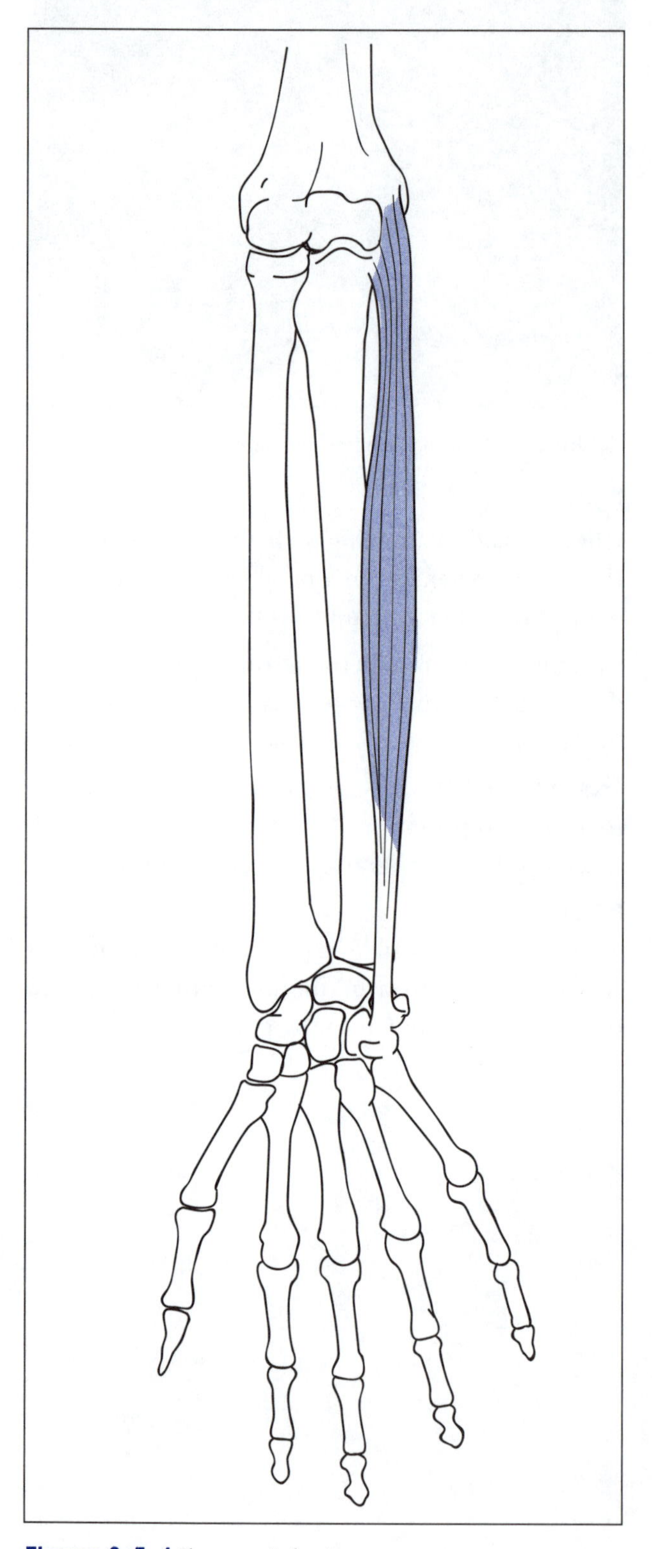

Figure 3-5-4 Flexor carpi ulnaris

Origin: Medial epicondyle, common flexor tendon, proximal ulna

Insertion: Pisiform bone

Innervation: Ulnar nerve

Action: Wrist flexion, wrist ulnar deviation

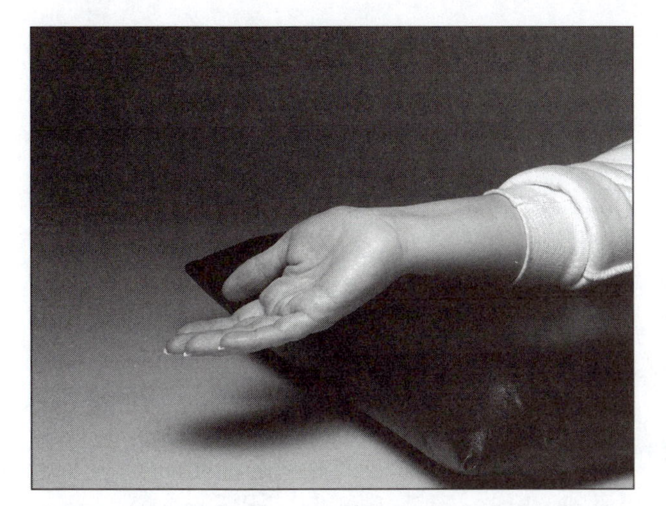

Figure 3-5-5 Start position for flexor carpi ulnaris.

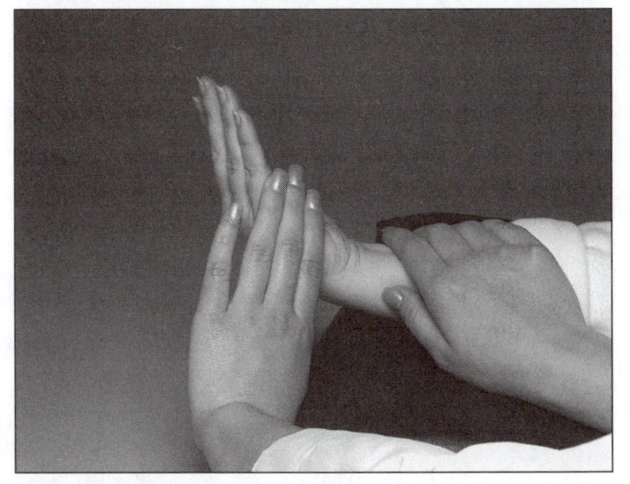

Figure 3-5-6 End position for flexor carpi ulnaris.

Normal, Good, Fair

Client Position: Starting—client is sitting with the testing extremity on a table with the forearm in supination, and the wrist over the edge of the table in slight extension (Figure 3-5-5).

Motion—client moves the testing extremity in the directions of both wrist flexion and wrist ulnar deviation (Figure 3-5-6).

Therapist Position: Stabilize at the distal forearm to avoid compensation. Resistance is applied at the fifth metacarpal in the directions of both extension and radial deviation when testing Normal or Good strengths. No resistance is applied when testing Fair strength.

Poor

Client Position: Starting—client is sitting with the testing extremity on a table with the wrist in neutral and the forearm in supination.

Motion—client moves the testing extremity in the directions of both wrist flexion and wrist ulnar deviation.

Therapist Position: Stabilize at the distal forearm to avoid compensation. No resistance is applied when testing in the gravity-eliminated position.

Trace

Flexor carpi ulnaris is palpated proximal to the pisiform bone on the anterior/distal forearm.

Wrist: *palmaris longus*

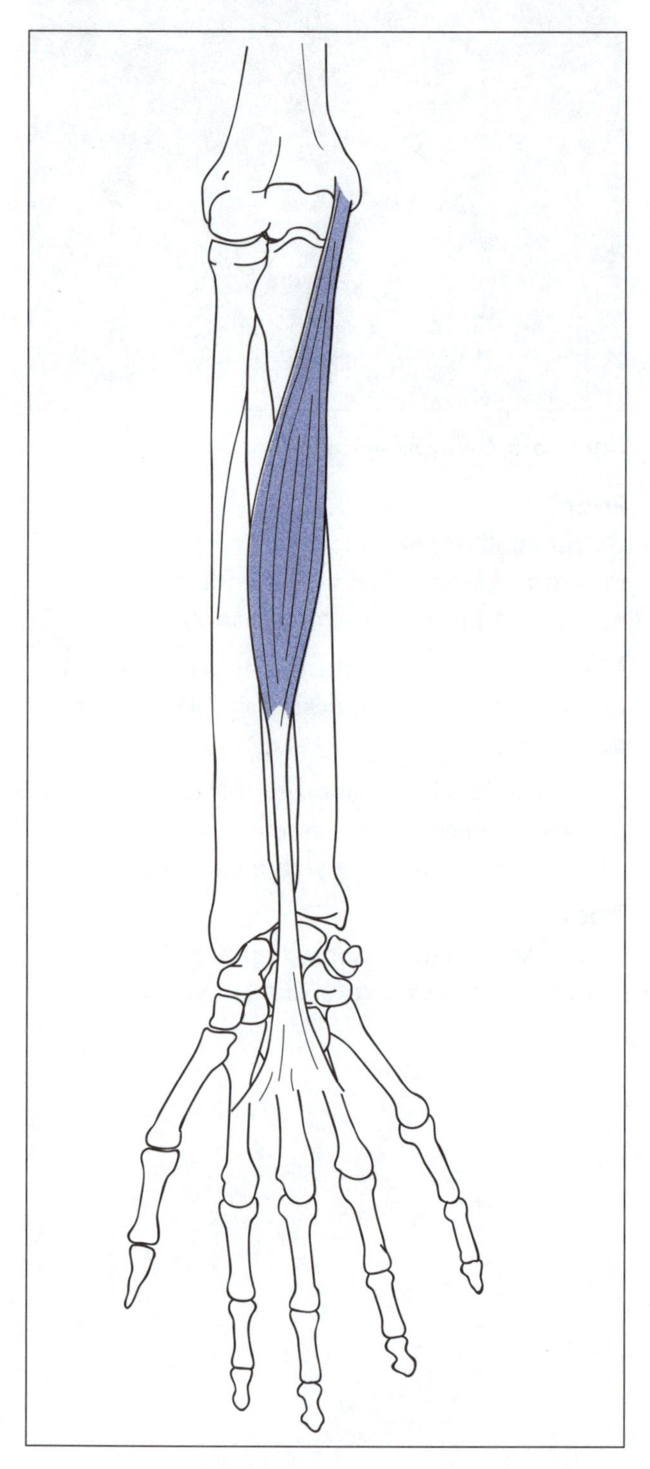

Figure 3-5-7 Palmaris longus

Origin: Medial epicondyle, common flexor tendon

Insertion: Palmar aponeurosis

Innervation: Median nerve

Action: Wrist flexion

Palmaris longus is not tested in isolation because it is a weak flexor, and only 80% of the population actually have this muscle. To determine if an individual has this muscle, ask the client to strongly flex the wrist while cupping all fingers together. Both the palmaris longus and the flexor carpi radialis should be prominent at the distal forearm.

Wrist: *extensor carpi radialus longus* (ECRL) and *brevis* (ECRB)

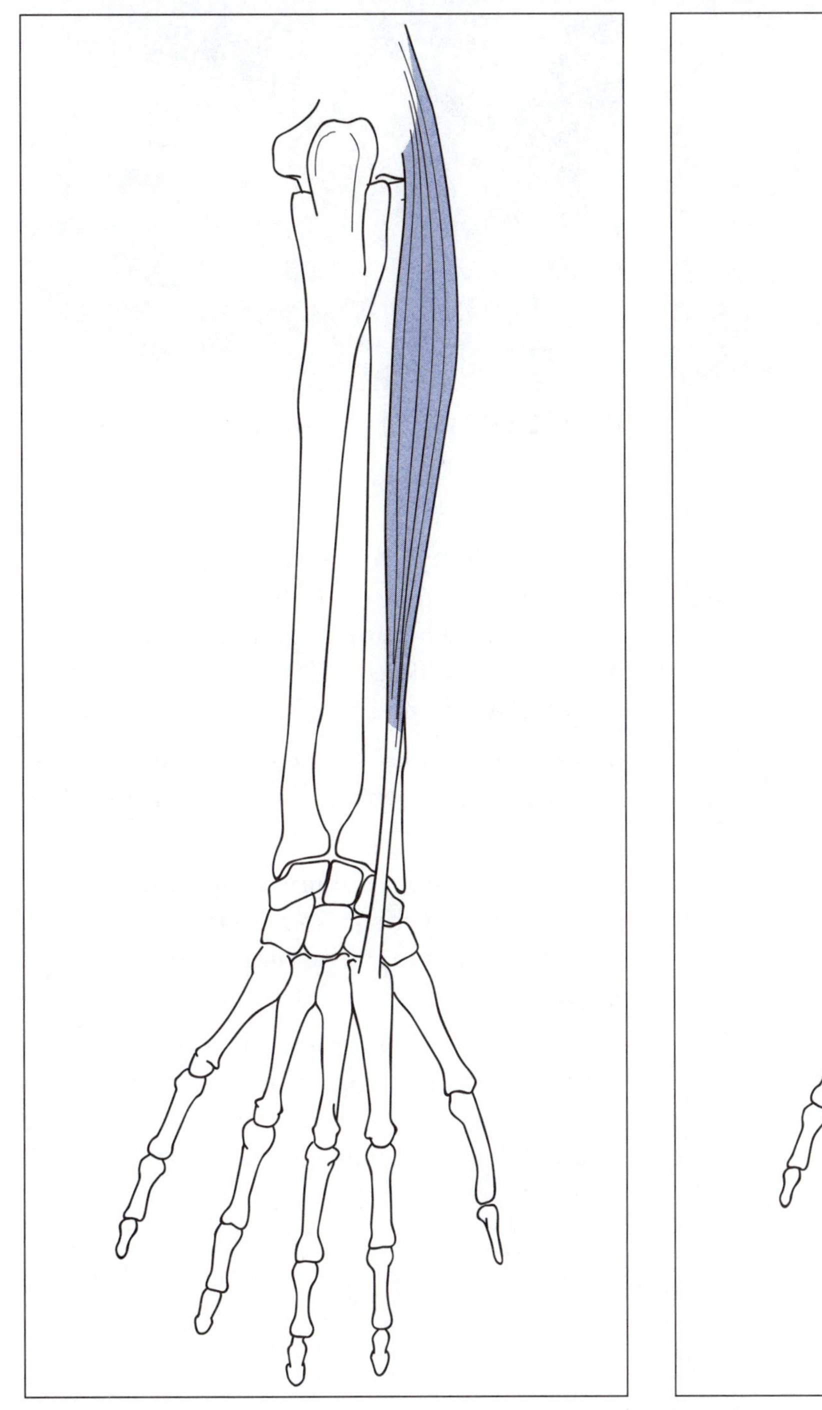

Figure 3-5-8 Extensor carpi radialis longus

ECRL

Origin: Lateral supracondylar ridge, lateral epicondyle, common extensor tendon

Insertion: Base of the second metacarpal

Innervation: Radial nerve

Action: Wrist extension and wrist radial deviation

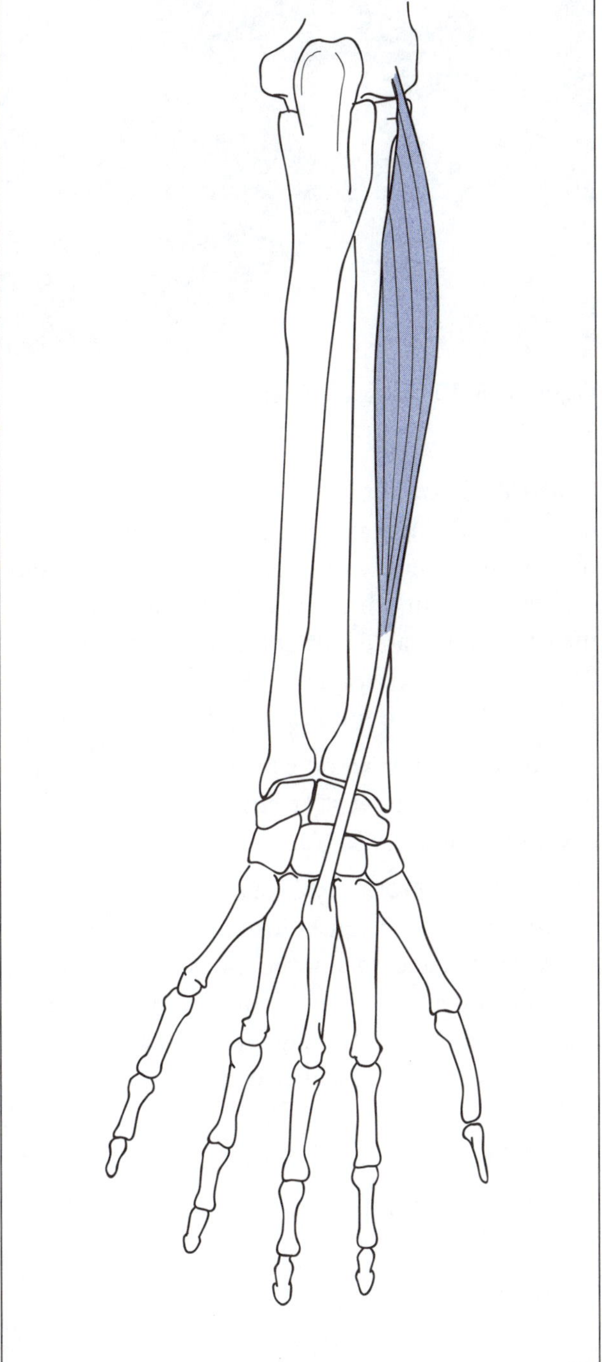

Figure 3-5-9 Extensor carpi radialis brevis

ECRB

Origin: Lateral epicondyle, common extensor tendon

Insertion: Base of the third metacarpal

Innervation: Radial nerve

Action: Wrist extension and wrist radial deviation

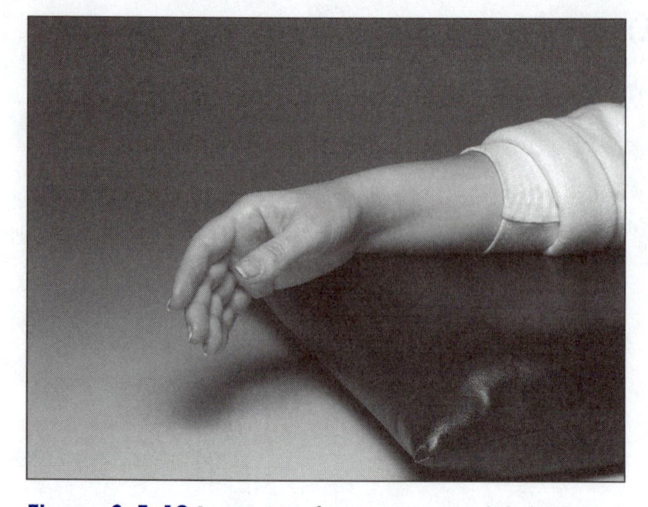

Figure 3-5-10 Start position for extensor carpi radialis longus and brevis.

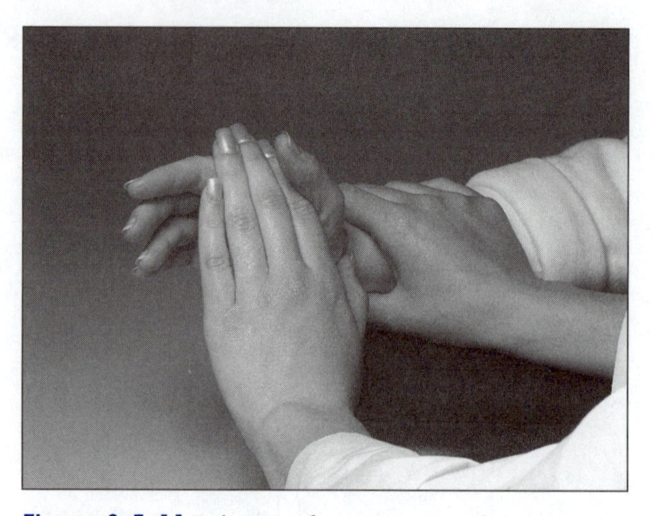

Figure 3-5-11 End position for extensor carpi radialis longus and brevis.

Normal, Good, Fair

Client Position: Starting—client is sitting with the testing extremity on a table with the forearm in slightly less than full pronation, and the wrist over the edge of the table in slight flexion. To isolate ECRL, elbow is flexed to 30 degrees, or to isolate ECRB, elbow is in full flexion (Figure 3-5-10).

Motion—client moves the testing extremity in the directions of both wrist extension and wrist radial deviation (Figure 3-5-11).

Therapist Position: Stabilize at the distal forearm to avoid compensation. Resistance is applied at the second metacarpal in the directions of both wrist flexion and wrist ulnar deviation when testing Normal or Good strengths. No resistance is applied when testing Fair strength.

Poor

Client Position: Starting—client is sitting with the testing extremity on a table with the wrist in neutral and the forearm in pronation. To isolate ECRL, elbow is flexed to 30 degrees, or to isolate ECRB, elbow is in full flexion (Figure 3-5-10).

Motion—client moves the testing extremity in the directions of both wrist extension and wrist radial deviation.

Therapist Position: Stabilize at the distal forearm to avoid compensation. No resistance is applied when testing in the gravity-eliminated position.

Trace

Extensor carpi radialis longus can be palpated at the distal/dorsal forearm, at the base of the second metacarpal. Extensor carpi radialis brevis can be palpated at the distal/dorsal forearm, at the base of the third metacarpal.

Wrist: *extensor carpi ulnaris*

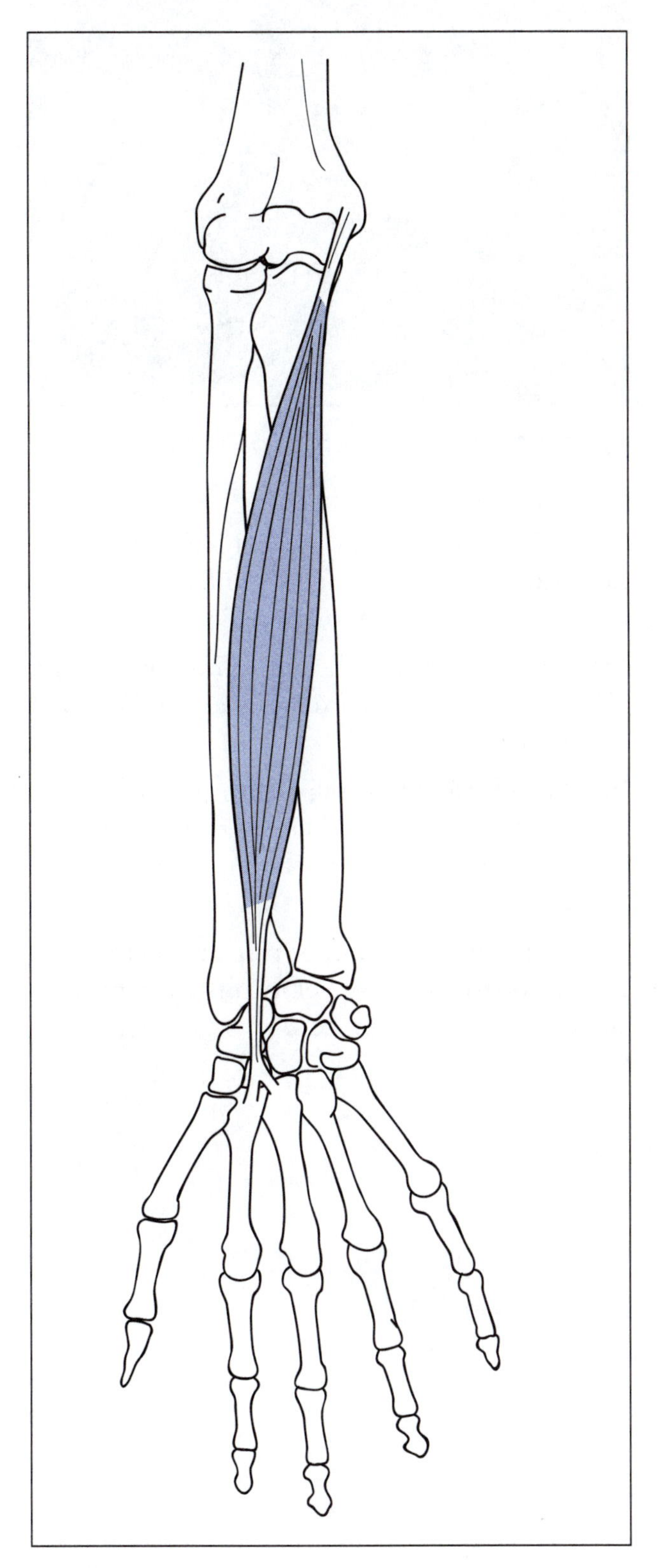

Figure 3-5-12 Extensor carpi ulnari

Origin: Lateral epicondyle, common extensor tendon, proximal ulna

Insertion: Base of the fifth metacarpal

Innervation: Radial nerve

Action: Wrist extension, wrist ulnar deviation

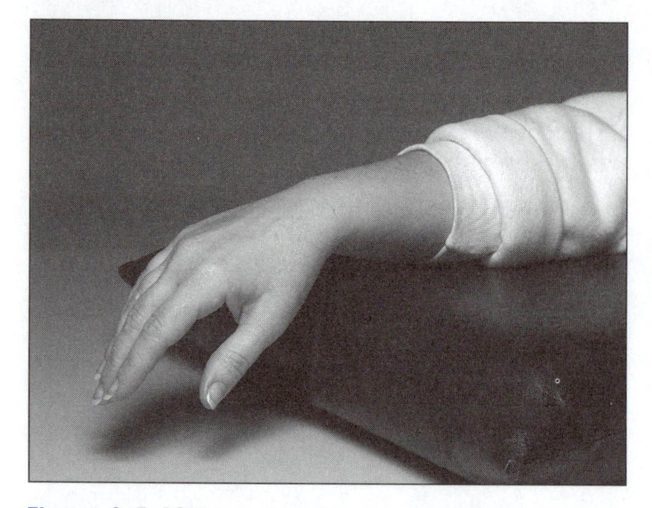

Figure 3-5-13 Start position for extensor carpi ulnaris.

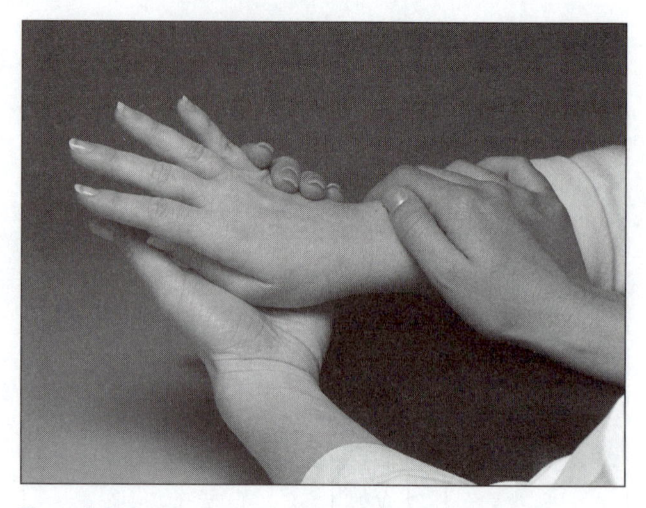

Figure 3-5-14 End position for extensor carpi ulnaris.

Normal, Good, Fair

Client Position: Starting—client is sitting with the testing extremity on a table with the forearm in pronation, and the wrist over the edge of the table in slight flexion (Figure 3-5-13).

Motion—client moves the testing extremity in the directions of both wrist extension and wrist ulnar deviation (Figure 3-5-14).

Therapist Position: Stabilize at the distal forearm to avoid compensation. Resistance is applied at the fifth metacarpal in the directions of both wrist flexion and wrist radial deviation when testing Normal or Good strengths. No resistance is applied when testing Fair strength.

Poor

Client Position: Starting—client is sitting with the testing extremity on a table with the wrist in neutral and the forearm in pronation.

Motion—client moves the testing extremity in the directions of both wrist extension and wrist ulnar deviation.

Therapist Position: Stabilize at the distal forearm to avoid compensation. No resistance is applied when testing in the gravity-eliminated position.

Trace

Extensor carpi ulnaris can be palpated on the dorsal wrist between the base of the fifth metacarpal and the ulnar styloid process.

Digit: *flexor digitorum superficialis*

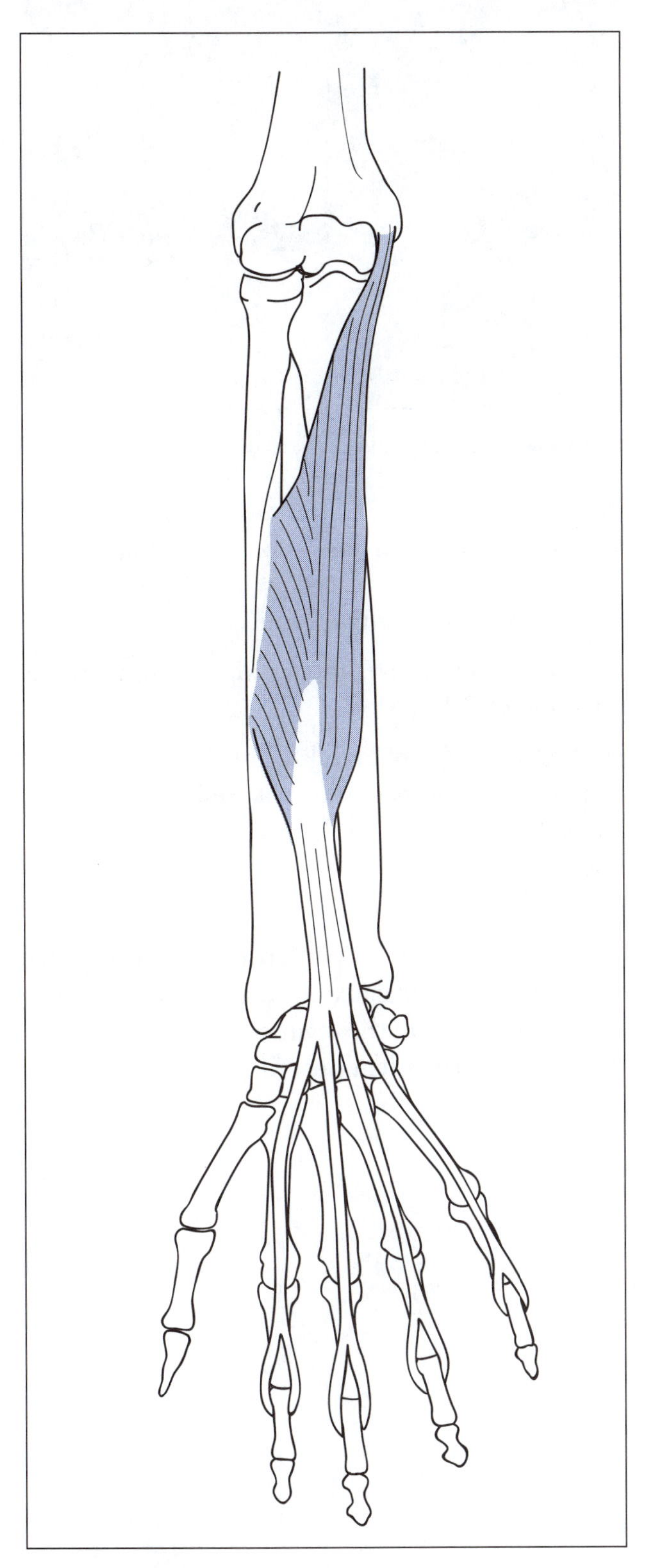

Figure 3-5-15 Flexor digitorum superficiali

Origin: Medial epicondyle, coronoid process, ulna, proximal radius

Insertion: Lateral and medial surface of the middle phalanx of digits 2–5

Innervation: Median nerve

Action: Flexion of the digit PIP joint

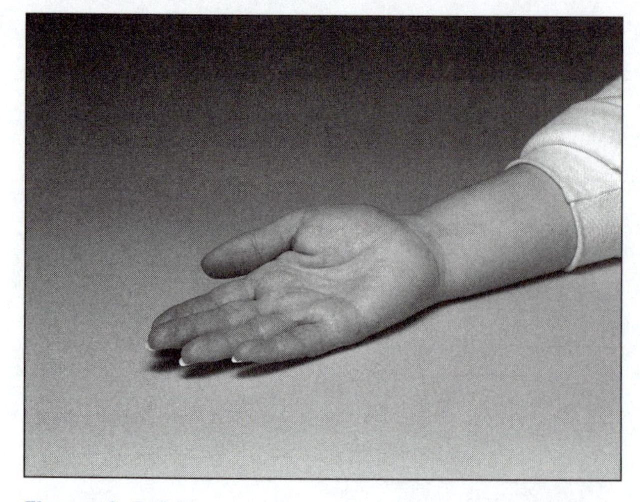

Figure 3-5-16 Start position for flexor digitorum superficialis.

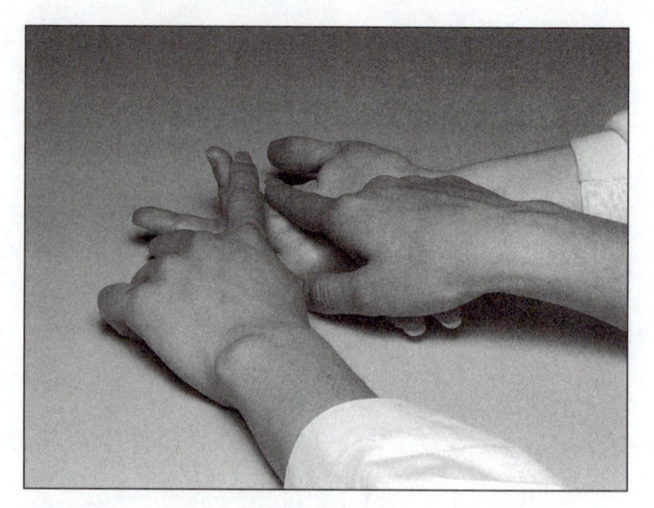

Figure 3-5-17 End position for flexor digitorum superficialis.

Normal, Good, Fair

Client Position: Starting—client is sitting with the testing extremity placed on the table in forearm supination and digit extension (Figure 3-5-16).

Motion—client moves the testing extremity in the direction of PIP flexion with MCPs remaining in extension (Figure 3-5-17).

Therapist Position: Stabilize at the proximal phalanx to avoid compensation. Resistance is applied at the middle phalanx in the direction of PIP extension when testing Normal or Good strengths. No resistance is applied when testing Fair strength.

Poor

Client Position: Starting—client is sitting with the testing extremity placed on a table in forearm neutral rotation and digit extension.

Motion—client moves the testing extremity in the direction of PIP flexion.

Therapist Position: Stabilize at the proximal phalanx to avoid compensation. No resistance is applied when testing in the gravity-eliminated position.

Trace

The flexor digitorum superficialis is palpated either on the proximal phalanx or on the volar surface of the wrist between the palmaris longus and the flexor carpi ulnaris tendons.

Digit: *flexor digitorum profundus*

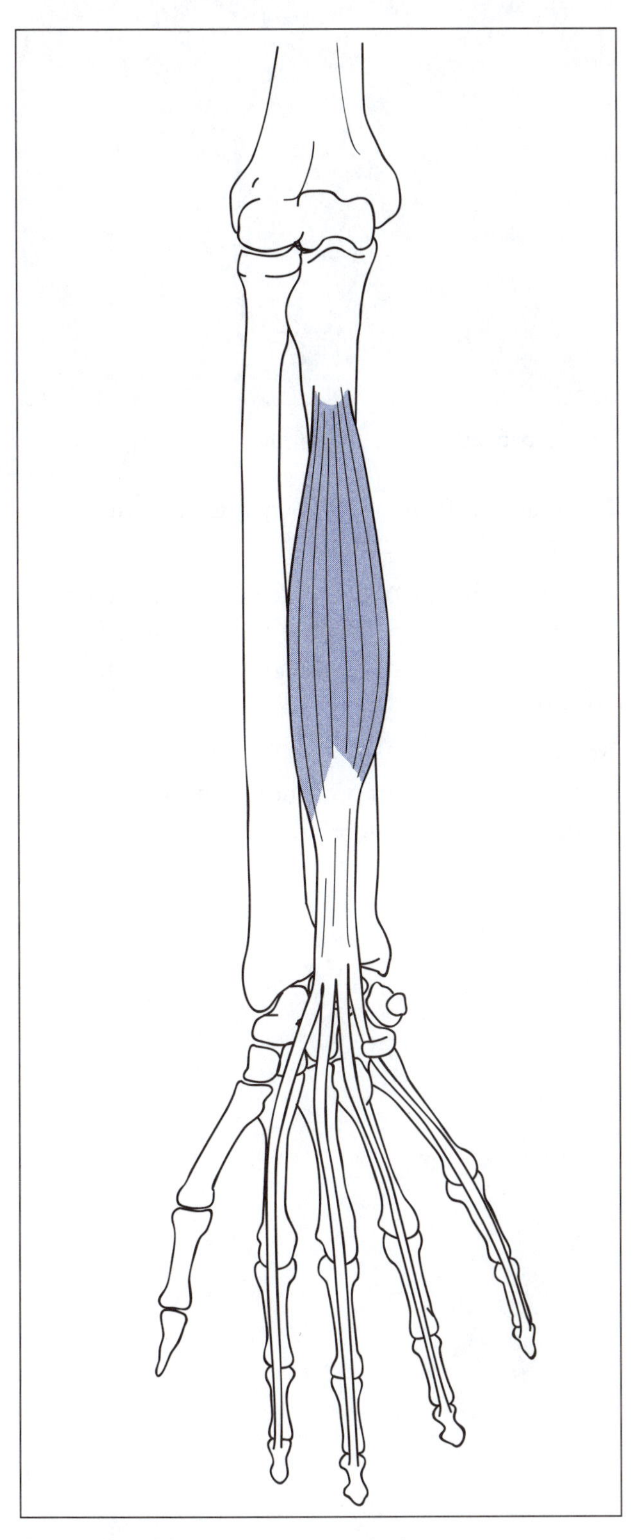

Figure 3-5-18 Flexor digitorum profundus

Origin: Body of the ulna

Insertion: Through the insertions of the flexor digitorum superficialis onto the distal phalanx of digits 2–5

Innervation: Ulnar nerve (digits 4 and 5), Median nerve (digits 2 and 3)

Action: Flexion of the digit DIP joint

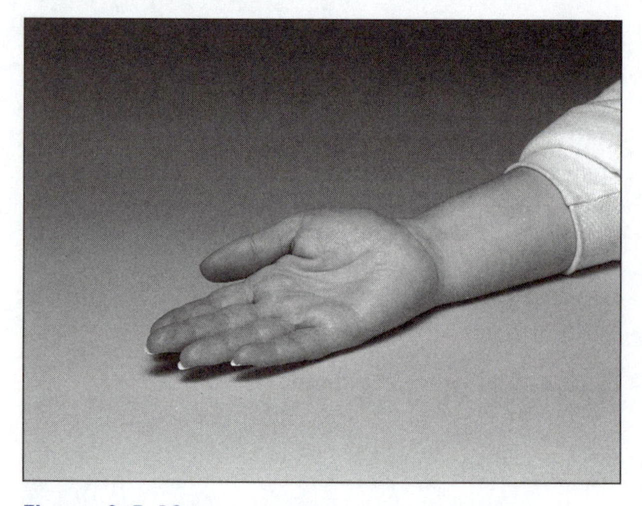

Figure 3-5-19 Start position for flexor digitorum profundus.

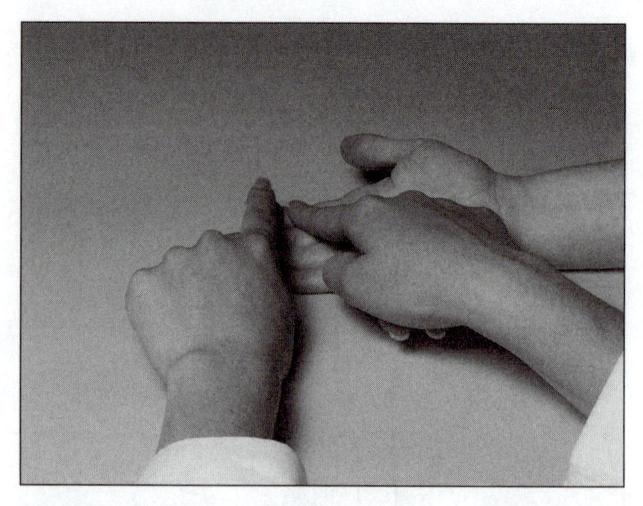

Figure 3-5-20 End position for flexor digitorum profundus.

Normal, Good, Fair

Client Position: Starting—client is sitting with the testing extremity placed on a table in forearm supination and digit extension (Figure 3-5-19).

Motion—client moves the testing extremity in the direction of DIP flexion with MCPs and PIPs remaining in extension (Figure 3-5-20).

Therapist Position: Stabilize at the middle phalanx to avoid compensation. Resistance is applied at the distal phalanx when testing Normal or Good strengths. No resistance is applied when testing Fair strength.

Poor

Client Position: Starting—client is sitting with the testing extremity placed on a table in forearm neutral rotation and digit extension.

Motion—client moves the testing extremity in the direction of DIP flexion.

Therapist Position: Stabilize at the middle phalanx to avoid compensation. No resistance is applied when testing in the gravity-eliminated position.

Trace

The flexor digitorum profundus tendon can be palpated over the middle phalanges of the digits, palmar surface.

Digit: *flexor digiti minimi*

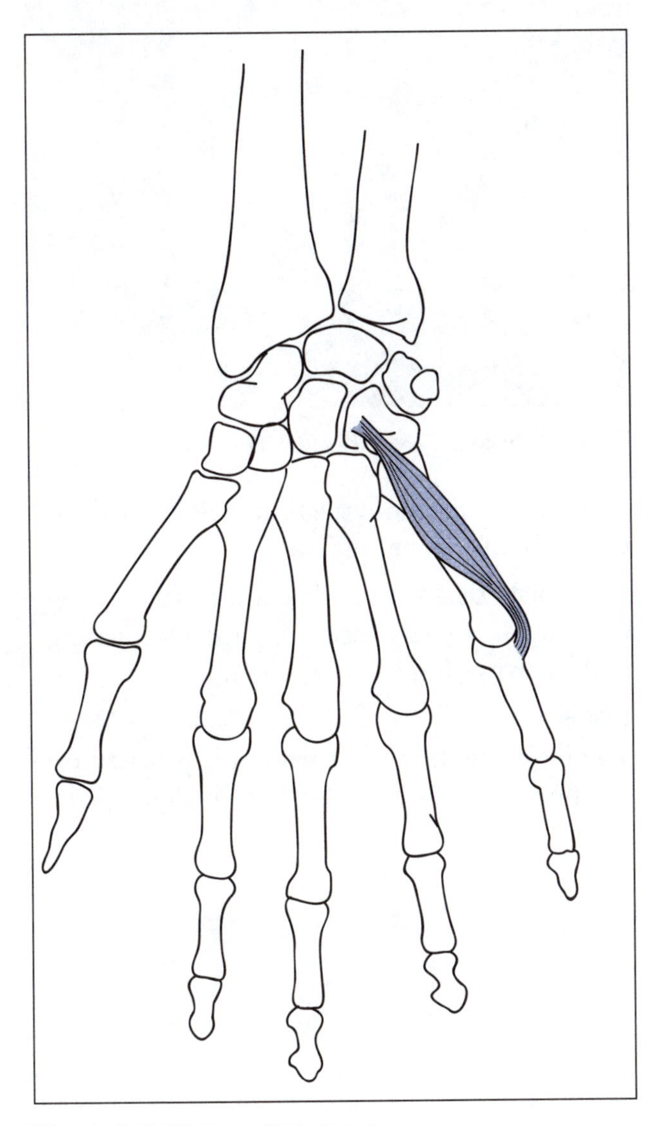

Figure 3-5-21 Flexor digiti minimi

Origin: Hook of hamate

Insertion: Base of the fifth digit proximal phalanx, ulnar side

Innervation: Ulnar nerve

Action: Fifth digit MCP flexion

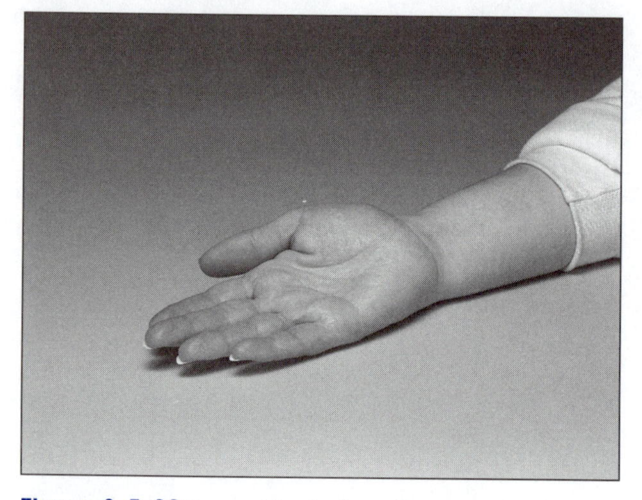

Figure 3-5-22 Start position for flexor digiti minimi.

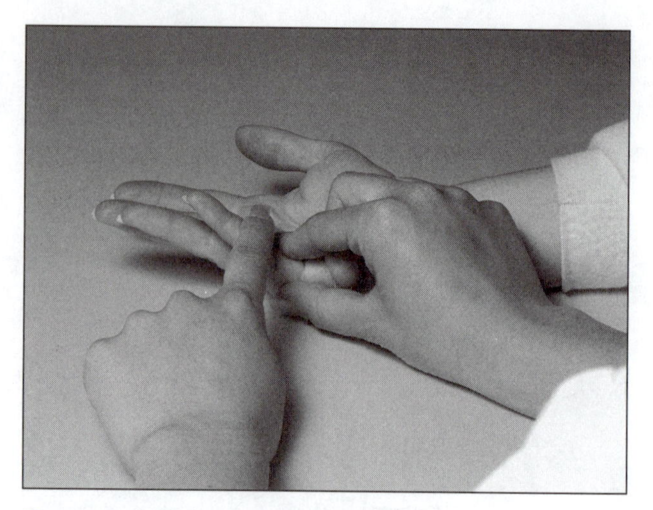

Figure 3-5-23 End position for flexor digiti minimi.

Normal, Good, Fair

Client Position: Starting—client is sitting with the testing extremity placed on the table with the forearm in supination (Figure 3-5-22).

Motion—client moves the fifth digit in the direction of MCP flexion (Figure 3-5-23).

Therapist Position: Stabilize at the fifth metacarpal. Resistance is applied at the fifth proximal phalanx in the direction of MCP extension when testing Normal or Good strengths. No resistance is applied when testing Fair strength.

Poor

Client Position: Starting—client is sitting with the testing extremity placed on the table with the forearm in neutral.

Motion—client moves the fifth digit in the direction of MCP flexion.

Therapist Position: Stabilize at the fifth metacarpal. No resistance is applied when testing in the gravity-eliminated position.

Trace

The flexor digiti minimi tendon is palpated over the proximal phalanx of the fifth digit, palmar surface.

Digit: *extensor digitorum*

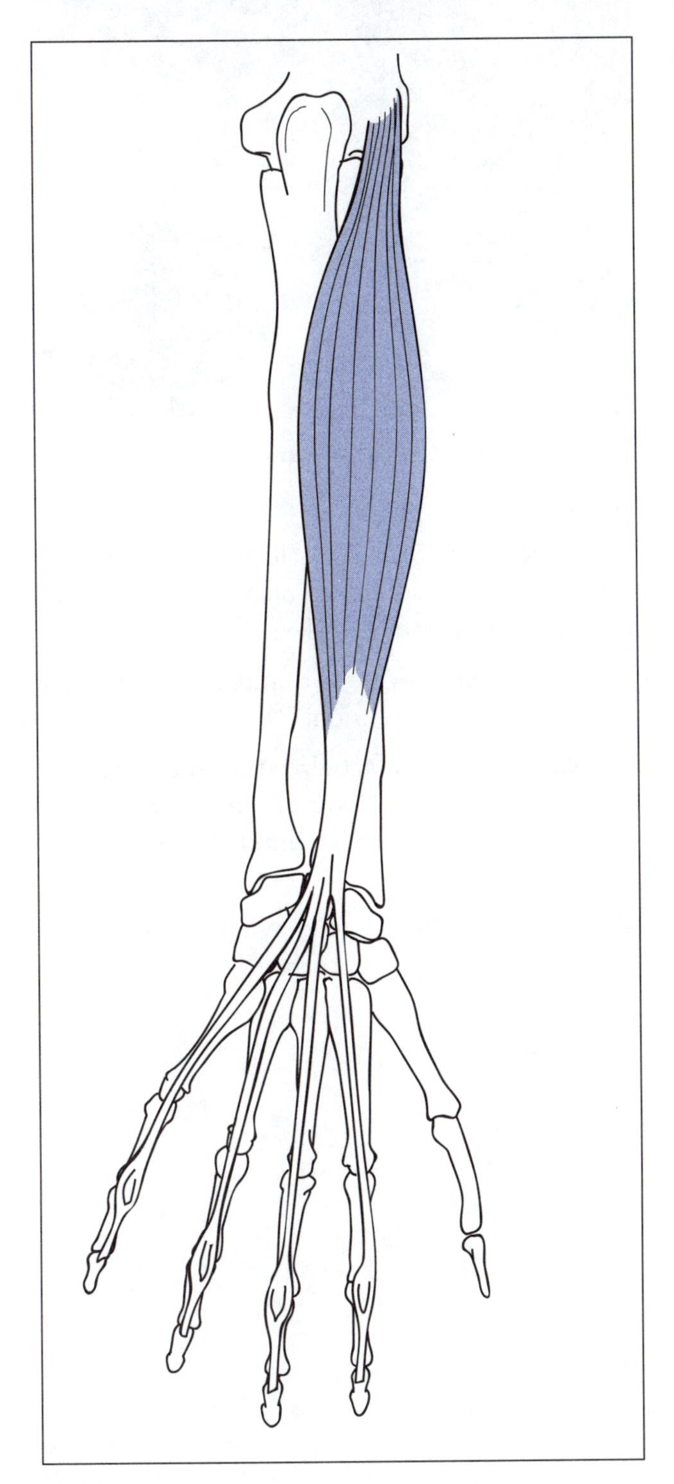

Figure 3-5-24 Extensor digitorum

Origin: Lateral epicondyle

Insertion: Base of the middle and distal phalanges digits 2–5

Innervation: Radial nerve

Action: Extension of the MCP of digits 2–5

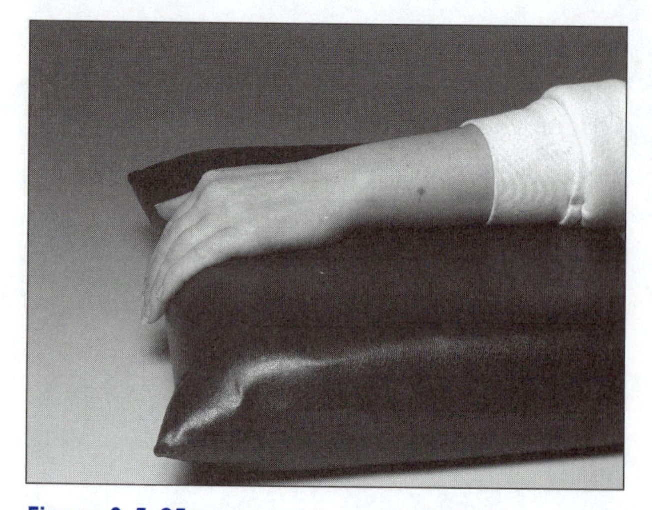

Figure 3-5-25 Start position for extensor digitorum.

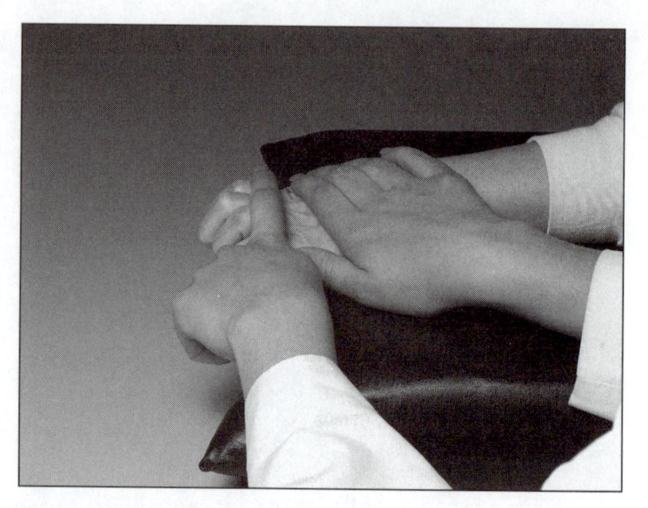

Figure 3-5-26 End position for extensor digitorum.

Normal, Good, Fair

Client Position: Starting—client is sitting with the testing extremity placed on a table edge (digits off the table) in forearm pronation and digit flexion (Figure 3-5-25).

Motion—client moves the testing extremity in the direction of digit MCP extension with PIP and DIP flexed (Figure 3-5-26).

Therapist Position: Stabilize at the metacarpals to avoid compensation. Resistance is applied at the proximal phalanges in the direction of digit MCP flexion when testing Normal or Good strengths. No resistance is applied when testing Fair strength.

Poor

Client Position: Starting—client is sitting with the testing extremity placed on a table in forearm neutral rotation and digit flexion.

Motion—client moves the testing extremity in the direction of digit extension.

Therapist Position: Stabilize at the metacarpals to avoid compensation. No resistance is applied when testing in the gravity-eliminated position.

Trace

The extensor digitorum tendon is palpated over the metacarpal heads, dorsal surface.

Digit: *extensor indicis*

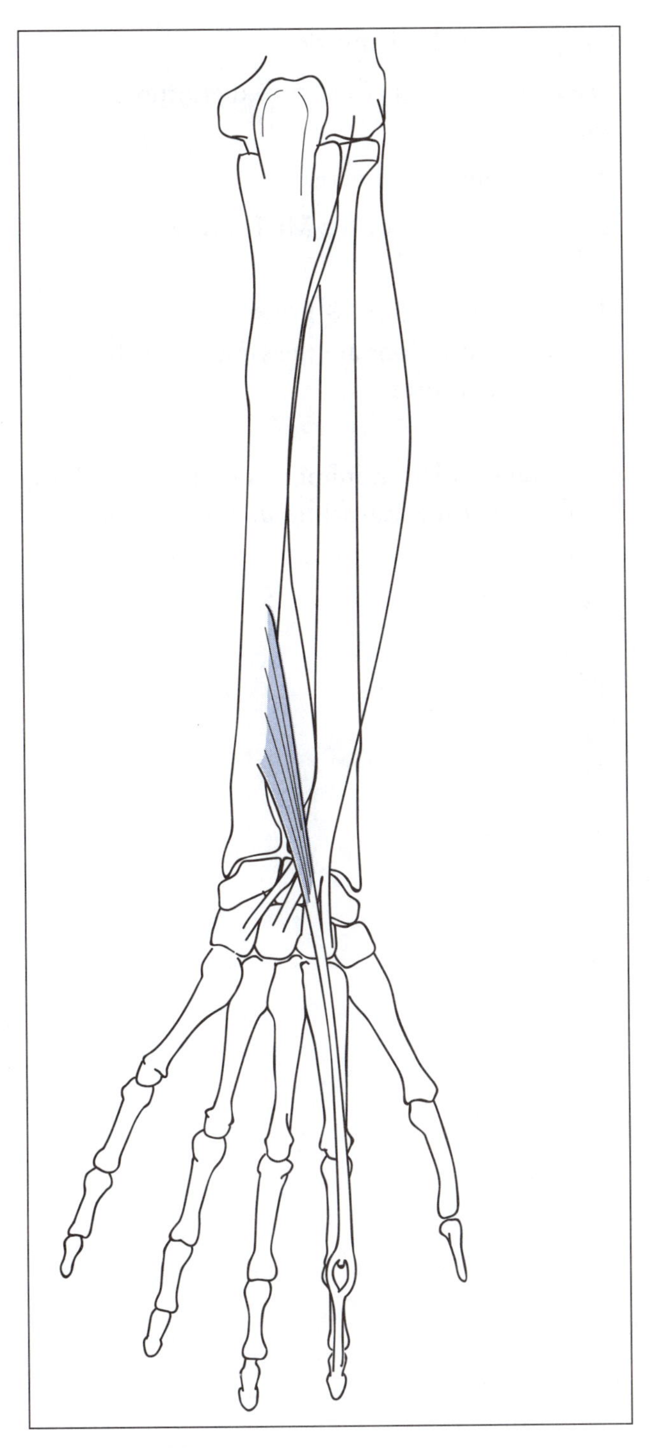

Figure 3-5-27 Extensor indicis

Origin: Posterior ulna

Insertion: Tendon of extensor digitorum, dorsal aponeurosis

Innervation: Radial nerve

Action: Extension of the MCP, PIP, DIP of the second digit

Normal, Good, Fair & Poor

The testing positions are the same as for the extensor digitorum.

Trace

The extensor indicis tendon is palpated over the second digit metacarpal head, dorsal surface.

Digit: *extensor digiti minimi*

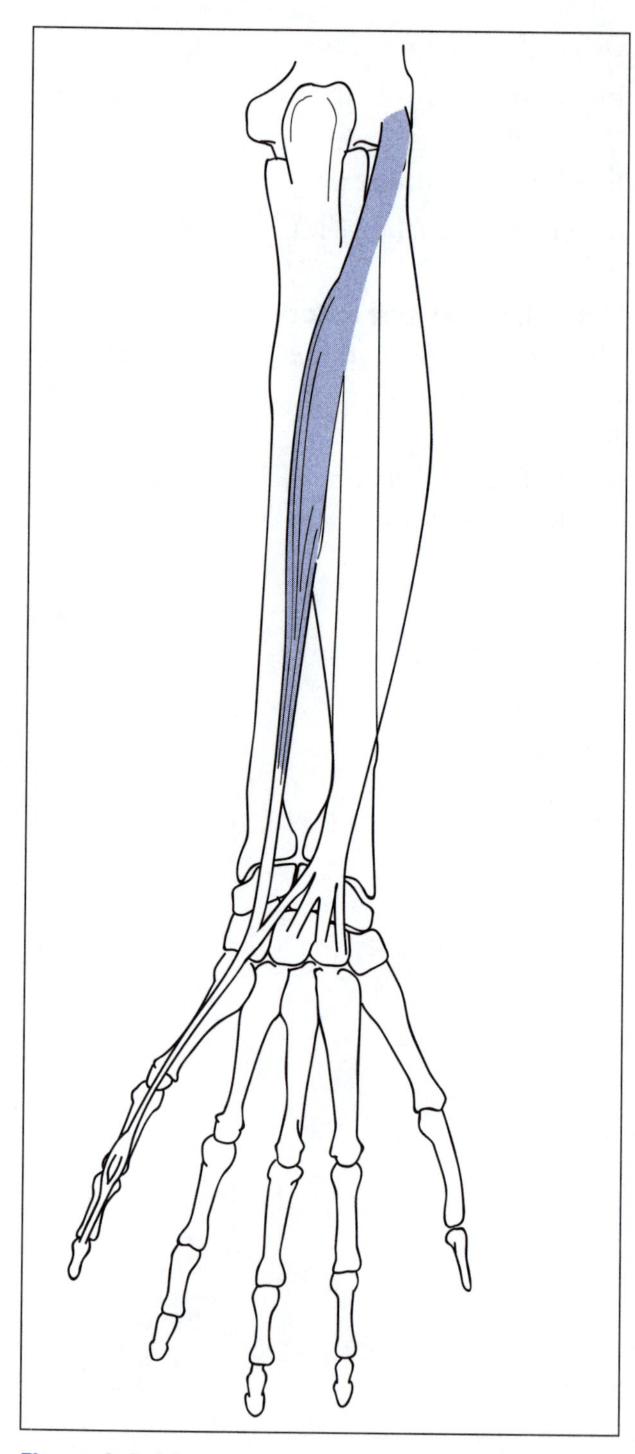

Figure 3-5-28 Extensor digiti minimi

Origin: Lateral epicondyle

Insertion: Tendon of extensor digitorum fifth digit

Innervation: Radial nerve

Action: Extension of the MCP, PIP, DIP of the fifth digit

Normal, Good, Fair, & Poor

The testing positions are the same as for the extensor digitorum.

Trace

The extensor digiti minimi tendon is palpated over the fifth digit metacarpal head, dorsal surface.

Digit: *lumbricals*

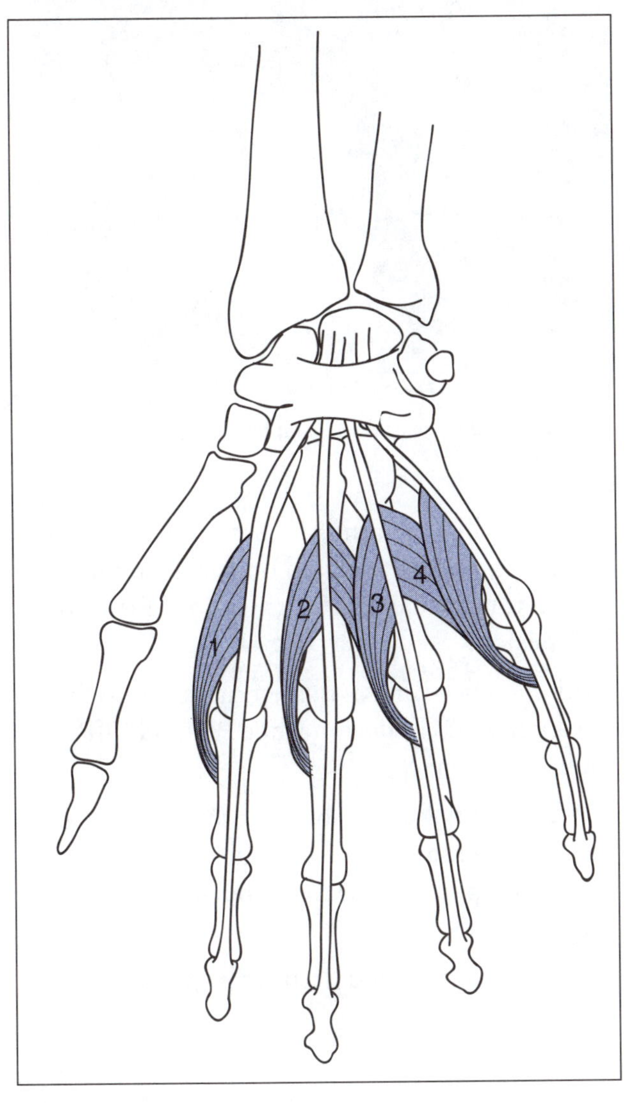

Figure 3-5-29 Lumbricals

Origin: First—FDP second digit tendon

Second—FDP third digit tendon

Third—FDP third and fourth digit tendons

Fourth—FDP fourth and fifth digit tendons

Insertion: Radial side dorsal aponeurosis

Innervation: First and second—median nerve, third and fourth—ulnar nerve

Action: MCP flexion and PIP/DIP extension

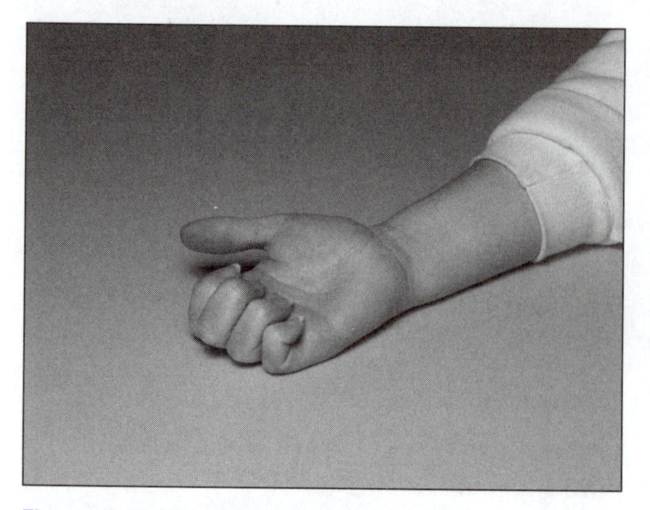

Figure 3-5-30 Start position for the lumbricals.

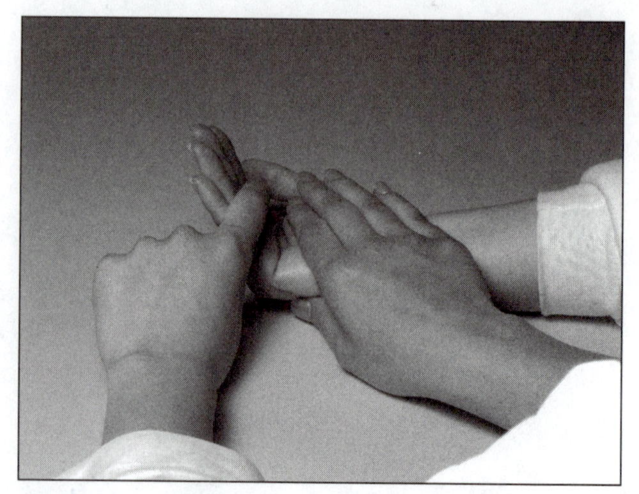

Figure 3-5-31 End position for the lumbricals.

Normal, Good, Fair

Client Position: Starting—client is sitting with the testing extremity placed on a table in forearm supination and MCP extension/ PIP and DIP flexion (Figure 3-5-30).

Motion—client moves the testing extremity in the direction of MCP flexion while PIP and DIP enter extension (Figure 3-5-31).

Therapist Position: Stabilize at the metacarpals to avoid compensation. Resistance is applied at the proximal phalanx in the direction of MCP extension when testing Normal or Good strengths. No resistance is applied when testing Fair strength.

Poor

Client Position: Starting—client is sitting with the testing extremity placed on a table in forearm neutral rotation, and MCP extension/ PIP and DIP flexion.

Motion—client moves the testing extremity in the direction of MCP flexion while PIP and DIP enter extension.

Therapist Position: Stabilize at the metacarpals to avoid compensation. No resistance is applied when testing in the gravity-eliminated position.

Trace

The lumbricals are too deep for palpation.

Digit: *palmar interossei*

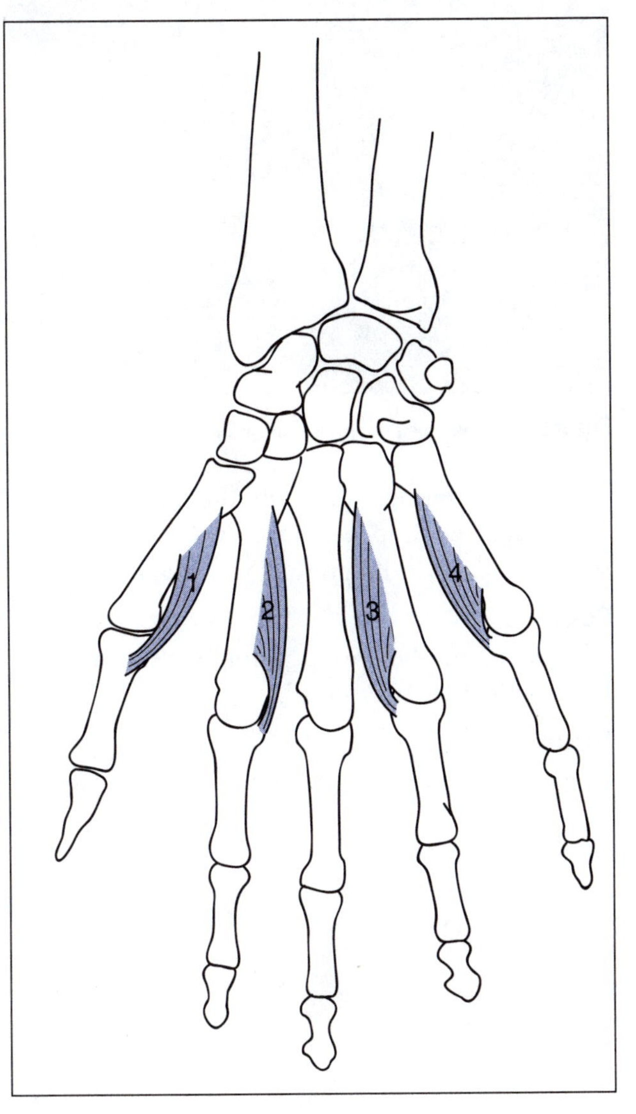

Figure 3-5-32 Palmar interossei

Origin: First interosseous—ulnar surface of second metacarpal

Second interossseous—ulnar surface of second metacarpal

Third interosseous—radial surface of fourth metacarpal

Fourth interosseous—radial surface of fifth metacarpal

Insertion: First interosseous—base of the first digit proximal phalanx, ulnar side

Second interosseous—base of the second digit proximal phalanx, ulnar side

Third interosseous—base of the fourth digit proximal phalanx, radial side

Fourth interosseous—base of the fifth digit proximal phalanx, radial side

Innervation: Ulnar nerve

Action: Digit MCP adduction

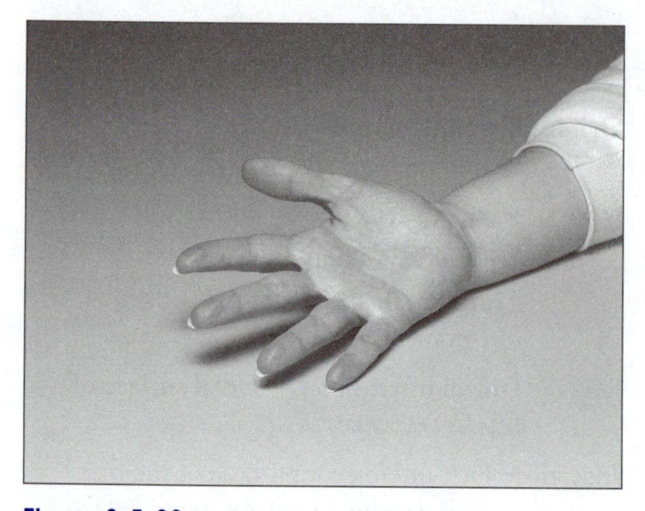

Figure 3-5-33 Start position for palmar interosseous.

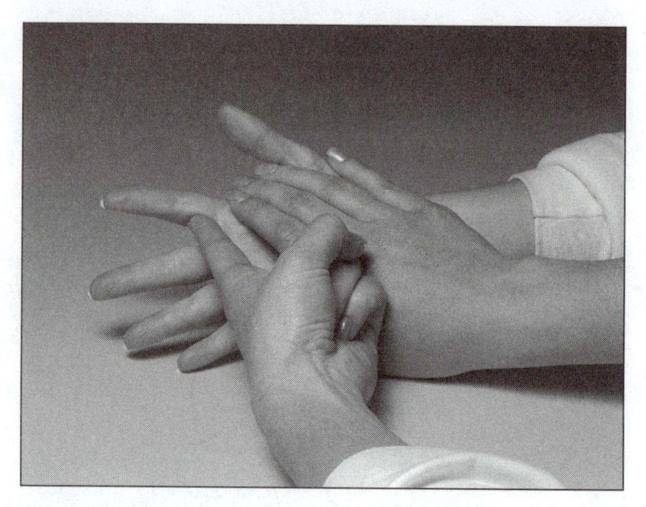

Figure 3-5-34 End position for palmar interosseous.

Normal, Good, Fair

Client Position: Starting—client is sitting with the testing extremity on a table in forearm supination and MCP abduction (Figure 3-5-33).

Motion—client moves the testing extremity in the direction of MCP adduction (Figure 3-5-34).

Therapist Position: Stabilize at the metacarpals to avoid compensation. Resistance is applied at the proximal phalanx on the ulnar side of the second digit, and the radial side of the fourth and fifth digits when testing Normal or Good strengths. No resistance is applied when testing Fair strength. The third digit does not adduct.

Poor

The client and therapist positions are the same and no resistance is applied.

Trace

The interossei are too deep for palpation.

Digit: *dorsal interossei*

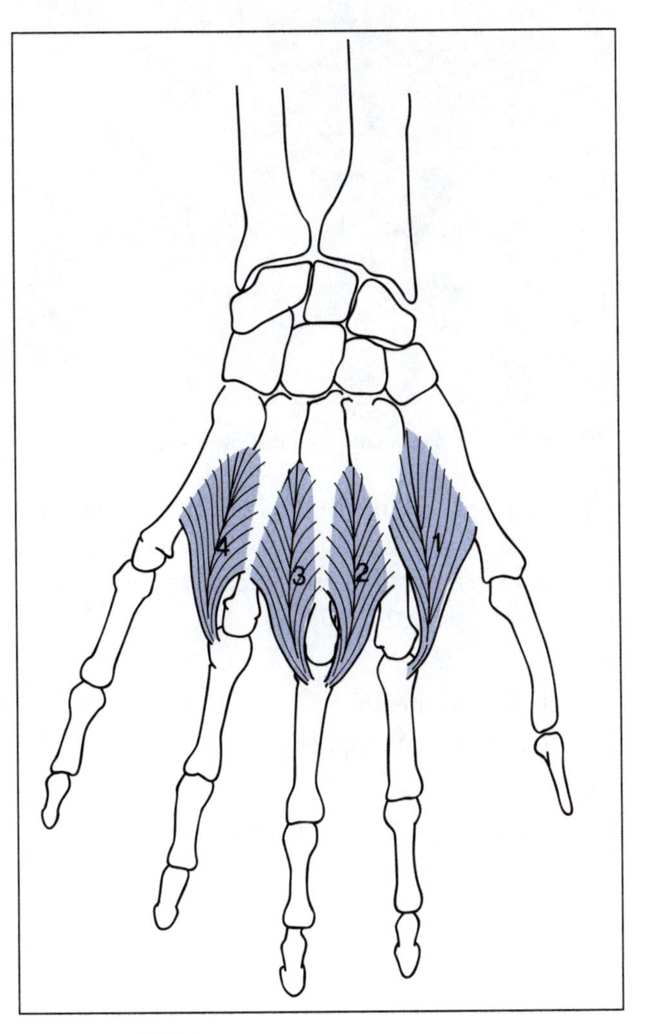

Figure 3-5-35 Dorsal interosse

Origin: Each interosseous has its origin on both of the adjacent metacarpals

Insertion: First interosseous—base of the second digit proximal phalanx, radial side

Second interosseous—base of the third digit proximal phalanx, radial side

Third interosseous—base of the third digit proximal phalanx, ulnar side

Fourth interosseous—base of the fourth digit proximal phalanx, ulnar side

Innervation: Ulnar nerve

Action: Digit MCP abduction

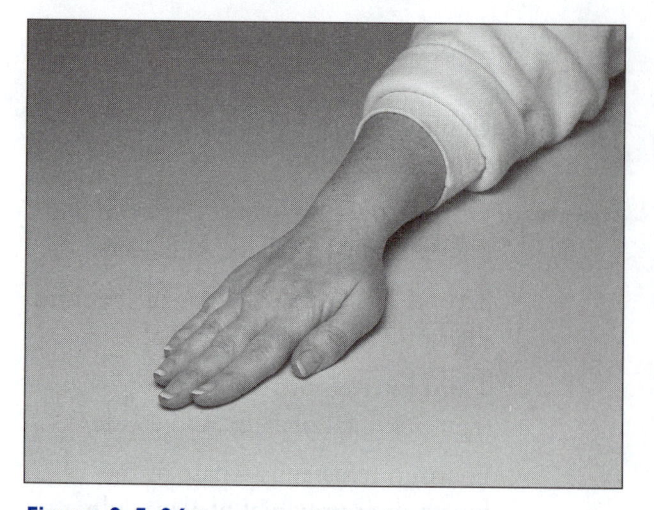

Figure 3-5-36 Start position for dorsal interosseous.

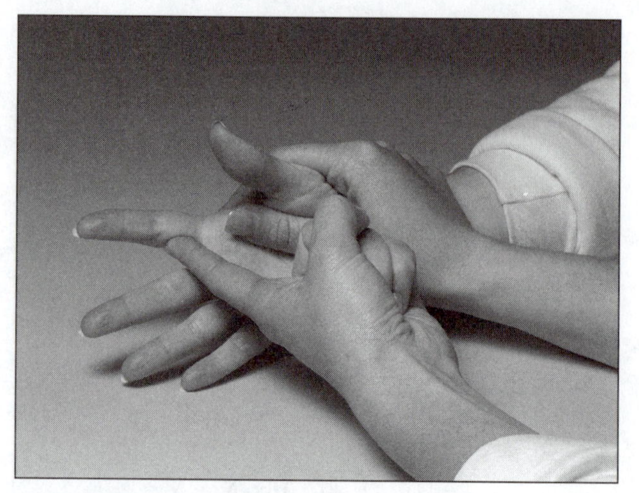

Figure 3-5-37 End position for dorsal interosseous.

Normal, Good, Fair

Client Position: Starting—client is sitting with the testing extremity on a table in forearm pronation and MCP adduction (Figure 3-5-36).

Motion—client moves the testing extremity in the direction of MCP abduction (Figure 3-5-37).

Therapist Position: Stabilize at the metacarpals to avoid compensation. Resistance is applied at the proximal phalanx on the radial side of the second digit, both the radial and ulnar side of the third digit as it abducts in two directions, the ulnar side of the fourth and fifth digits when testing Normal or Good strengths. No resistance is applied when testing Fair strength.

Poor

The client and therapist positions are the same and no resistance is applied.

Trace

The interossei are too deep for palpation.

Digit: *abductor digiti minimi* (can be tested with dorsal interossei)

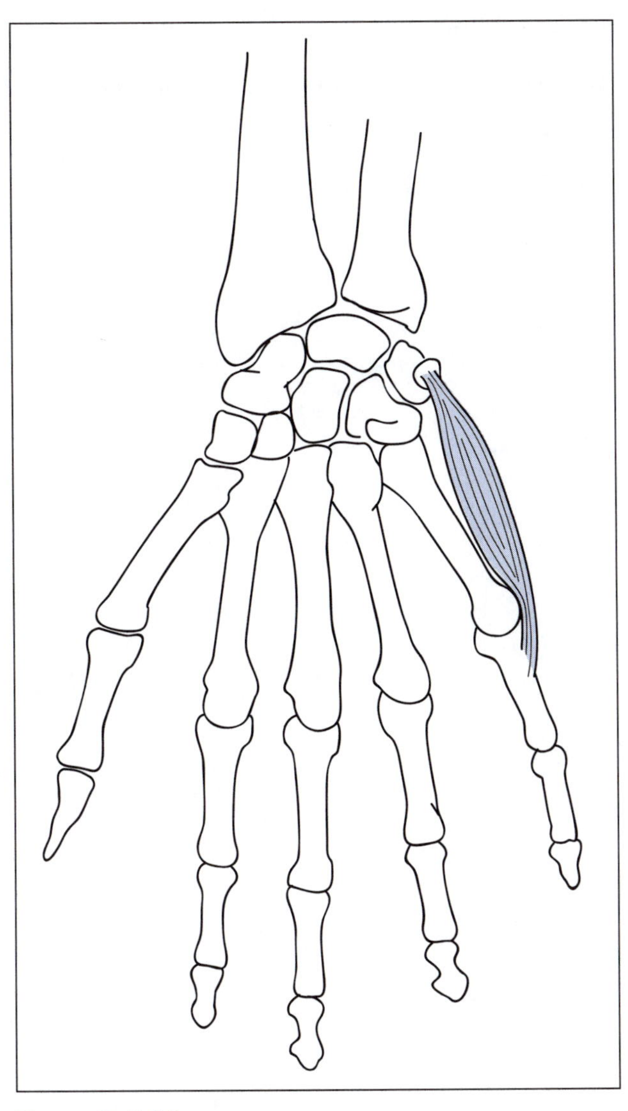

Figure 3-5-38 Abductor digiti minimi

Origin: Pisiform

Insertion: Base of the fifth digit proximal phalanx, ulnar side

Innervation: Ulnar nerve

Action: MCP abduction of the fifth digit

Normal, Good, Fair, & Poor

The testing positions are the same as for the dorsal interosseous.

Trace

The abductor digiti minimi is palpated on the lateral aspect of the fifth digit metacarpal.

Digit: *opponens digiti minimi*

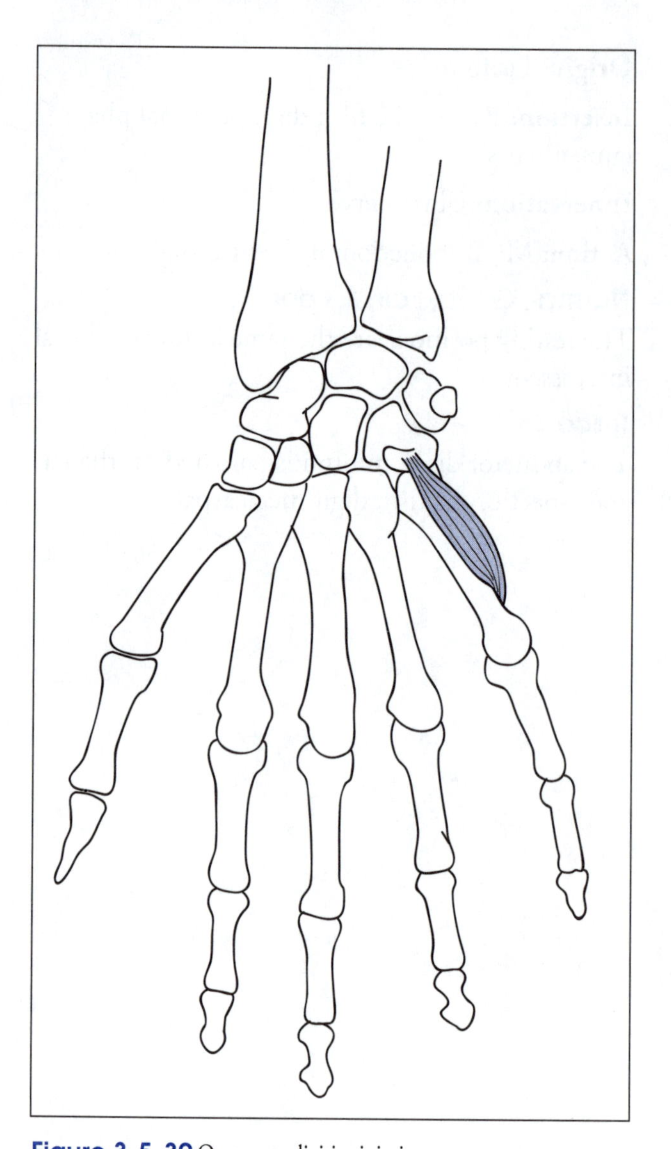

Figure 3-5-39 Opponens digiti minimi

Origin: Hamate

Insertion: Fifth digit metacarpal, ulnar side

Innervation: Ulnar nerve

Action: Fifth digit opposition

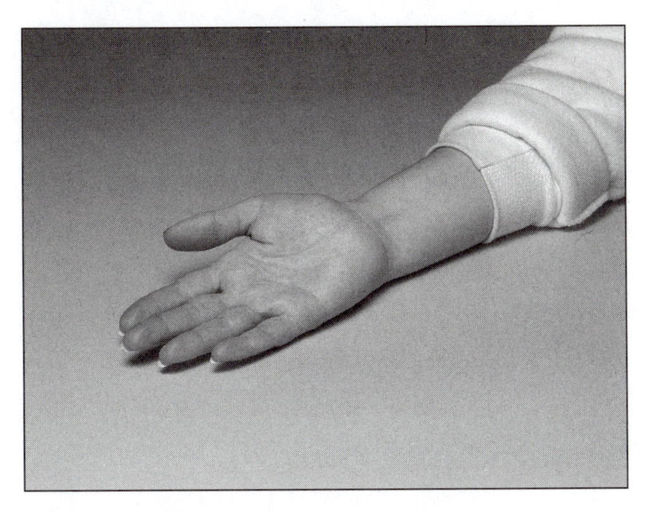

Figure 3-5-40 Start position for opponens digiti minimi.

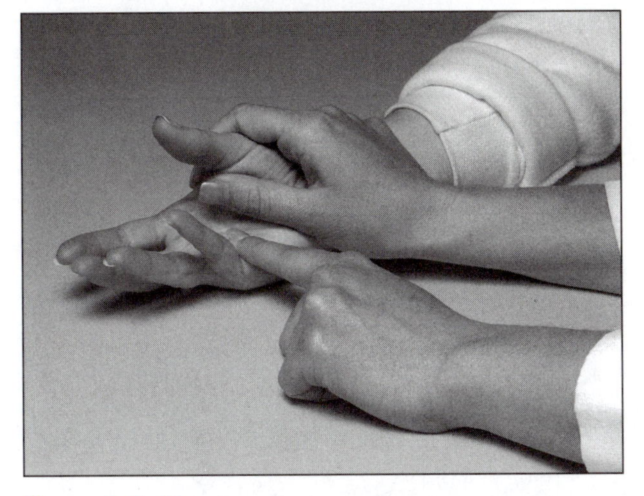

Figure 3-5-41 End position for opponens digiti minimi.

Normal, Good, Fair

Client Position: Starting—client is sitting with the testing extremity on a table in forearm supination (Figure 3-5-40).

Motion—Client moves the testing extremity in the direction of opposition (flexion and adduction) (Figure 3-5-41).

Therapist Position: Stabilize at the first metacarpal. Resistance is applied at the fifth metacarpal in the opposite direction of opposition (extension and abduction) when testing Normal or Good strengths. No resistance is applied when testing Fair strength.

Poor

The client and therapist positions are the same and no resistance is applied. A grade of poor is given when the client is unable to move through the complete ROM.

Trace

Opponens digiti minimi is palpated on the hypothenar eminence.

Thumb: *opponens pollicis*

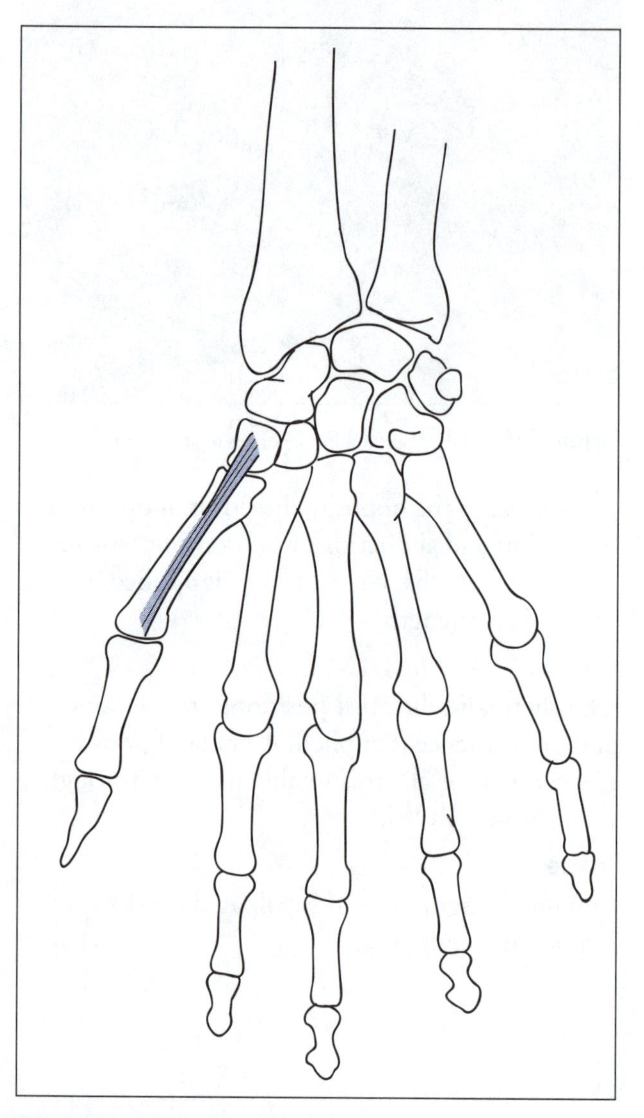

Figure 3-5-42 Opponens pollicis

Origin: Trapezium

Insertion: First digit metacarpal, radial side

Innervation: Median nerve

Action: First digit opposition

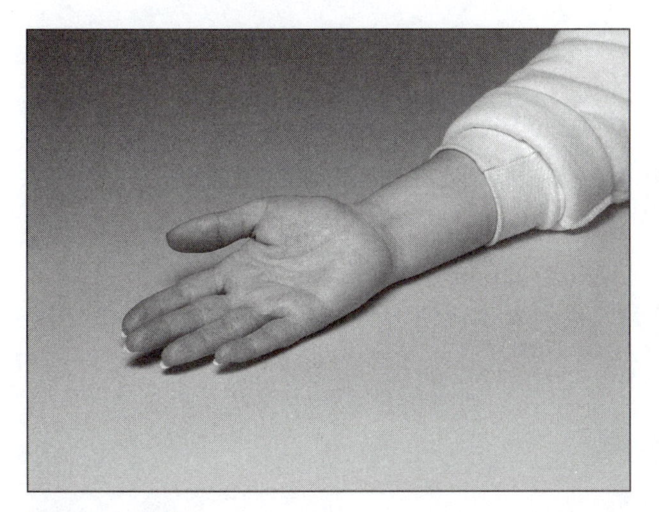

Figure 3-5-43 Start position for opponens pollicis.

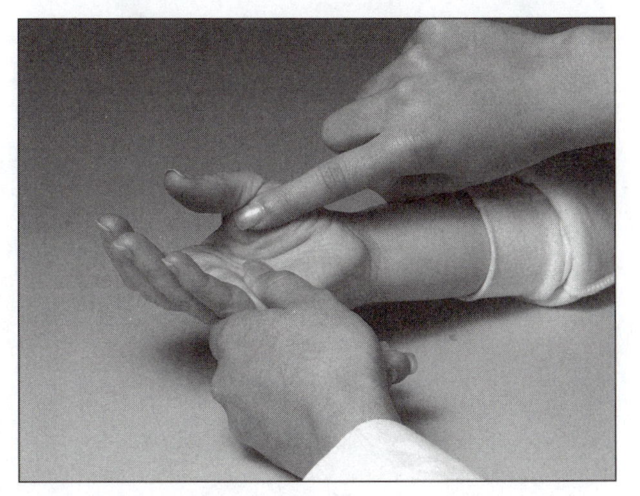

Figure 3-5-44 End position for opponens pollicis.

Normal, Good, Fair

Client Position: Starting—client is sitting with the testing extremity placed on the table in forearm supination (Figure 3-5-43).

Motion—client moves the testing extremity in the direction of thumb opposition (CMC flexion and abduction) (Figure 3-5-44).

Therapist Position: Stabilize at the fifth metacarpal to avoid compensation. Resistance is applied at the first metacarpal in the opposite direction from opposition (CMC extension and adduction) when testing Normal or Good strengths. No resistance is applied when testing Fair strength.

Poor

The testing positions are the same as above. A grade of poor is given when the client can move through only a small portion of the range in this position.

Trace

Opponens pollicis is palpated in the thenar eminence, lateral to the abductor pollicis.

Thumb: *flexor pollicis brevis*

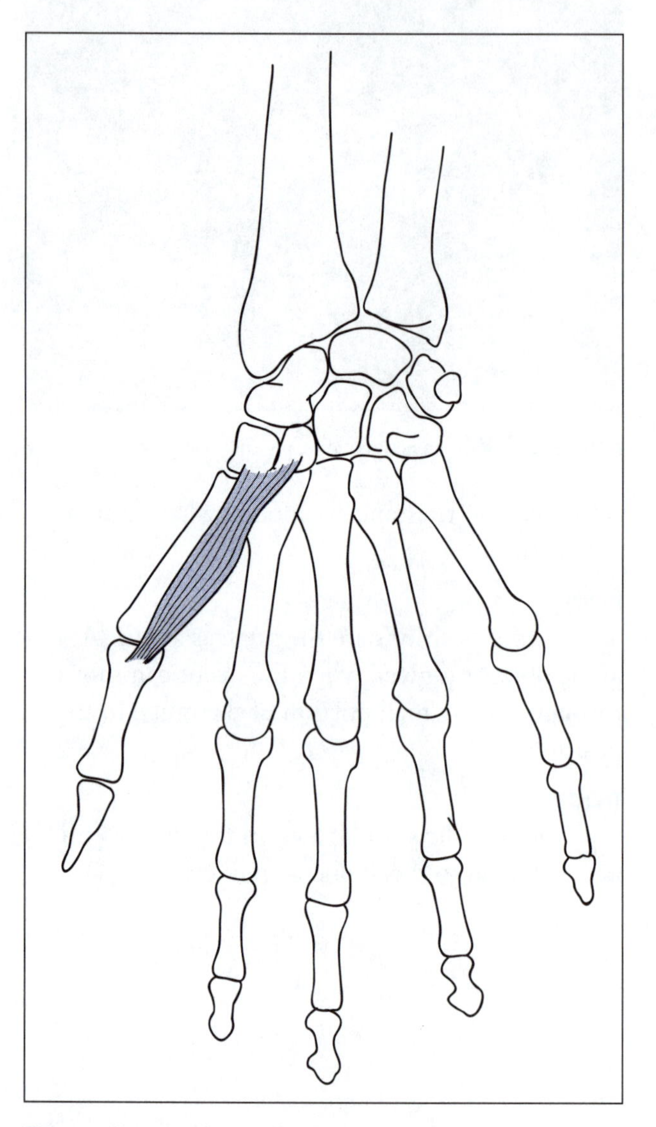

Figure 3-5-45 Flexor pollicis brevis

Origin: Trapezium, trapezoid

Insertion: Base of the first digit proximal phalanx

Innervation: Median and ulnar nerves

Action: Thumb MCP flexion, and assist with CMC flexion

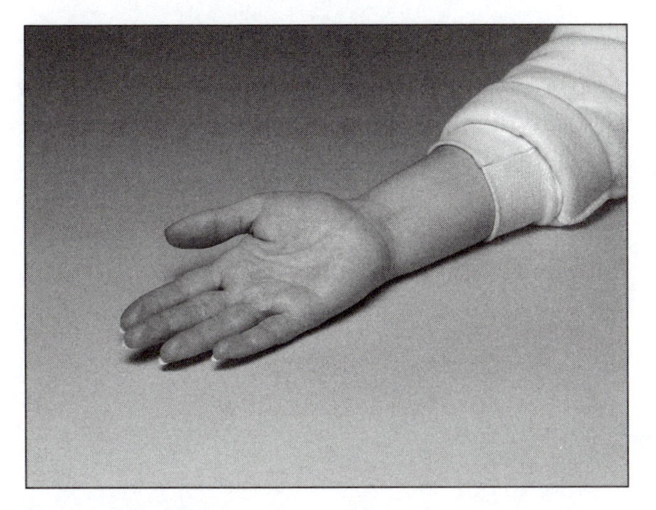

Figure 3-5-46 Start position for flexor pollicis brevis.

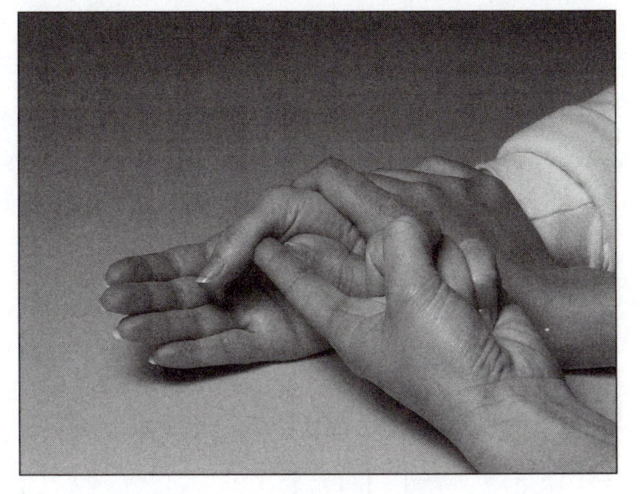

Figure 3-5-47 End position for flexor pollicis brevis.

Normal, Good, Fair

Client Position: Starting—client is sitting with the testing extremity placed on the table in forearm supination (Figure 3-5-46).

Motion—client moves the testing extremity in the direction of thumb MCP flexion (Figure 3-5-47).

Therapist Position: Stabilize at the metacarpal to eliminate any compensation. Resistance is applied at the proximal phalanx of the thumb in the direction of MCP extension when testing Normal or Good strengths. No resistance is applied when testing Fair strength.

Poor

The testing positions are the same as above. A grade of poor is given when the client can move the testing extremity through only a small portion of the range in this position.

Trace

Flexor pollicis brevis is palpated over the first metacarpal, palmar surface.

Thumb: *flexor pollicis longus*

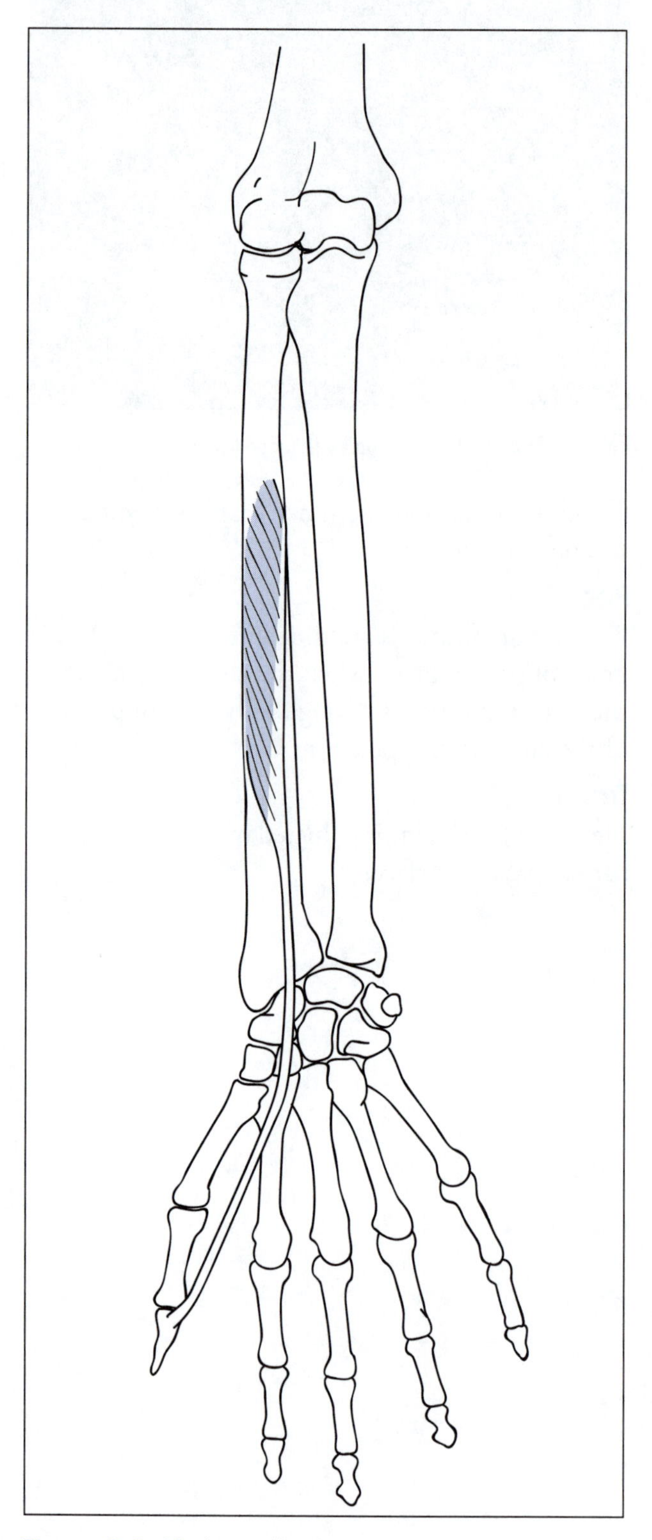

Figure 3-5-48 Flexor pollicis longus

Origin: Anterior radius

Insertion: Base of the first digit distal phalanx

Innervation: Median nerve

Action: Thumb IP flexion

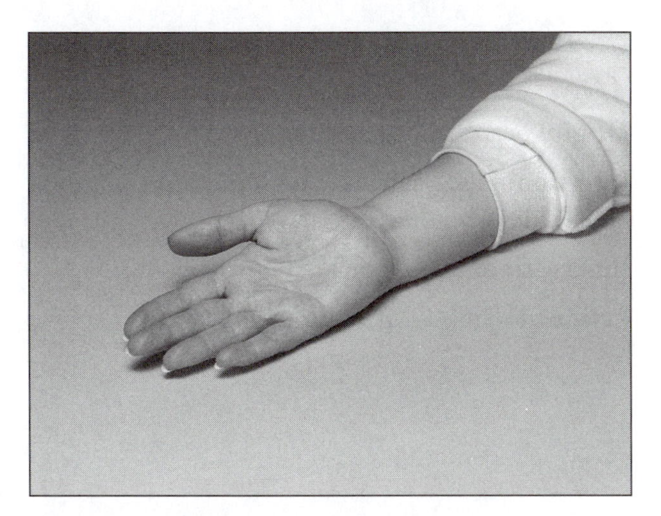

Figure 3-5-49 Start position for flexor pollicis longus.

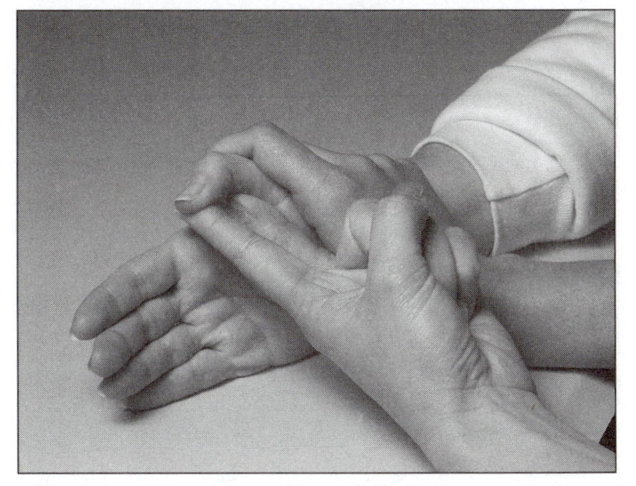

Figure 3-5-50 End position for flexor pollicis longus.

Normal, Good, Fair

Client Position: Starting—client is sitting with the testing extremity placed on the table in forearm supination (Figure 3-5-49).

Motion—client moves the testing extremity in the direction of thumb IP flexion while maintaining thumb MCP extension (Figure 3-5-50).

Therapist Position: Stabilize at the proximal phalanx to eliminate any compensation. Resistance is applied at the distal phalanx of the thumb in the direction of IP extension when testing Normal or Good strengths. No resistance is applied when testing Fair strength.

Poor

The testing positions are the same as above. A grade of poor is given when the client can move the testing extremity through only a small portion of the range in this position.

Trace

Flexor pollicis brevis tendon is palpated over the first proximal phalanx, palmar surface.

Thumb: *abductor pollicis brevis*

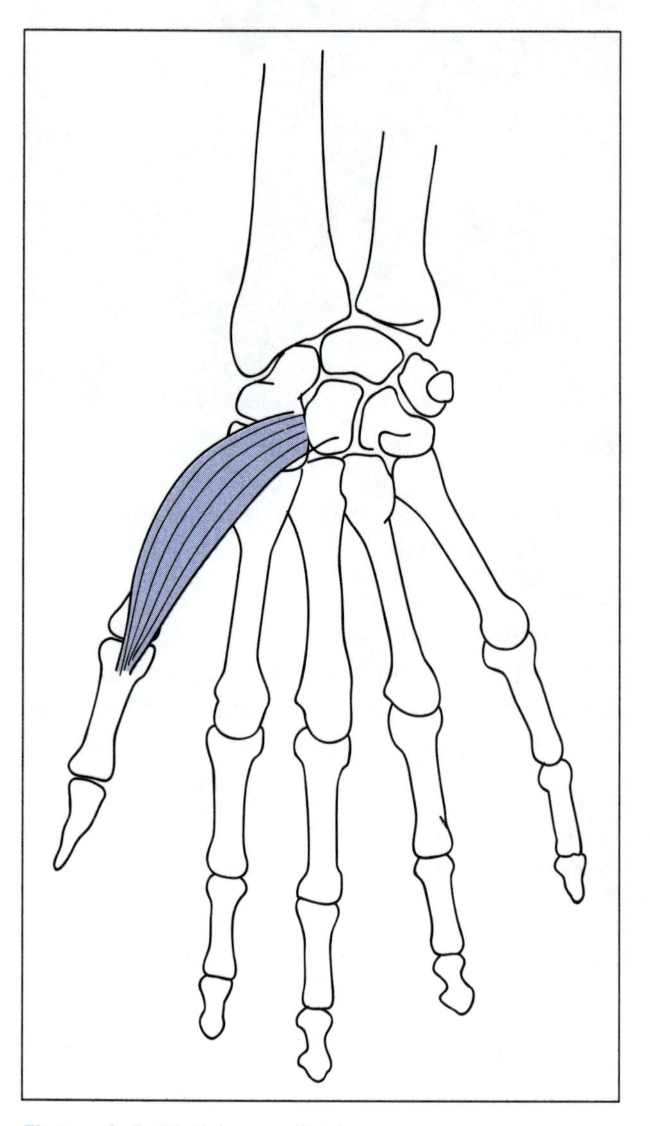

Figure 3-5-51 Abductor pollicis brevis

Origin: Scaphoid, trapezium

Insertion: Base of the first digit proximal phalanx, radial side

Innervation: Median nerve

Action: Thumb CMC abduction

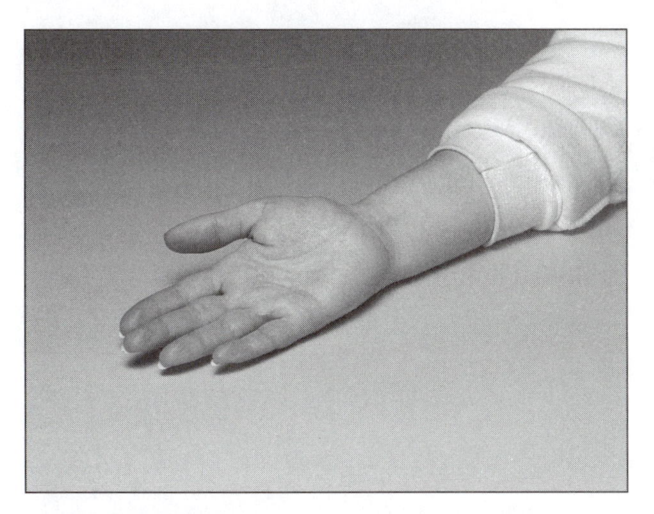

Figure 3-5-52 Start position for abductor pollicis brevis.

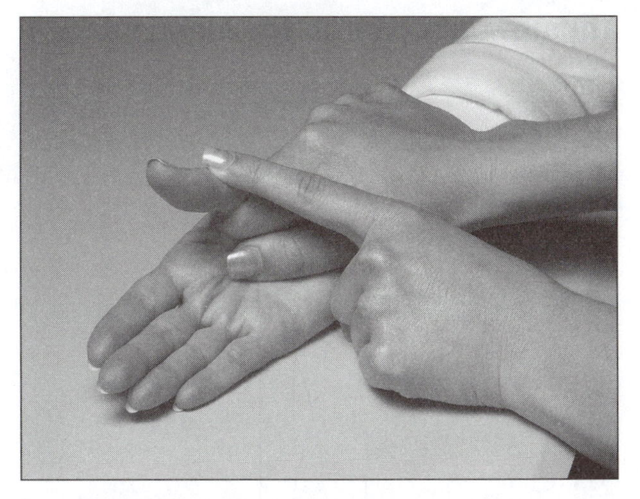

Figure 3-5-53 End position for abductor pollicis brevis.

Normal, Good, Fair

Client Position: Starting—client is sitting with the testing extremity placed on the table in forearm supination (Figure 3-5-52).

Motion—client moves the testing extremity in the direction of thumb CMC abduction (Figure 3-5-53).

Therapist Position: Stabilize the hand to eliminate any compensation. Resistance is applied at the proximal phalanx of the thumb in the direction of CMC adduction when testing Normal or Good strengths. No resistance is applied when testing Fair strength.

Poor

The testing positions are the same as above. A grade of poor is given when the client can move the testing extremity through only a small portion of the range in this position.

Trace

Abductor pollicis brevis is palpated over the first digit metacarpal, lateral surface.

Thumb: *abductor pollicis longus*

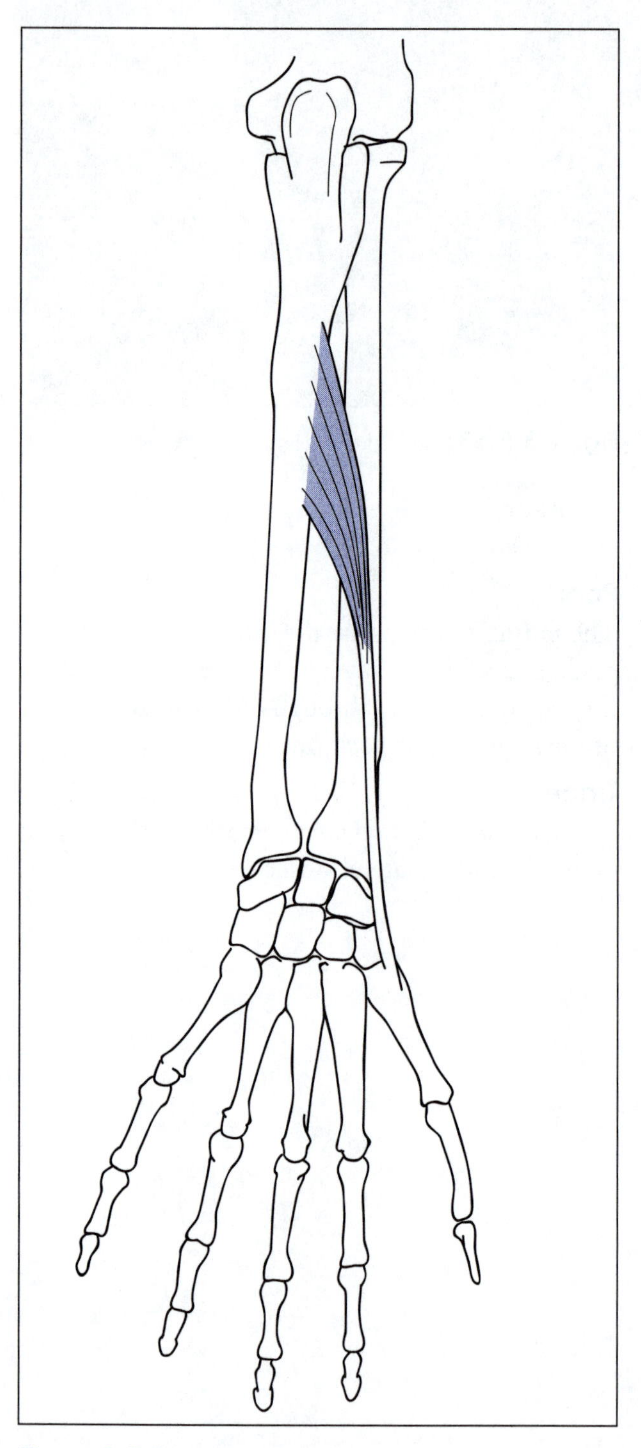

Figure 3-5-54 Abductor pollicis longus

Origin: Posterior, middle radius and ulna

Insertion: Base of the first digit metacarpal

Innervation: Radial nerve

Action: Thumb CMC abduction

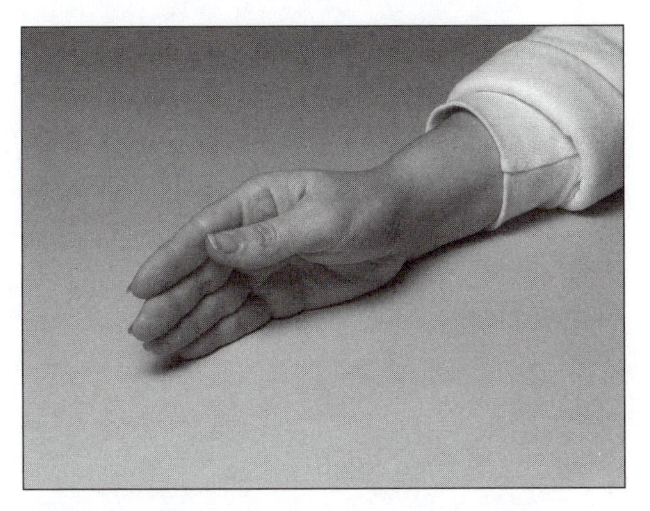

Figure 3-5-55 Start position for abductor pollicis longus.

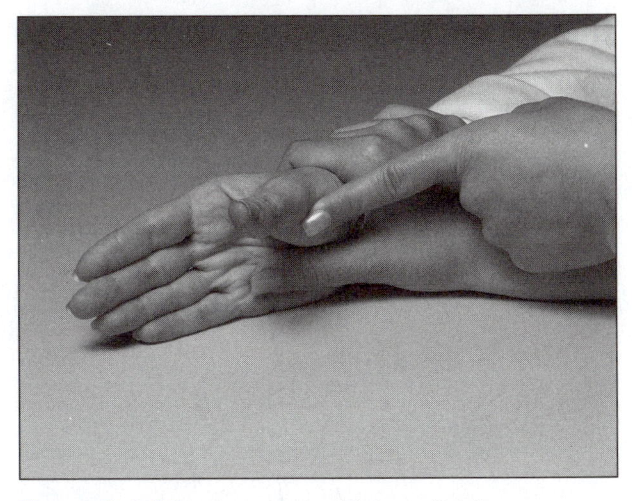

Figure 3-5-56 End position for abductor pollicis longus.

Normal, Good, Fair

Client Position: Starting—client is sitting with the testing extremity placed on the table with the forearm in neutral (Figure 3-5-55).

Motion—client moves the testing extremity in the direction of thumb CMC abduction (Figure 3-5-56).

Therapist Position: Stabilize at the wrist to eliminate any compensation. Resistance is applied at the thumb metacarpal in the direction of CMC adduction when testing Normal or Good strengths. No resistance is applied when testing Fair strength.

Poor

The testing positions are the same as above. A grade of poor is given when the client can move the testing extremity through only a small portion of the range in this position.

Trace

Abductor pollicis longus tendon is palpated at the base of the first digit metacarpal, lateral surface.

Thumb: *adductor pollicis*

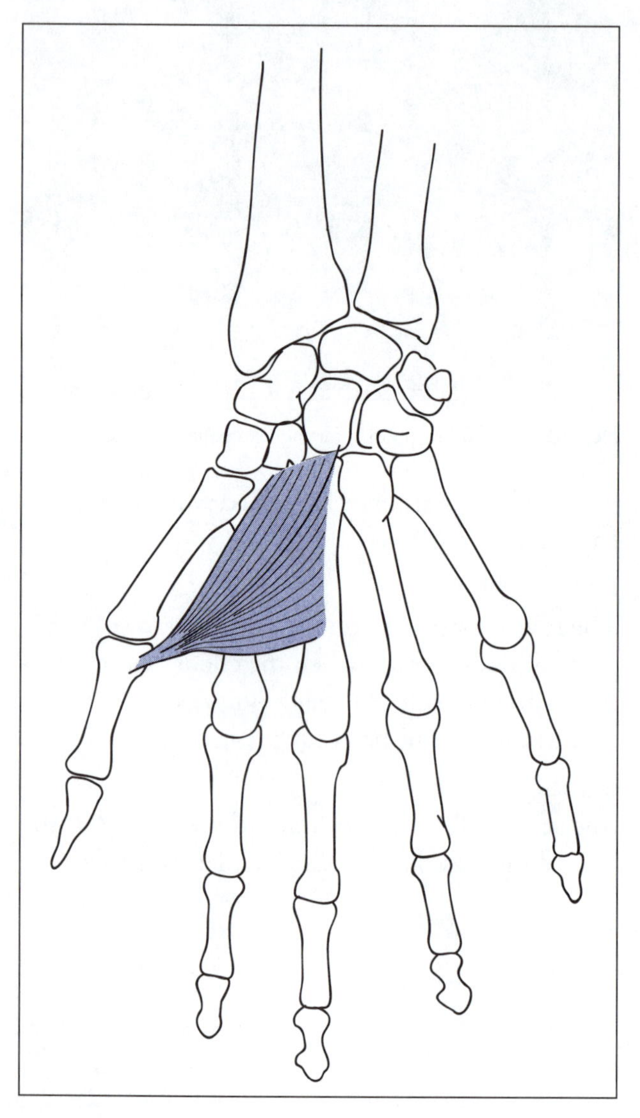

Figure 3-5-57 Adductor pollicis

Origin: Third digit metacarpal, capitate, traezoid

Insertion: Base of the first digit proximal phalanx, ulnar side

Innervation: Ulnar nerve

Action: Thumb CMC adduction

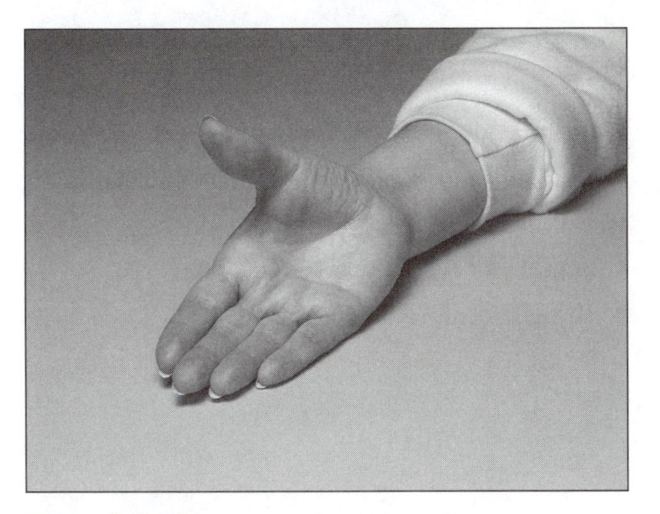

Figure 3-5-58 Start position for adductor pollicis.

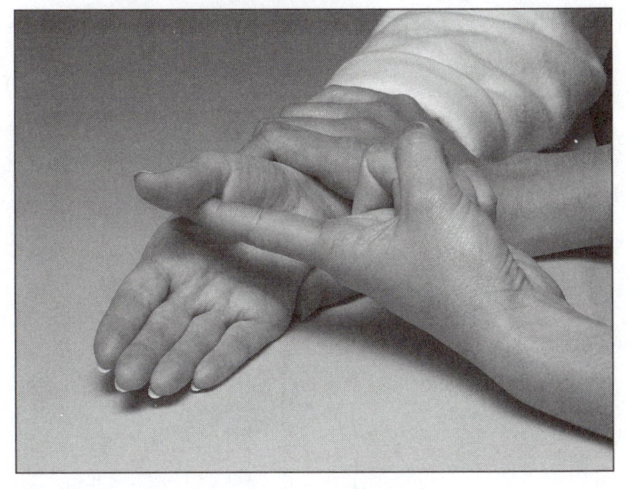

Figure 3-5-59 End position for adductor pollicis.

Normal, Good, Fair

Client Position: Starting—client is sitting with the testing extremity placed on the table in forearm supination. Thumb is placed in CMC abduction (Figure 3-5-58).

Motion—client moves the testing extremity in the direction of thumb CMC adduction (Figure 3-5-59).

Therapist Position: Stabilize at the wrist to eliminate any compensation. Resistance is applied at the proximal phalanx of the thumb in the direction of CMC abduction when testing Normal or Good strengths. No resistance is applied when testing Fair strength.

Poor

The testing positions are the same as above. A grade of poor is given when the client can move the testing extremity through only a small portion of the range in this position.

Trace

Adductor pollicis is palpated between the first and second metacarpals, palmar surface.

Thumb: *extensor pollicis longus*

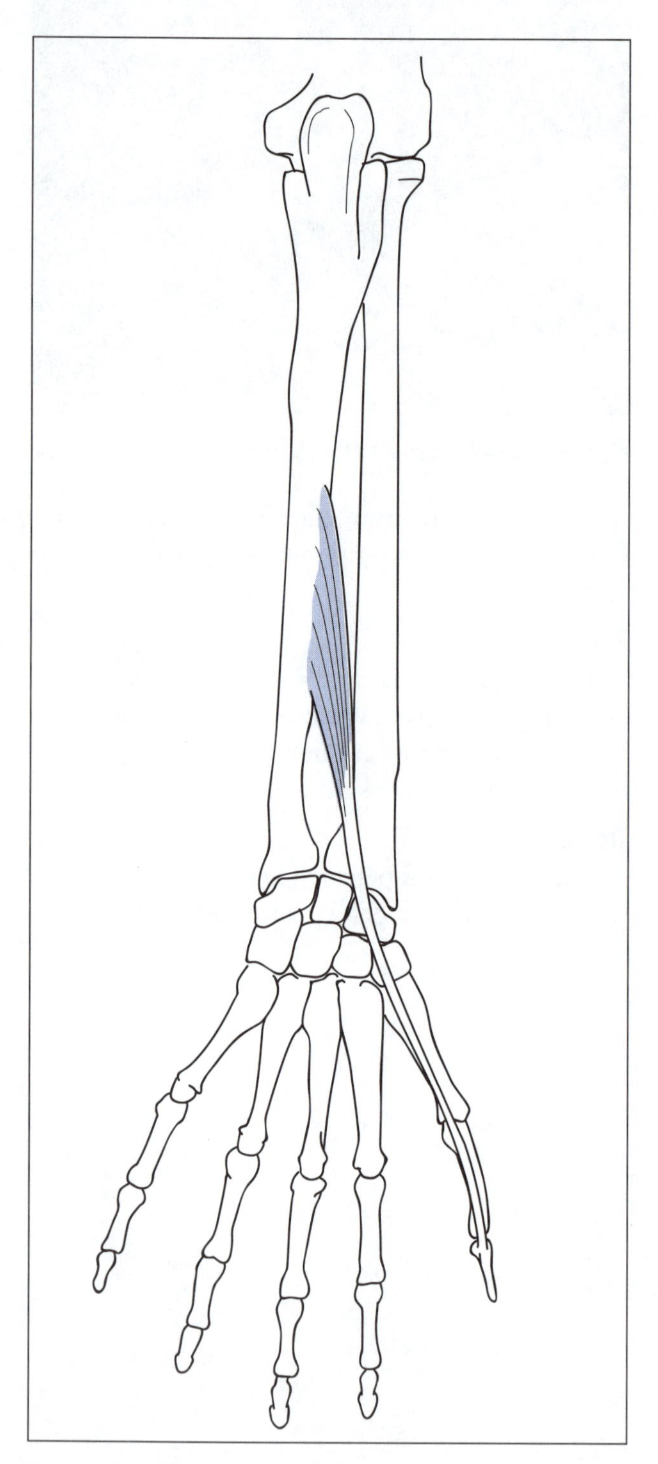

Figure 3-5-60 Extensor pollicis longus

Origin: Middle, posterior ulna

Insertion: Base of the first digit distal phalanx, dorsal surface

Innervation: Radial nerve

Action: Thumb IP extension

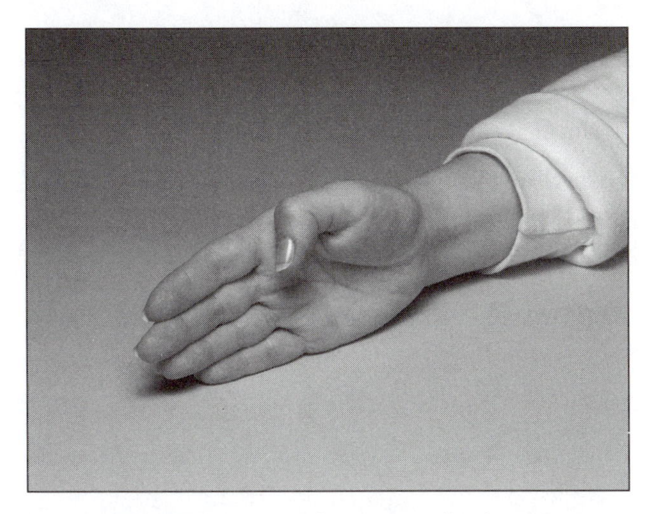

Figure 3-5-61 Start position for extensor pollicis longus.

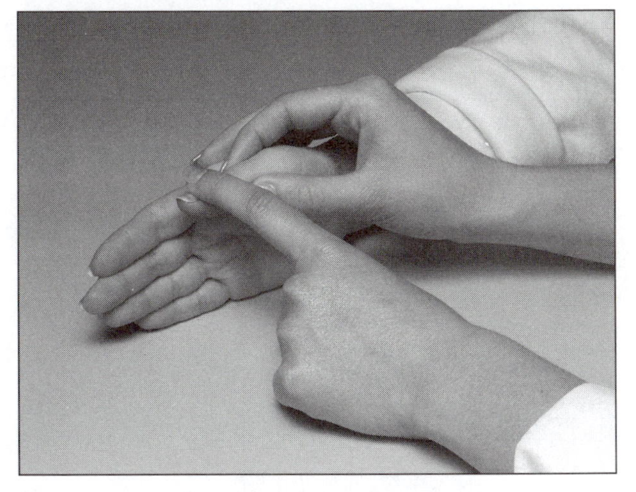

Figure 3-5-62 End position for extensor pollicis longus.

Normal, Good, Fair

Client Position: Starting—client is sitting with the testing extremity placed on the table with the forearm in neutral and thumb IP flexed (Figure 3-5-61).

Motion—client moves the testing extremity in the direction of thumb IP extension (Figure 3-5-62).

Therapist Position: Stabilize at the thumb proximal phalanx to eliminate any compensation. Resistance is applied at the distal phalanx of the thumb in the direction of thumb IP flexion when testing Normal or Good strengths. No resistance is applied when testing Fair strength.

Poor

The testing positions are the same as above. A grade of poor is given when the client can move the testing extremity through only a small portion of the range in this position.

Trace

Extensor pollicis longus tendon is palpated over the first proximal phalanx, dorsal surface.

Thumb: *extensor pollicis brevis*

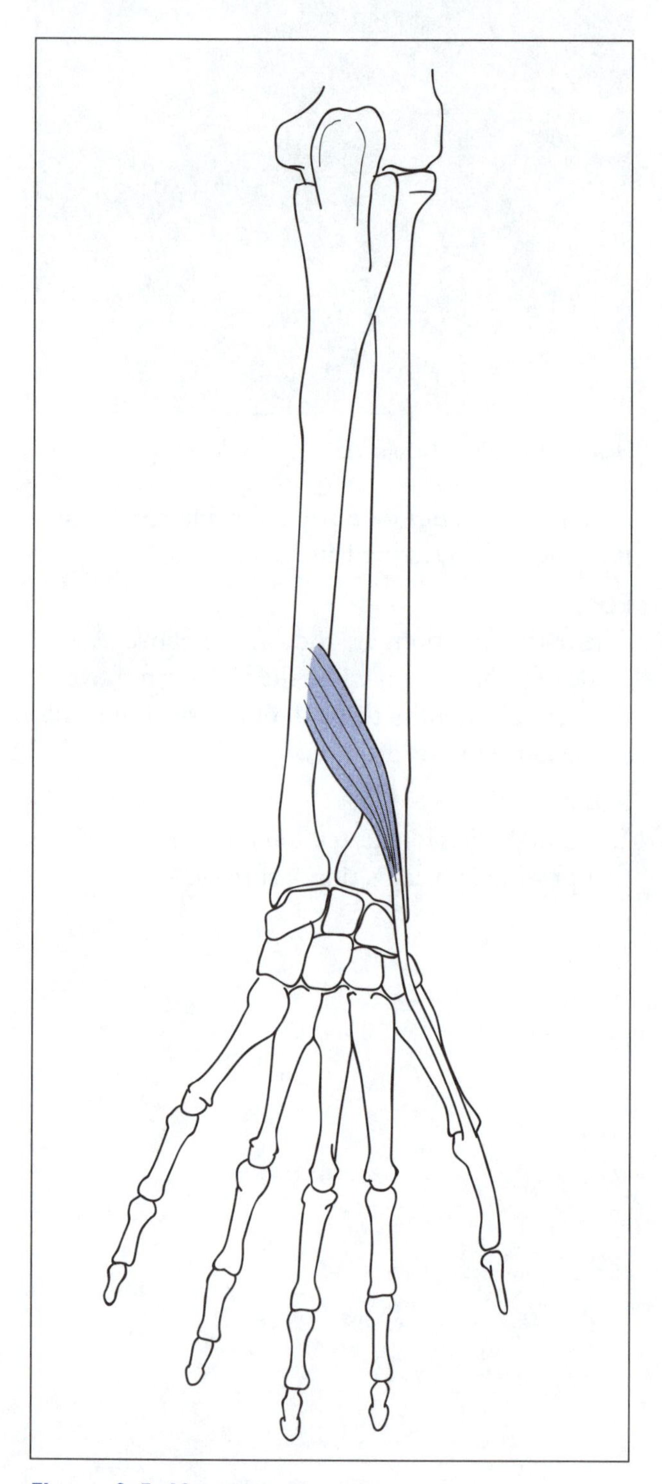

Figure 3-5-63 Extensor pollicis brevis

Origin: Posterior radius and ulna

Insertion: Base of the first digit proximal phalanx, dorsal surface

Innervation: Radial nerve

Action: MCP and assists CMC extension

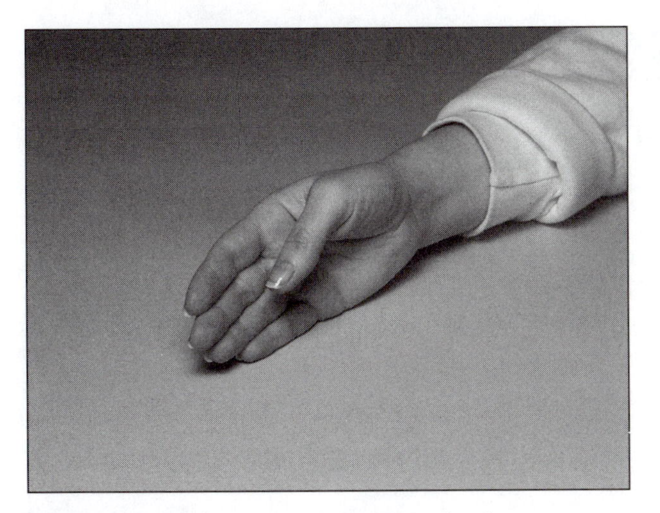

Figure 3-5-64 Start position for extensor pollicis brevis.

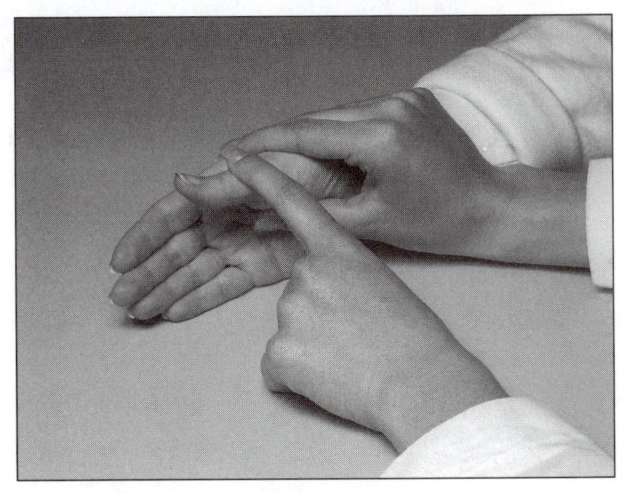

Figure 3-5-65 End position for extensor pollicis brevis.

Normal, Good, Fair

Client Position: Starting—client is sitting with the testing extremity placed on the table with the forearm in neutral and thumb in slight MCP flexion (Figure 3-5-64).

Motion—client moves the testing extremity in the direction of thumb MCP extension (Figure 3-5-65).

Therapist Position: Stabilize at the thumb metacarpal to eliminate any compensation. Resistance is applied at the proximal phalanx of the thumb in the direction of thumb MCP flexion when testing Normal or Good strengths. No resistance is applied when testing Fair strength.

Poor

The testing positions are the same as above. A grade of poor is given when the client can move the testing extremity through only a small portion of the range in this position.

Trace

Extensor pollicis brevis tendon is palpated at the base of the first metacarpal, dorsal surface.

SECTION 3-6: Isolated Manual Muscle Testing of the Hip and Knee

Hip: *iliacus* and *psoas major* (*Iliacus* and *psoas major* may be referred to as the *iliopsoas.*) (tested together)

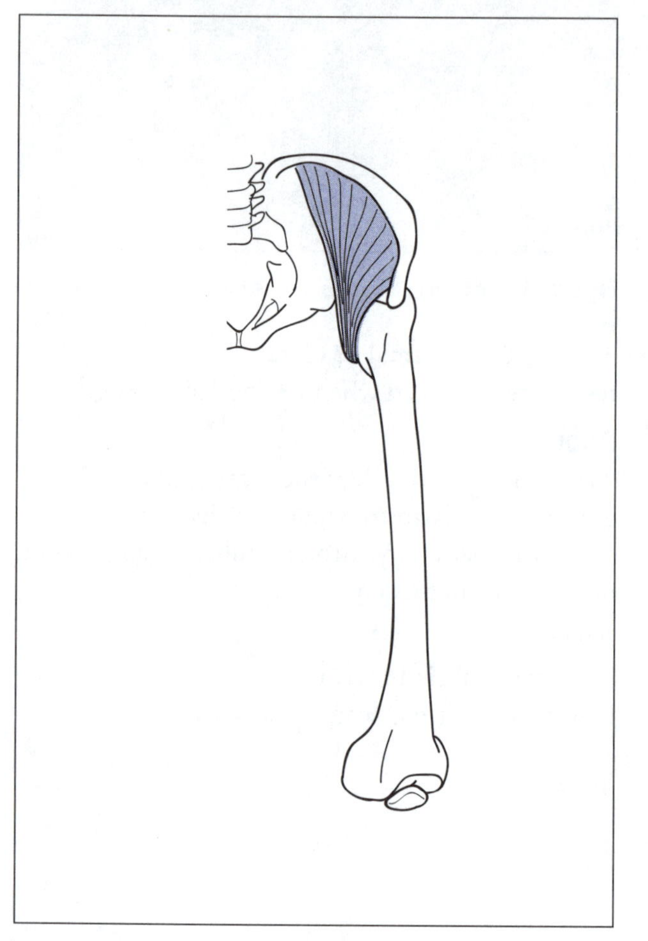

Figure 3-6-1 Iliacus

Iliacus

Origin: Superior 2/3 of ilium, anterior iliac crest

Insertion: Lesser trochanter of femur

Innervation: Femoral nerve

Action: Hip flexion

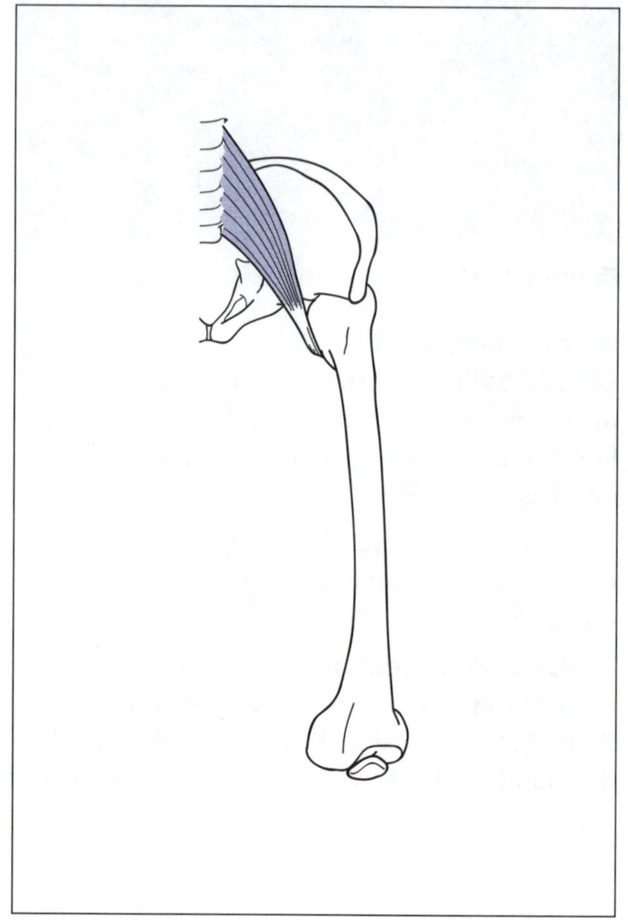

Figure 3-6-2 Psoas major

Psoas major

Origin: Transverse processes of L1–L5, vertebral bodies of T12–L5

Insertion: Lesser trochanter of femur

Innervation: Lumbar plexus L2–L4

Action: Hip flexion

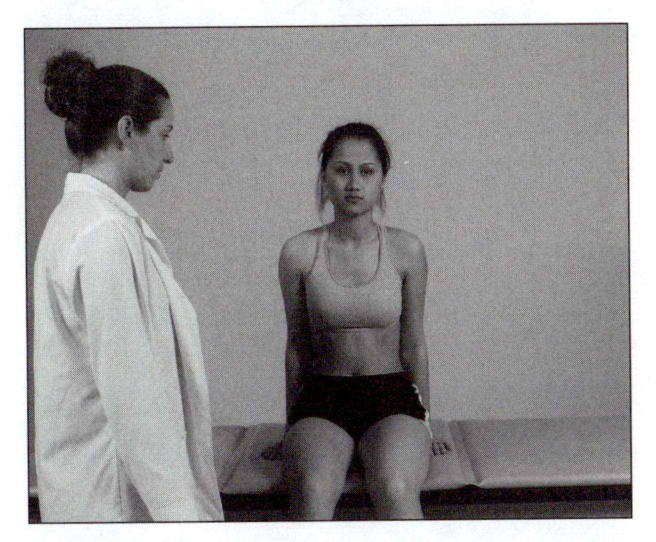

Figure 3-6-3 Start position for iliacus and psoas major (iliopsoas).

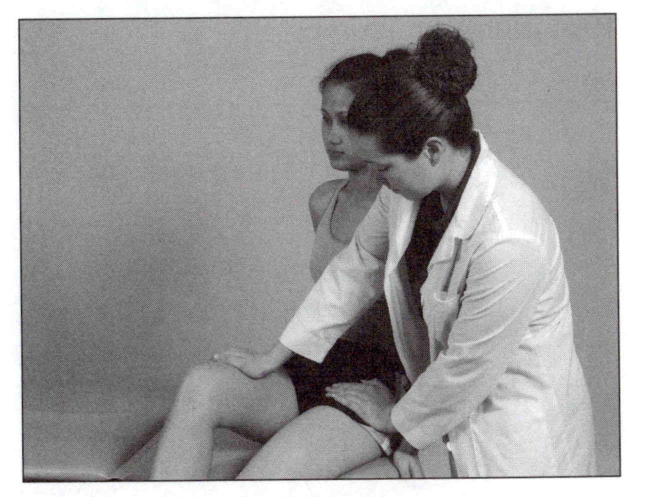

Figure 3-6-4 End position for iliacus and psoas major (iliopsoas).

Normal, Good, Fair

Client Position: Starting—client is sitting with the testing extremity in 90 degrees of hip flexion, neutral hip rotation, and the lower leg over the edge of the testing surface. The knee is flexed and the foot is unsupported (Figure 3-6-3).

Motion—client moves the testing extremity in the direction of hip flexion while allowing the knee to follow into flexion (Figure 3-6-4).

Therapist Position: Stabilize at the contralateral iliac crest of the pelvis. Resistance is applied over the anterior aspect of the thigh proximal to the knee in the direction of hip extension when testing Normal or Good strengths. No resistance is applied when testing Fair strength.

Poor

Client Position: Starting—client is lying on nontest side. Client holds nontest extremity in maximal hip and knee flexion. The testing extremity is in hip extension and knee flexion.

Motion—client moves the testing extremity into maximal hip flexion.

Therapist Position: While standing behind the client, stabilize the side-lying position and the pelvis. Therapist supports the testing extremity to eliminate gravity without assisting the motion. No resistance is applied in the gravity-eliminated position.

Trace

The iliopsoas cannot be palpated.

Hip: *gluteus maximus*

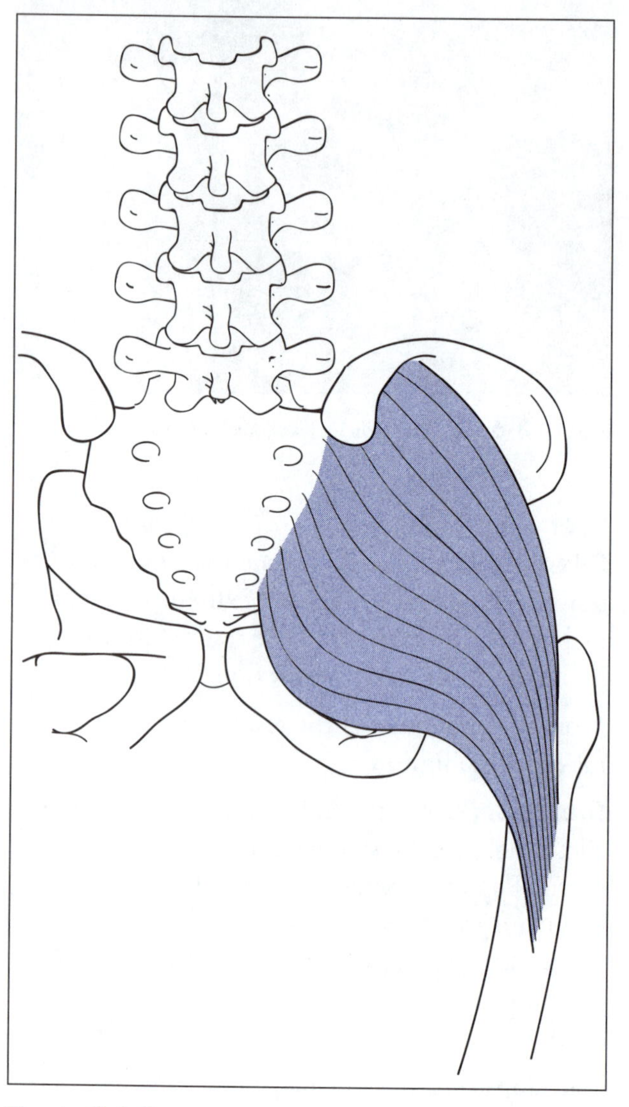

Figure 3-6-5 Gluteus maximus

Origin: Lateral surface of the ilium at posterior gluteal line, posterior surface of sacrum, posterior coccyx, and sacrotuberous ligaments

Insertion: Iliotibial tract of fascia latae and gluteal tuberosity of femur

Innervation: Inferior gluteal nerve

Action: Hip extension

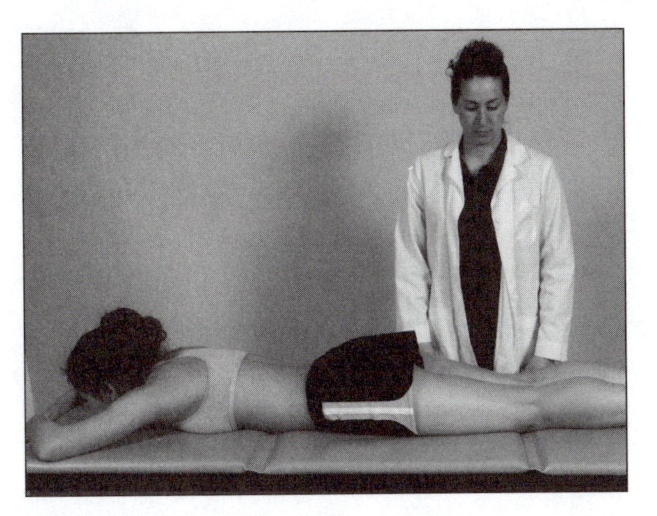

Figure 3-6-6 Start position for gluteus maximus.

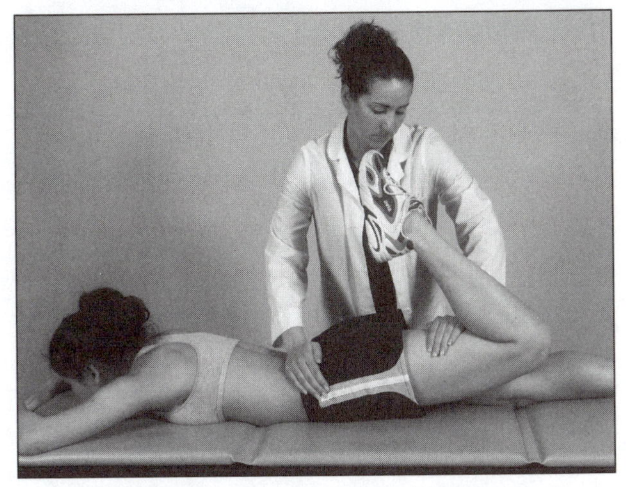

Figure 3-6-7 End position for gluteus maximus.

Normal, Good, Fair

Client Position: Starting—client is prone with both legs extended and resting on testing surface. Client is asked to hold onto edge of testing surface as resistance is applied (Figure 3-6-6).

Motion—client moves the testing extremity in the direction of hip extension while knee remains flexed (Figure 3-6-7).

Therapist Position: Stabilize at the pelvis. Resistance is applied over the posterior aspect of the thigh proximal to the knee in the direction of flexion when testing Normal or Good strengths. No resistance is applied when testing Fair strength.

Poor

Client Position: Starting—client is lying on non-test side. The client holds the nontest extremity in maximal hip and knee flexion. Testing hip is in neutral and knee is flexed.

Motion—client moves the testing extremity into maximal hip extension.

Therapist Position: While standing behind the client, stabilize the side-lying position and the pelvis. Therapist supports the testing extremity to eliminate gravity without assisting the motion. No resistance is applied in the gravity-eliminated position.

Trace

The gluteus maximus is palpated medial to its insertion on the gluteal tuberosity.

Alternate Position

If hip flexors are tight, client may stand with trunk flexed and trunk in prone position, resting on testing surface.

Hip: *sartorius*

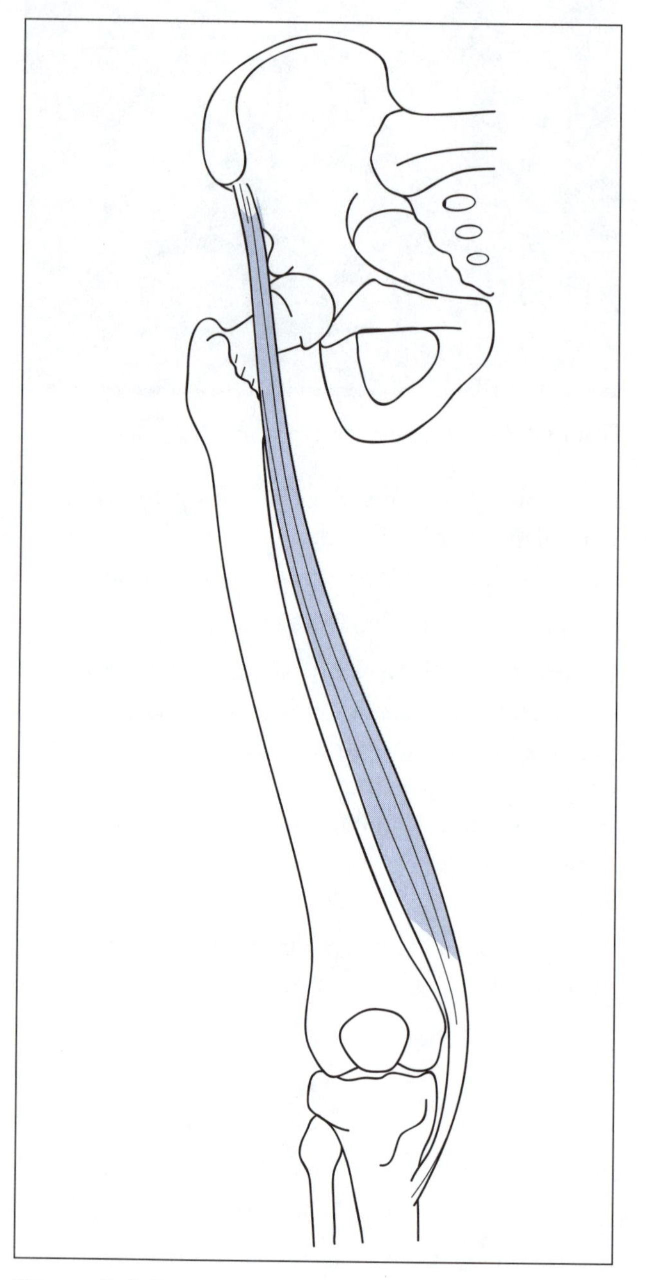

Figure 3-6-8 Sartorius

Origin: Anterior superior iliac spine (ASIS)

Insertion: Proximal aspect of the medial surface of tibia

Innervation: Femoral nerve

Action: Hip flexion, hip abduction, and hip external rotation

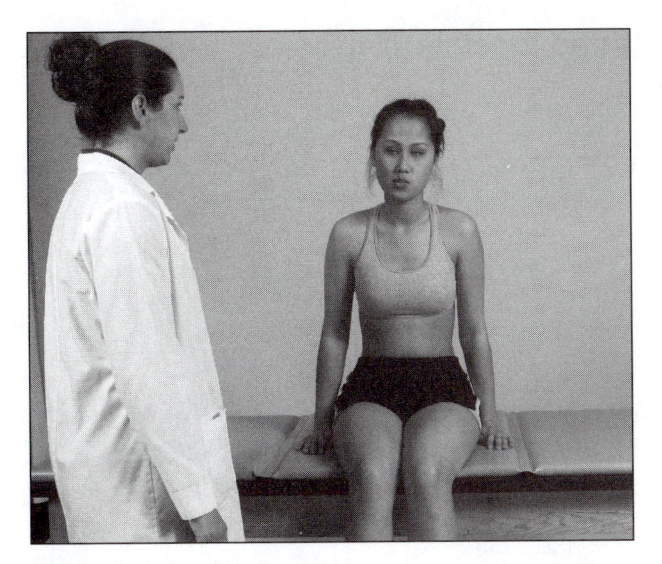

Figure 3-6-9 Start position for sartorius.

Normal, Good, Fair

Client Position: Starting—client is sitting with knee flexed and over edge of testing surface (Figure 3-6-9).

Motion—client moves testing extremity into maximal hip flexion, abduction, and external rotation while the knee remains flexed (Figure 3-6-10).

Therapist Position: Resistance is applied over the anterolateral aspect of the thigh proximal to the knee and the posterior aspect of the lower leg proximal to the ankle in the direction of hip extension, adduction, and internal rotation when testing Normal or Good strengths. No resistance is applied when testing Fair strength.

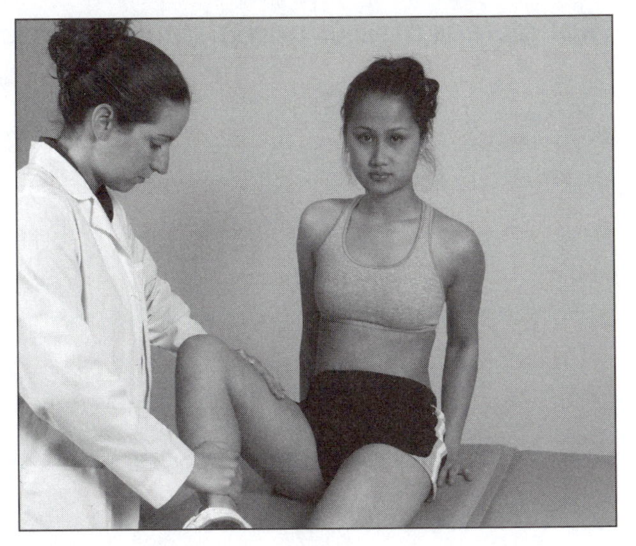

Figure 3-6-10 End position for sartorius.

Poor

Client Position: Starting—client is supine with both legs extended and resting on testing surface.

Motion—client moves the testing extremity in the direction of hip flexion, abduction, and external rotation while knee flexes.

Therapist Position: Therapist supports the testing extremity to eliminate gravity without assisting the motion. No resistance is applied in the gravity-eliminated position.

Trace

The sartorius is palpated on the anterior aspect of the thigh medial to tensor fascia latae, above the medial aspect of the knee.

Hip: *gluteus medius* and *gluteus minimus* (tested together)

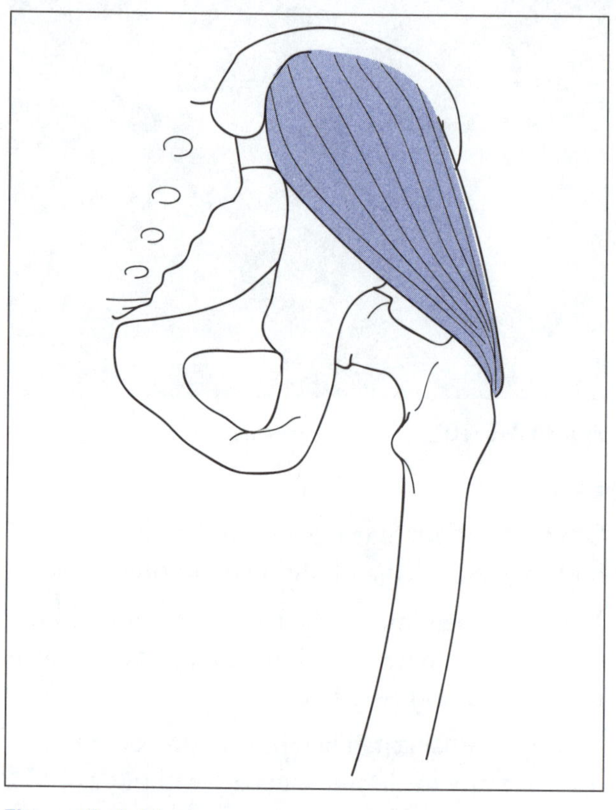

Figure 3-6-11 Gluteus medius

Gluteus medius

Origin: Lateral surface of the ilium, anterior and posterior to the gluteal line

Insertion: Greater trochanter of femur

Innervation: Superior gluteal nerve

Action: Hip abduction and hip internal rotation

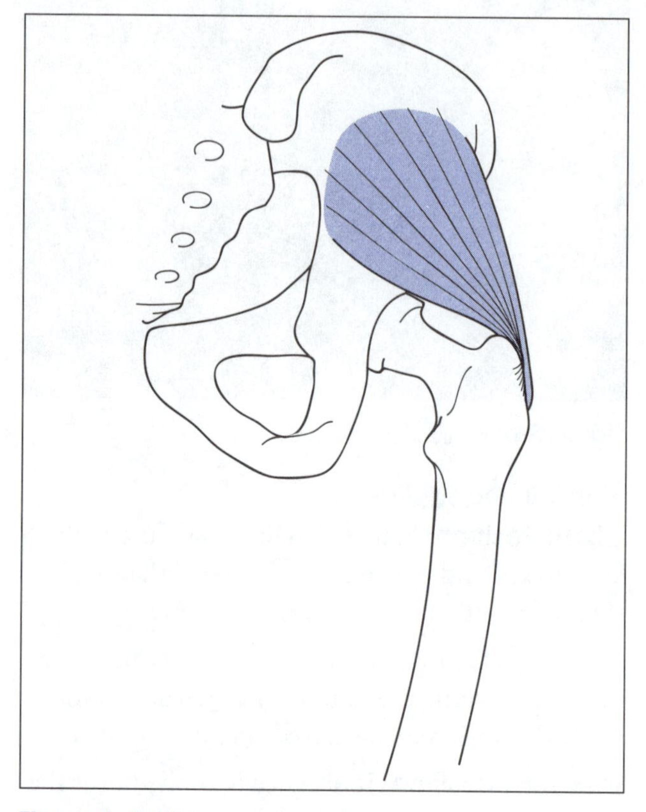

Figure 3-6-12 Gluteus minimus

Gluteus minimus

Origin: Lateral surface of the ilium between the anterior and inferior gluteal lines

Insertion: Greater trochanter of femur

Innervation: Superior gluteal nerve

Action: Hip abduction and internal rotation

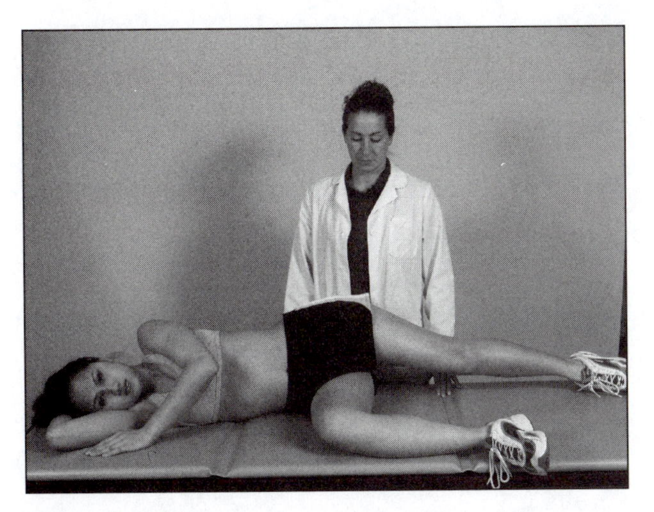

Figure 3-6-13 Start position for gluteus medius and gluteus minimus.

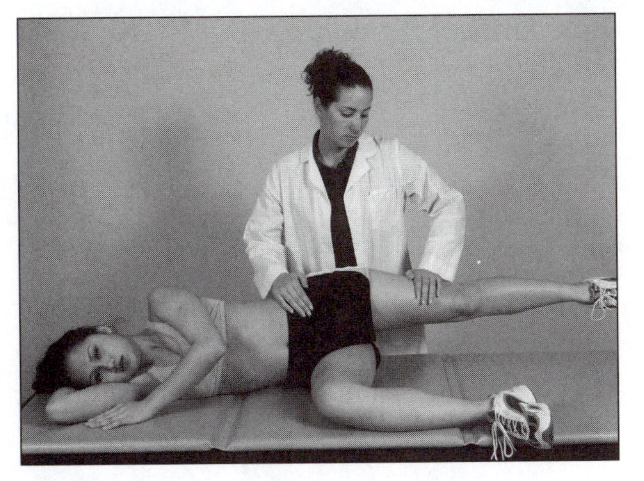

Figure 3-6-14 End position for gluteus medius and gluteus minimus.

Normal, Good, Fair

Client Position: Starting—client is lying on nontest side. Client holds nontest extremity in maximal hip and knee flexion. Testing extremity is in slight hip extension, neutral rotation, and knee extension. The pelvis is rotated slightly forward (Figure 3-6-13).

Motion—client moves the testing extremity in the direction of hip abduction (Figure 3-6-14).

Therapist Position: Stabilize at the pelvis. Resistance is applied over the lateral aspect of the thigh proximal to the knee in the direction of adduction when testing Normal or Good strengths. No resistance is applied when testing Fair strength.

Poor

Client Position: Starting—client is supine with hip and knees extended resting on testing surface.

Motion—client moves the testing extremity into maximal hip abduction.

Therapist Position: Stabilize the pelvis on the contralateral side. Therapist supports the testing extremity to eliminate gravity without assisting the motion. No resistance is applied in the gravity-eliminated position.

Trace

The gluteus medius is palpated distal to the lateral lip of the iliac crest or proximal to the greater trochanter of the femur. The gluteus minumus is too deep to be palpated.

Hip: *tensor fascia latae*

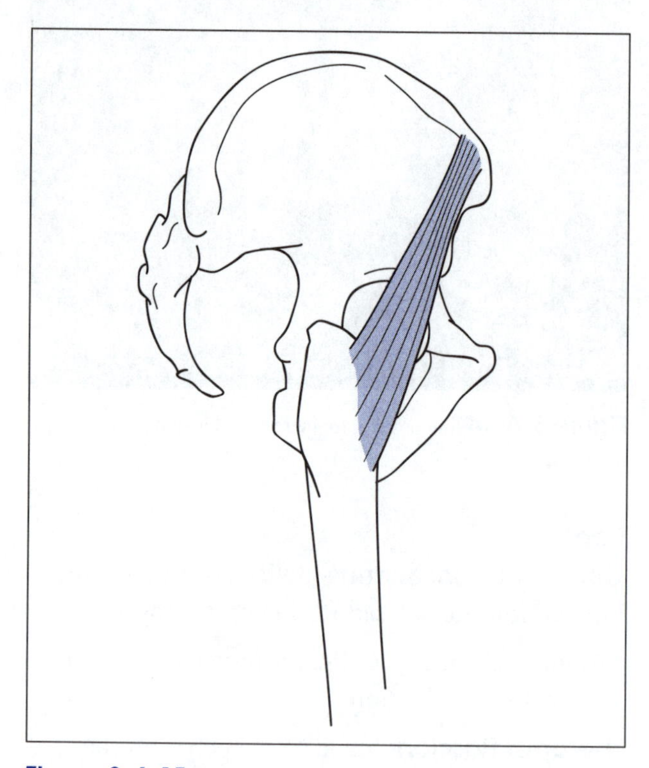

Figure 3-6-15 Tensor fascia latae

Origin: Iliac crest posterior to the ASIS

Insertion: Iliotibial tract

Innervation: Superior gluteal nerve

Action: Hip flexion, hip abduction, and hip internal rotation

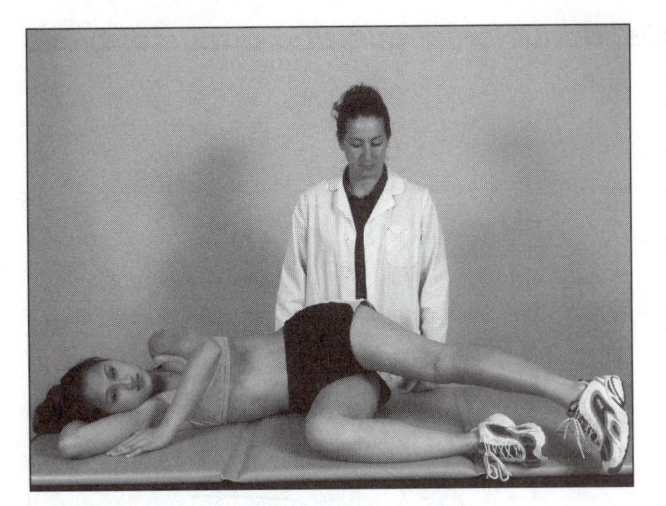

Figure 3-6-16 Start position for tensor fascia latae.

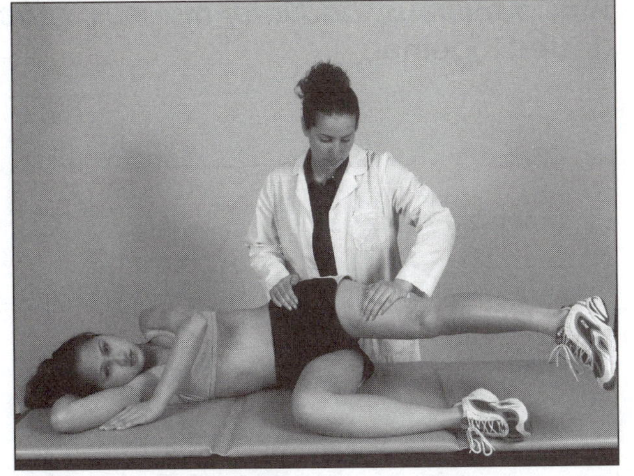

Figure 3-6-17 End position for tensor fascia latae.

Normal, Good, Fair

Client Position: Starting—client is lying on nontest side. Client holds nontest extremity in maximal hip and knee flexion. Testing extremity is in 45 degrees of hip flexion, and in internal rotation and knee extension. The pelvis is rolled backward (Figure 3-6-16).

Motion—client moves the testing extremity in the direction of hip abduction while maintaining hip flexion (Figure 3-6-17).

Therapist Position: Stabilize at the pelvis. Resistance is applied on the anterolateral aspect of the thigh proximal to the knee in the direction of hip adduction and extension when testing Normal or Good strengths. No resistance is applied when testing Fair strength.

Poor

Client Position: Starting—client is supine with hip and knees extended resting on testing surface.

Motion—client moves the testing extremity into maximal hip abduction and slight hip flexion.

Therapist Position: Stabilize the pelvis. Therapist supports the testing extremity to eliminate gravity without assisting the motion. No resistance is applied in the gravity-eliminated position.

Trace

The tensor fascia latae is palpated lateral to the upper portion of the sartorius or distal to the greater trochanter on the iliotibial band.

Hip: *pectineus*, *adductor magnus*, *gracilis*, *adductor longus*, and *adductor brevis* (tested together)

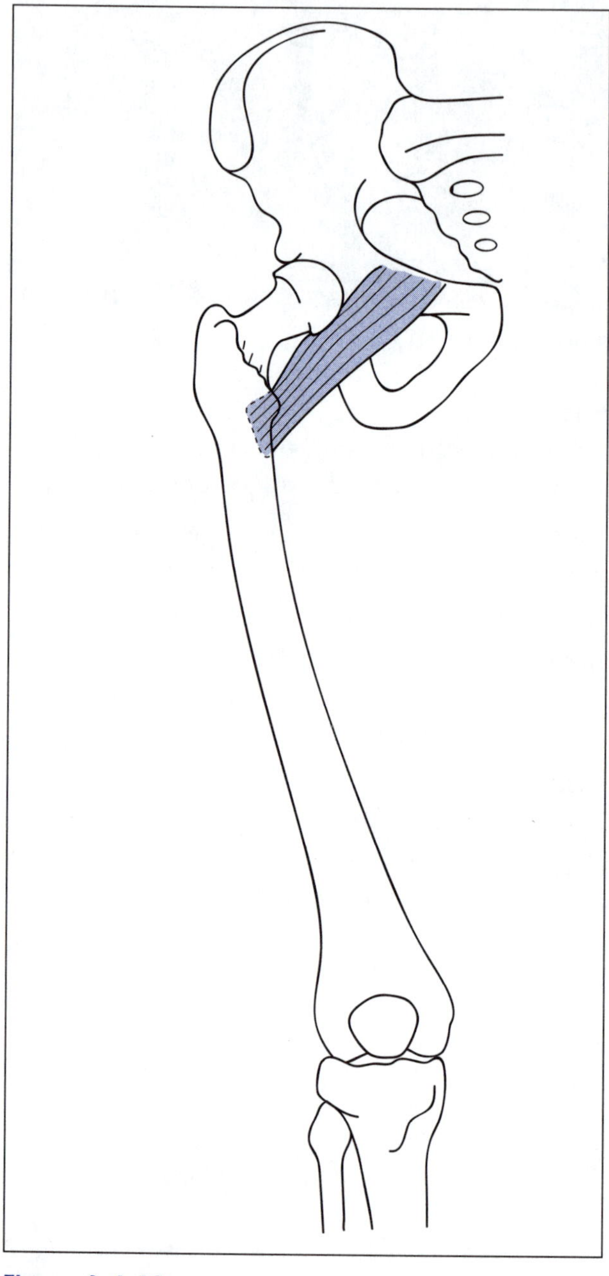

Figure 3-6-18 Pectineus

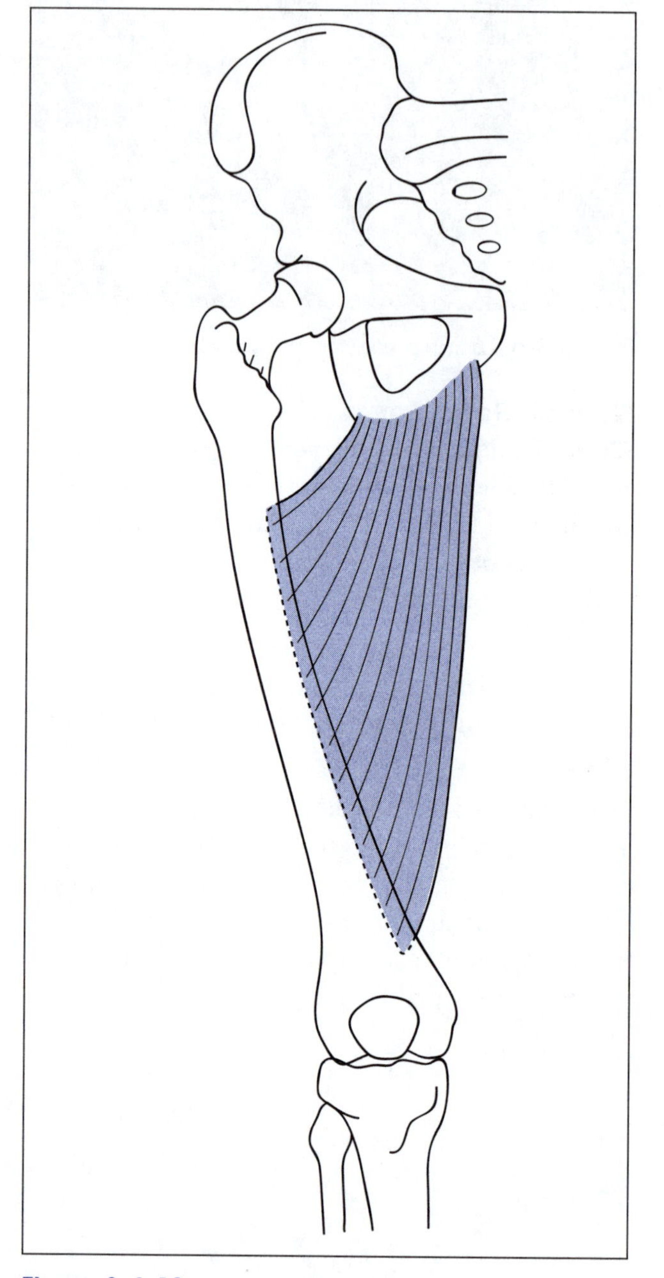

Figure 3-6-19 Adductor magnus

Pectineus

Origin: Superior ramus of the pubis

Insertion: Between the lesser trochanter and the linea aspera of the posterior femur

Innervation: Femoral and obturator nerves

Action: Hip adduction

Adductor magnus

Origin: Inferior pubic ramus, ramus of the ischium, and ischial tuberosity

Insertion: Linea aspera and the adductor tubercle on the medial condyle of the femur

Innervation: Obturator and sciatic nerves

Action: Hip adduction

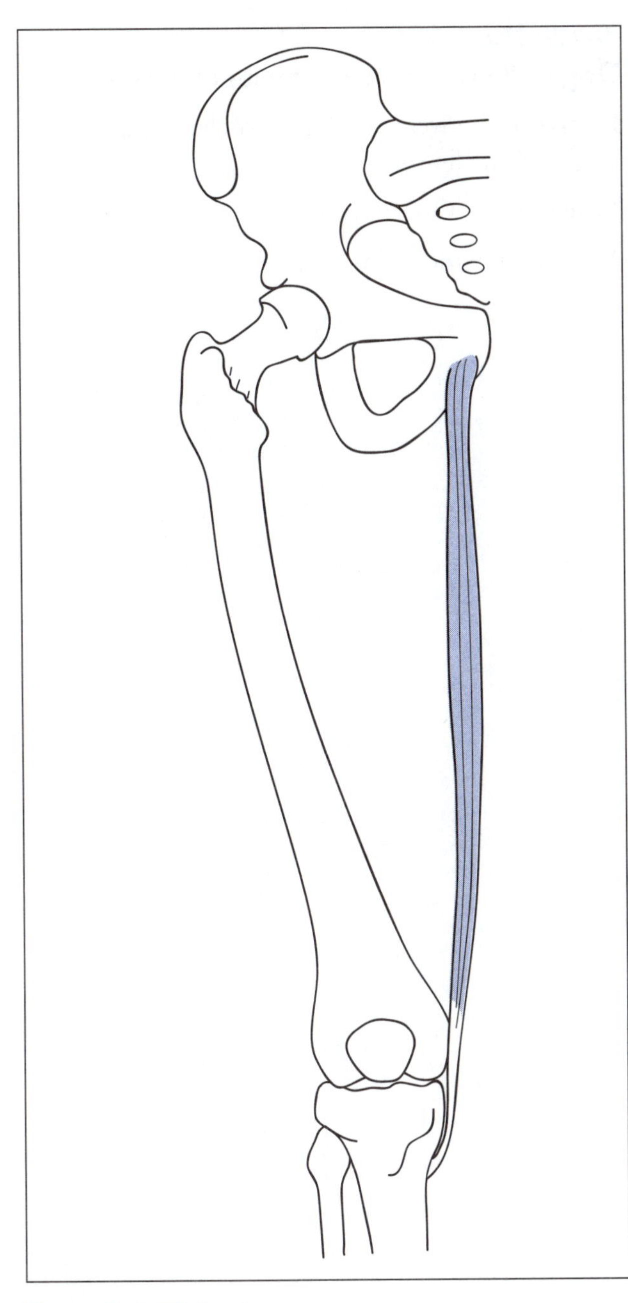

Figure 3-6-20 Gracilis

Gracilis

Origin: Inferior ramus of the pubis and ischium

Insertion: Proximal aspect of the tibia distal to the medial condyle

Innervation: Obturator nerve

Action: Hip adduction

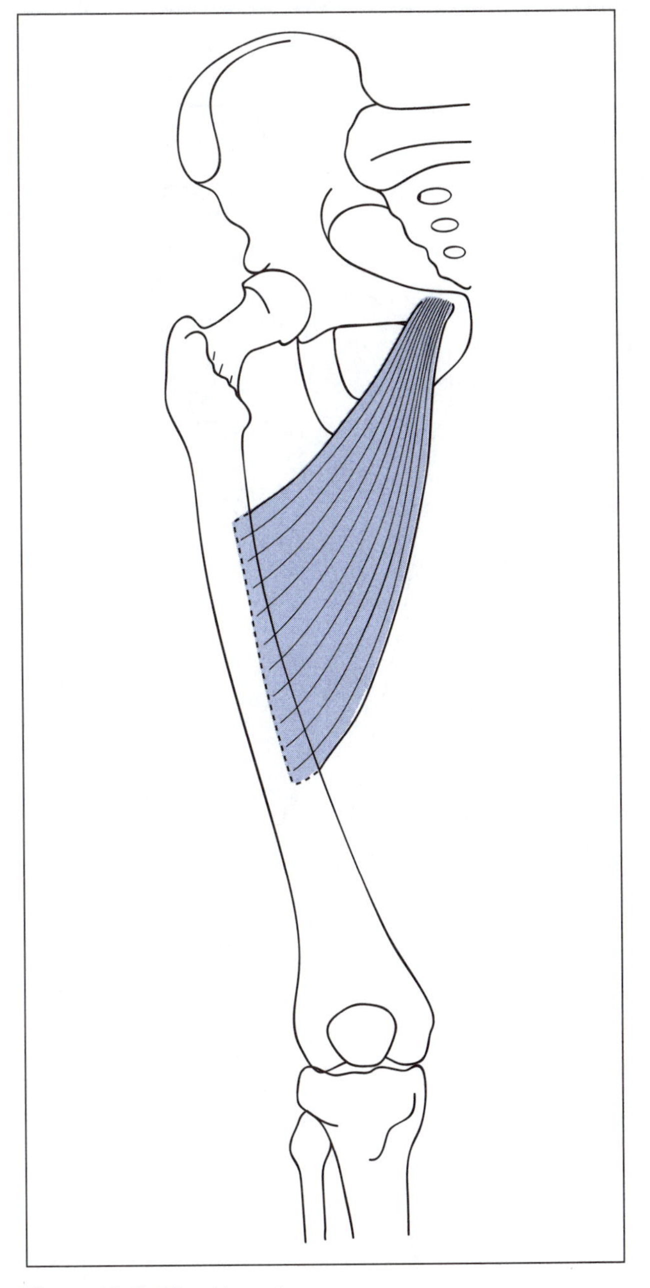

Figure 3-6-21 Adductor longus

Adductor longus

Origin: Pubic tubercle/anterior crest of pubis

Insertion: Medial lip of linea aspera of femur

Innervation: Obturator nerve

Action: Hip adduction

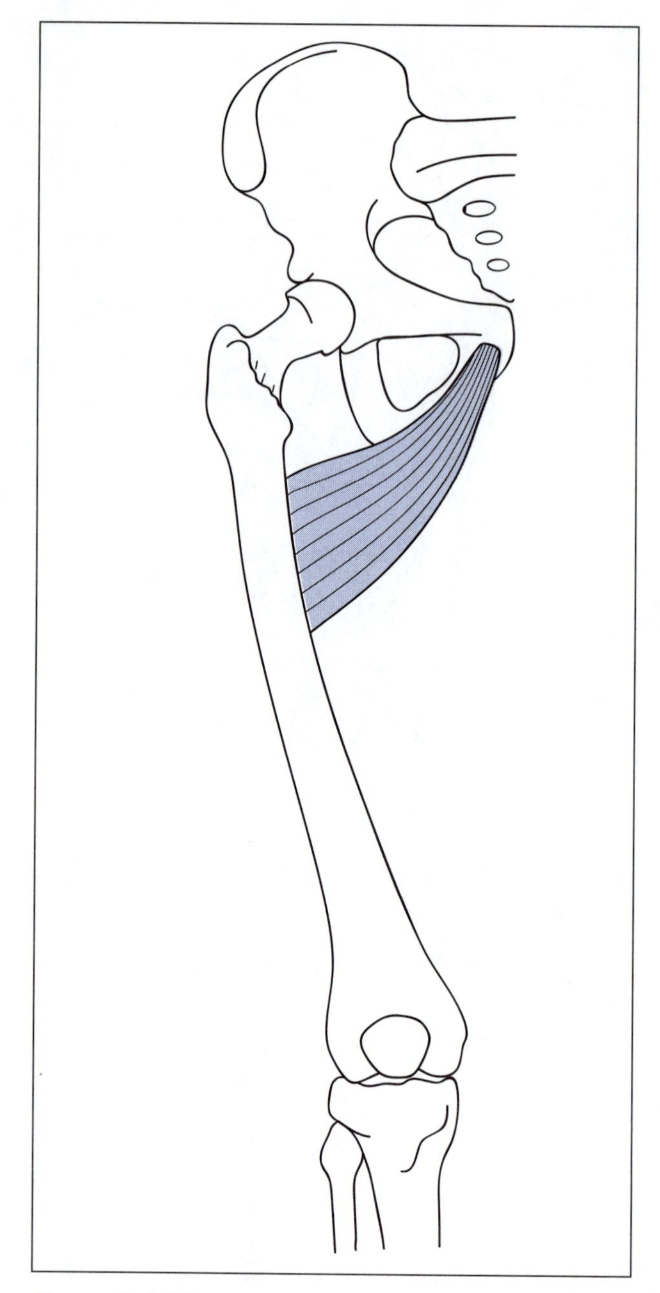

Figure 3-6-22 Adductor brevis

Adductor brevis

Origin: Body and inferior ramus of the pubis

Insertion: Between the lesser trochanter and linea aspera of the femur

Innervation: Obturator nerve

Action: Hip adduction

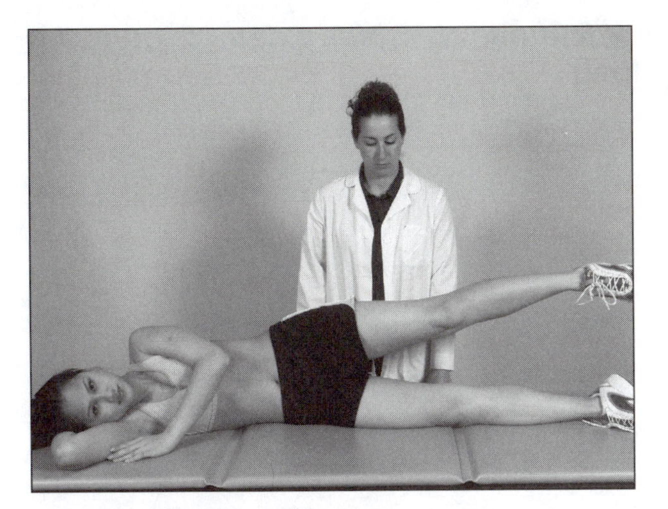

Figure 3-6-23 Start position for pectineus, adductor magnus, gracilis, adductor longus, and adductor brevis.

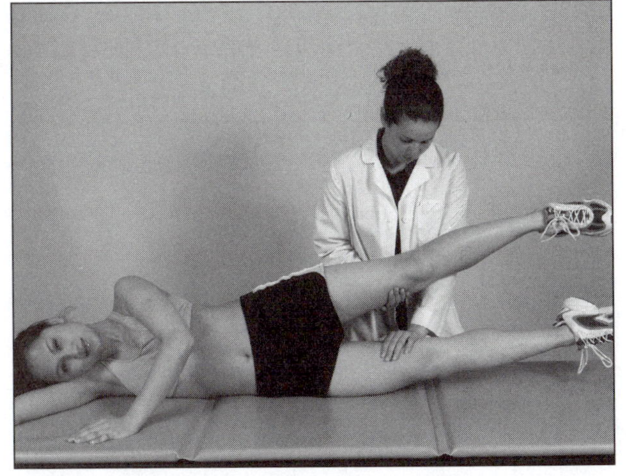

Figure 3-6-24 End position for pectineus, adductor magnus, gracilis, adductor longus, and adductor brevis.

Normal, Good, Fair

Client Position: Starting—client is lying on side on testing extremity with hip in neutral and knee extended on testing surface. Nontest extremity is in abduction and knee is extended (Figure 3-6-23).

Motion—client moves the testing extremity in the direction of hip adduction toward the nontest extremity (Figure 3-6-24).

Therapist Position: Support the nontest extremity in hip abduction. Resistance is applied over the medial aspect of the thigh proximal to the knee in the direction of abduction when testing Normal or Good strengths. No resistance is applied when testing Fair strength.

Poor

Client Position: Starting—client is supine with hip in abduction and knee extended on testing surface.

Motion—client moves the testing extremity into maximal hip adduction.

Therapist Position: Stabilize the pelvis. Therapist supports the testing extremity to eliminate gravity without assisting the motion. No resistance is applied in the gravity-eliminated position.

Trace

The adductors are palpated as a group on the medial and proximal aspect of the thigh.

Hip: *piriformis, quadratus femoris, obturator internis, obturator externus, gemellus superior,* and *gemellus inferior* (tested together)

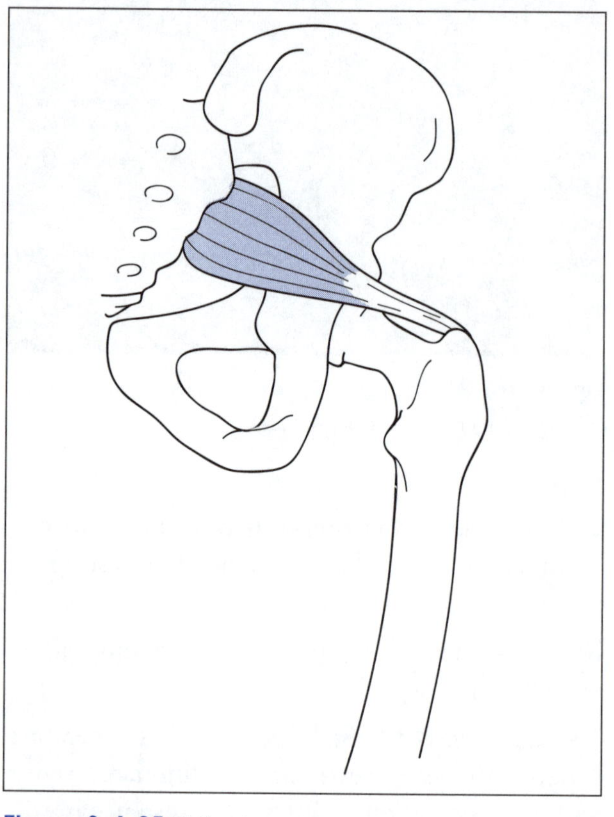

Figure 3-6-25 Piriformis

Piriformis

Origin: Anterior sacrum and sciatic notch of ilium

Insertion: Superior border of the greater trochanter of the femur

Innervation: Sacral plexus

Action: Hip external rotation

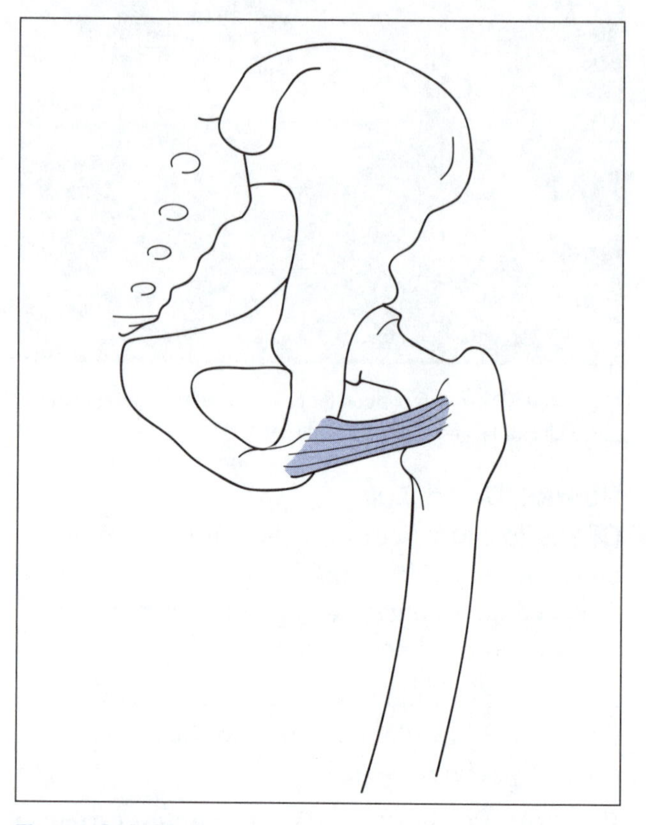

Figure 3-6-26 Quadratus femoris

Quadratus femoris

Origin: Lateral border of ischial tuberosity

Insertion: Posterior surface of the femur between the greater and lesser trochanters

Innervation: Sacral plexus

Action: Hip external rotation

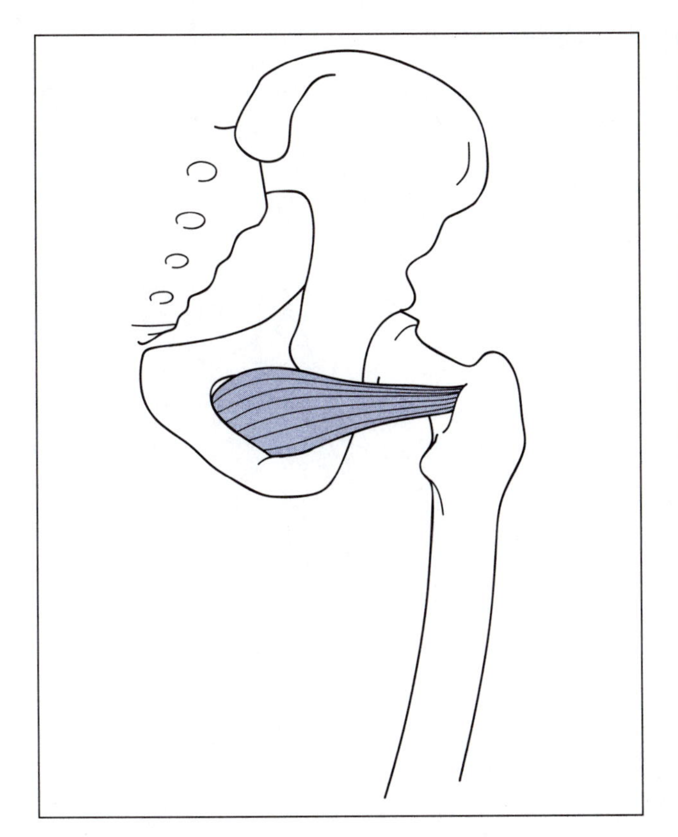

Figure 3-6-27 Obturator internis

Obturator internis

Origin: Obturator membrane, margin of obturator foramin, and internal surface of the pelvis

Insertion: Medial surface of the greater trochanter proximal to the trochanter fossa

Innervation: Sacral plexus

Action: Hip external rotation

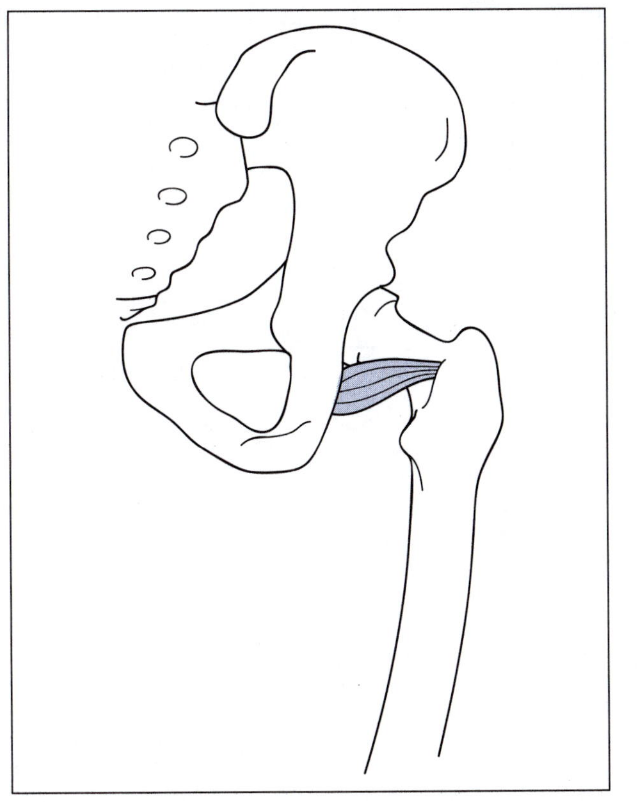

Figure 3-6-28 Obturator externus

Obturator externus

Origin: Obturator membrane: bone around foramen on external surface of pelvis

Insertion: Trochanteric fossa of the femur

Innervation: Obturator nerve

Action: Hip external rotation

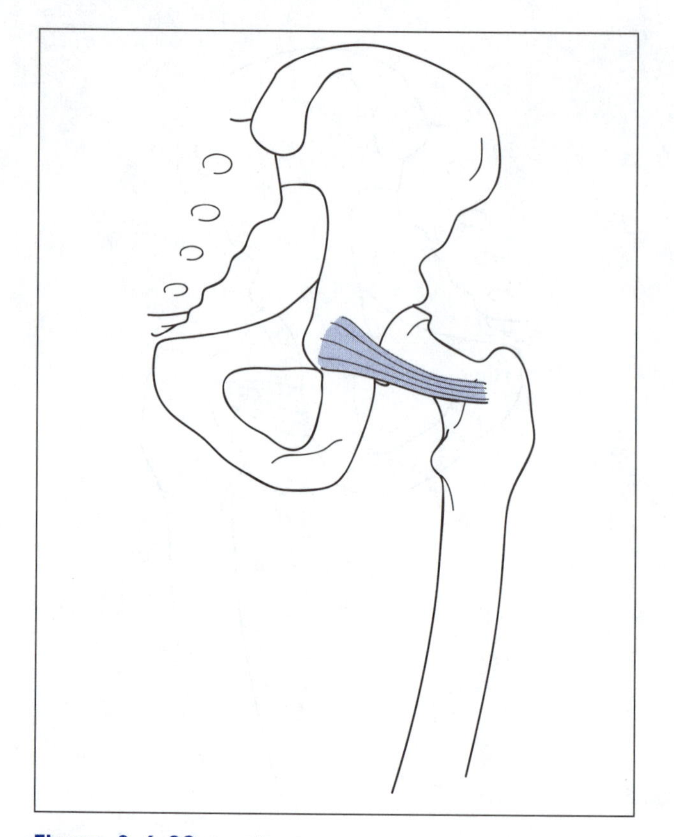

Figure 3-6-29 Gemellus superior

Gemellus superior

Origin: Dorsal aspect of the spine of ischium

Insertion: Greater trochanter of the femur

Innervation: Sacral plexus

Action: Hip external rotation

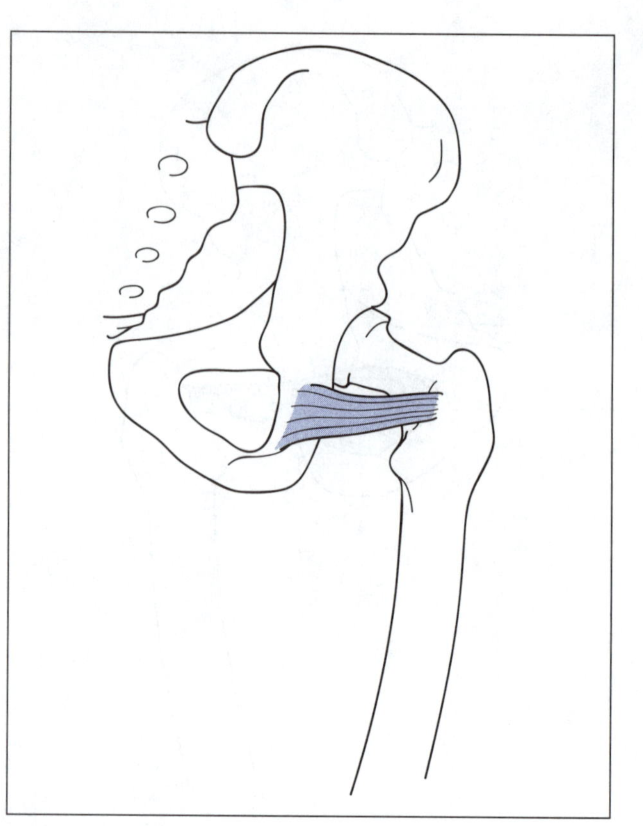

Figure 3-6-30 Gemellus inferior

Gemellus inferior

Origin: Proximal aspect of the ischial tuberosity

Insertion: Greater trochanter of the femur

Innervation: Obturator nerve

Action: Hip external rotation

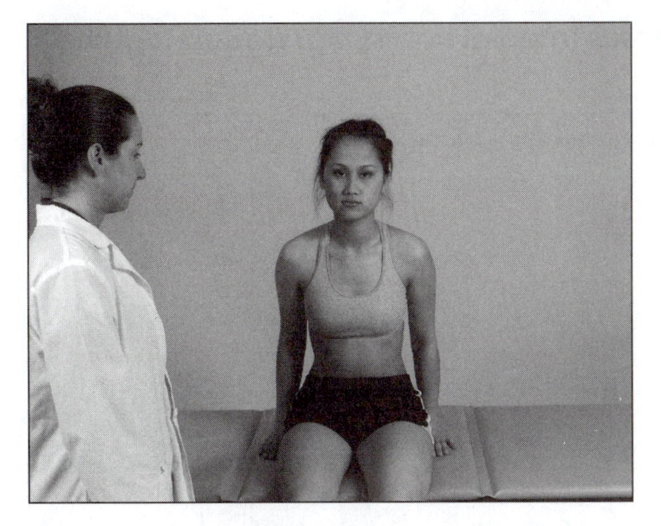

Figure 3-6-31 Start position for piriformis, quadratus femoris, obturator internis, obturator externus, gemellus superior, and gemellus inferior.

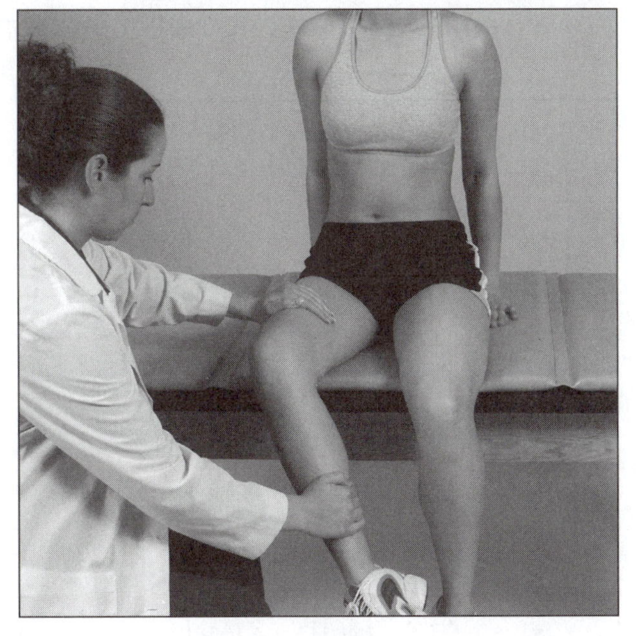

Figure 3-6-32 End position for piriformis, quadratus femoris, obturator internis, obturator externus, gemellus superior, and gemellus inferior.

Normal, Good, Fair

Client Position: Starting—client is sitting with testing hip in 90 degrees of flexion, knee flexed at edge of testing surface. The midpoint of patella is aligned with the ASIS (Figure 3-6-31).

Motion—client moves the testing extremity in the direction of hip external rotation (Figure 3-6-32).

Therapist Position: The stabilizing hand applies counterpressure at the anterolateral aspect of the distal thigh while resistance is applied by the other hand. Resistance is applied over the medial aspect of the lower leg proximal to the ankle in the direction of internal rotation when testing Normal or Good strengths. No resistance is applied when testing Fair strength.

Poor

Client Position: Starting—client is supine with testing hip in internal rotation and knee extension.

Motion—client moves the testing extremity into maximal hip external rotation.

Therapist Position: Stabilize the medial aspect of the thigh. No resistance is applied in the gravity-eliminated position.

Trace

The external rotators are too deep to palpate.

Knee: *semitendinosus* and *semimembranosus* (medial hamstring) (tested together)

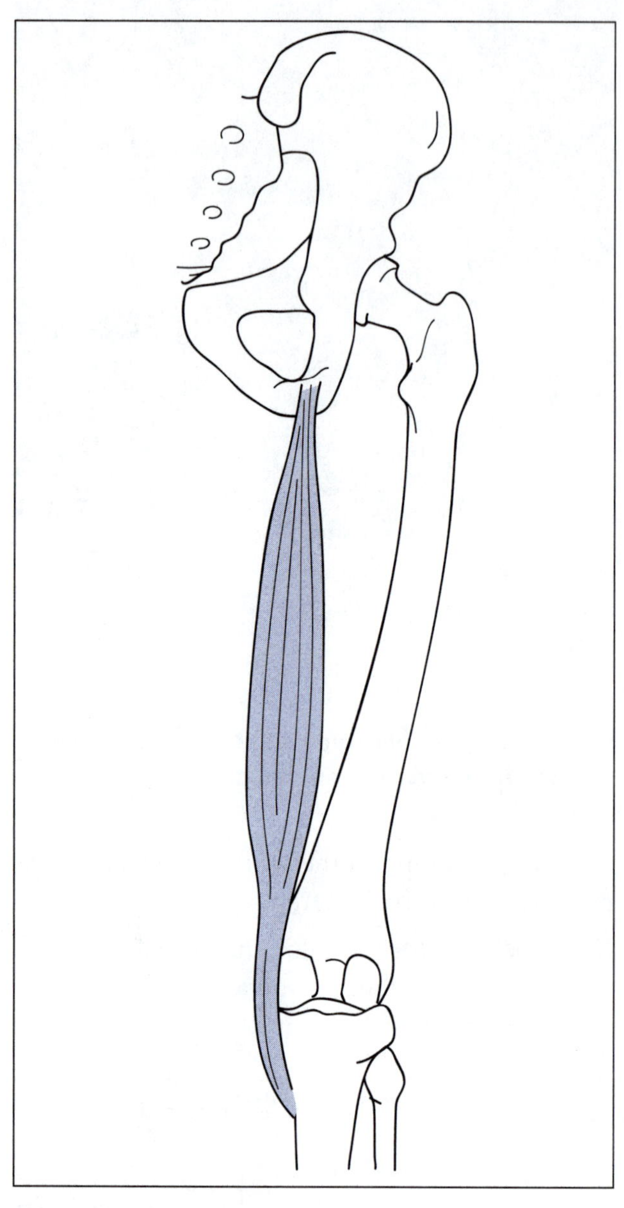

Figure 3-6-33 Semitendinosis

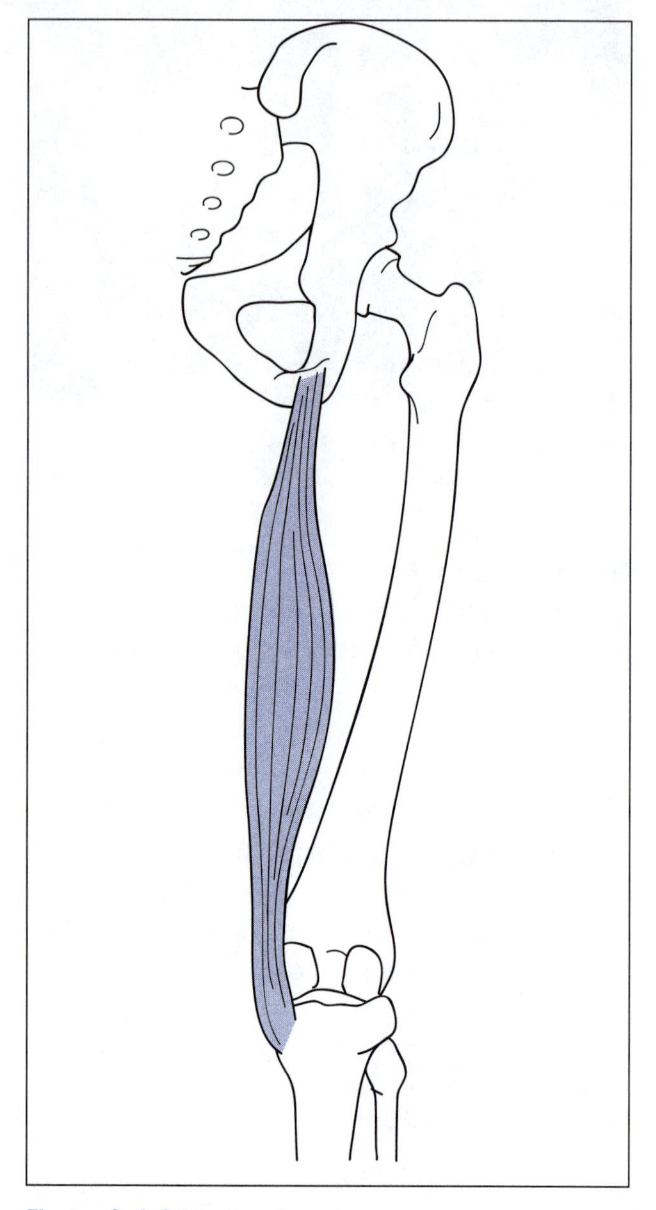

Figure 3-6-34 Semimembranosis

Semitendinosus

Origin: Superior aspect of the ischial tuberosity

Insertion: Proximal aspect of the medial surface of the tibia

Innervation: Sciatic nerve (tibial branch)

Action: Knee flexion and knee internal rotation of tibia during flexion, hip extension when knee is flexed

Semimembranosus

Origin: Superolateral aspect of the ischial tuberosity

Insertion: Medial tibial condyle and medial condyle of the femur

Innervation: Sciatic nerve (tibial branch)

Action: Knee flexion and knee internal rotation of tibia during flexion, hip extension when knee is flexed

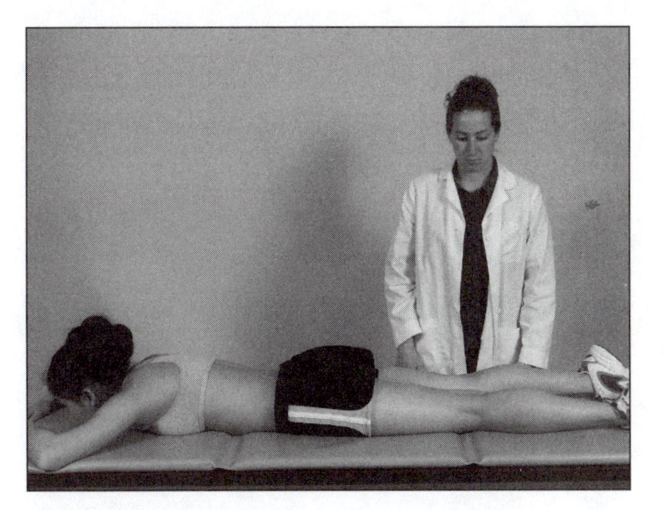

Figure 3-6-35 Start position for semitendinosis and semimembranosis.

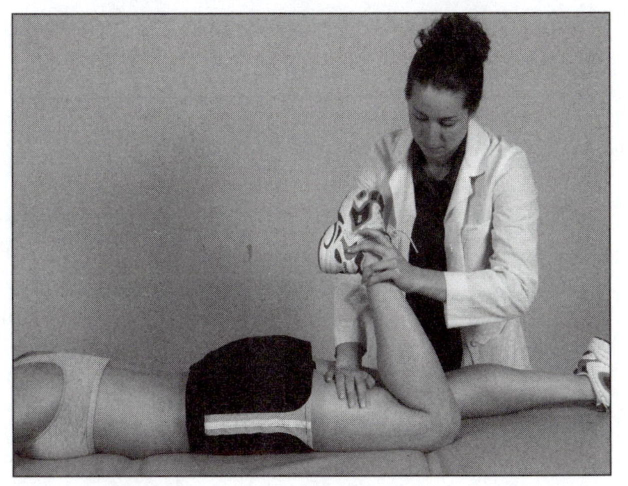

Figure 3-6-36 End position for semitendinosis and semimembranosis.

Normal, Good, Fair

Client Position: Starting—client is prone. The testing knee is slightly flexed and internally rotated (toes are pointed toward nontest side) (Figure 3-3-35).

Motion—while maintaining knee internal rotation of the tibia, the client flexes the knee in a diagonal motion toward the lateral aspect of the testing extremity buttocks (Figure 3-3-36).

Therapist Position: Stabilize the testing thigh. Resistance is applied proximal to the ankle in the direction of knee extension and external rotation when testing Normal or Good strengths. No resistance is applied when testing Fair strength.

Poor

Client Position: Starting—client is lying on nontest side. The testing hip and knee are extended.

Motion—client moves the testing extremity into maximal knee flexion.

Therapist Position: Stabilize the thigh. Therapist supports the testing extremity to eliminate gravity without assisting the motion. No resistance is applied in the gravity-eliminated position.

Trace

The semitendinosus is palpated proximal to the knee joint on the medial aspect of the popliteal fossa.

The semimembranosus is palpated proximal to the knee joint on either side of the tendon.

Knee: *biceps femoris* (lateral hamstring)

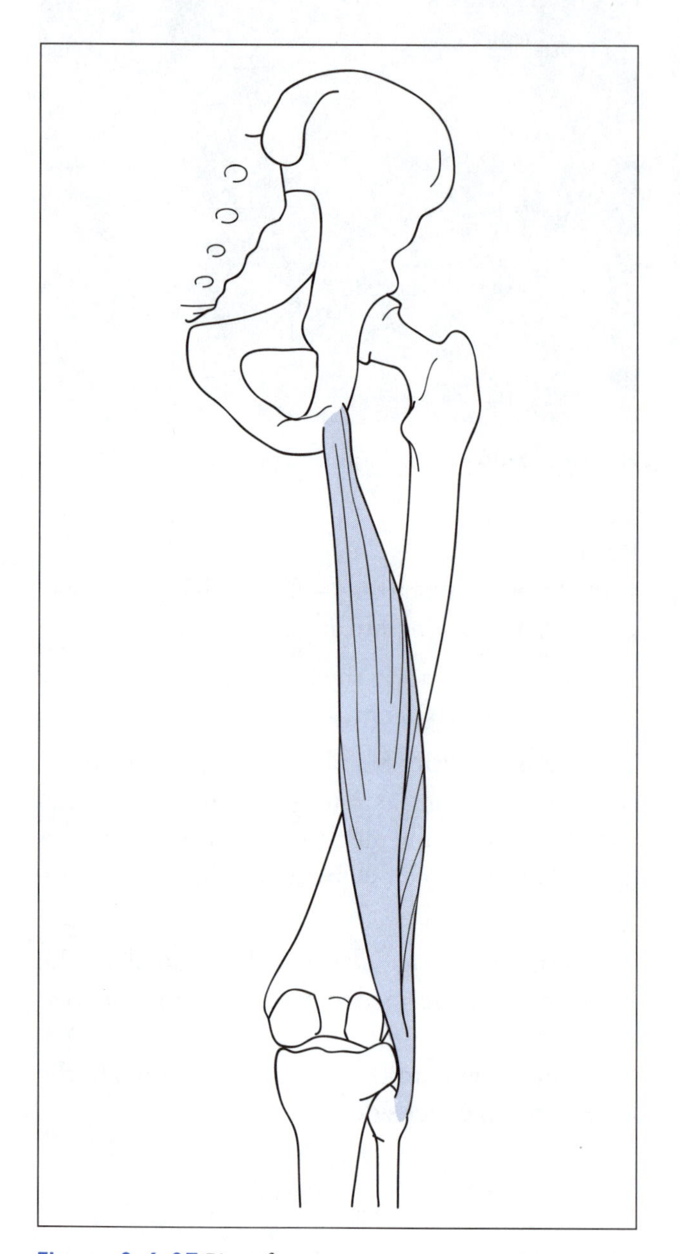

Figure 3-6-37 Biceps femoris

Origin: Long head—ischial tuberosity. Short head—posterior, distal femur

Insertion: Lateral head of the fibula and lateral condyle of the tibia

Innervation: Sciatic nerve (tibial and peroneal branches)

Action: Knee flexion and knee external rotation of tibia during flexion

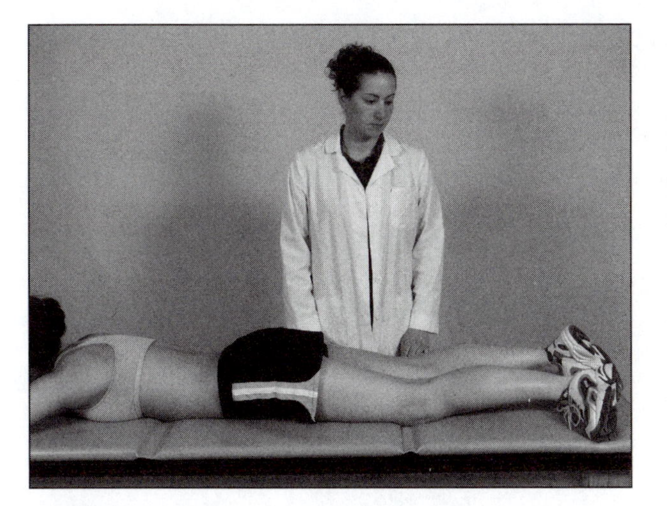

Figure 3-6-38 Start position for biceps femoris.

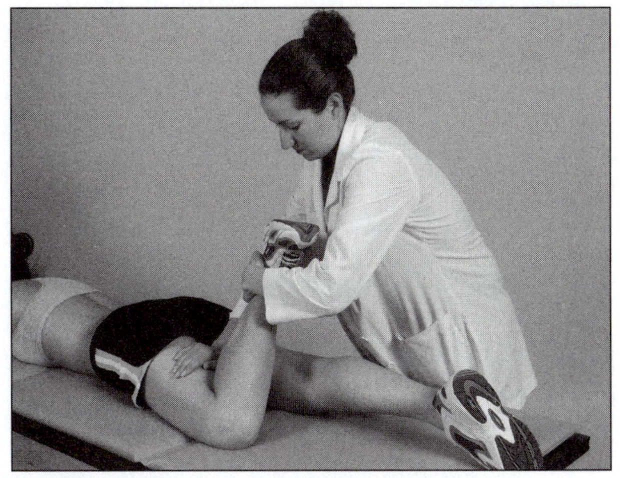

Figure 3-6-39 End position for biceps femoris.

Normal, Good, Fair

Client Position: Starting—client is prone. The testing knee is slightly flexed and externally rotated (toes are pointed away from nontest side) (Figure 3-6-38).

Motion—while maintaining knee external rotation of the tibia, the client flexes the knee in a diagonal motion toward the contralateral buttocks (Figure 3-6-39).

Therapist Position: Stabilize the testing thigh. Resistance is applied proximal to the ankle on the posterior aspect of the leg in the direction of knee extension and internal rotation when testing Normal or Good strengths. No resistance is applied when testing Fair strength.

Poor

Client Position: Starting—client is lying on nontest side. The testing hip and knee are extended.

Motion—client moves the testing extremity into maximal knee flexion.

Therapist Position: Stabilize the thigh. Therapist supports the testing extremity to eliminate gravity without assisting the motion. No resistance is applied in the gravity-eliminated position.

Trace

The biceps femoris is palpated proximal to the knee joint on the lateral margin of the popliteal fossa.

Knee: *rectus femoris*, *vastus intermedius*, *vastus lateralis*, and *vastus medialis* (tested together)

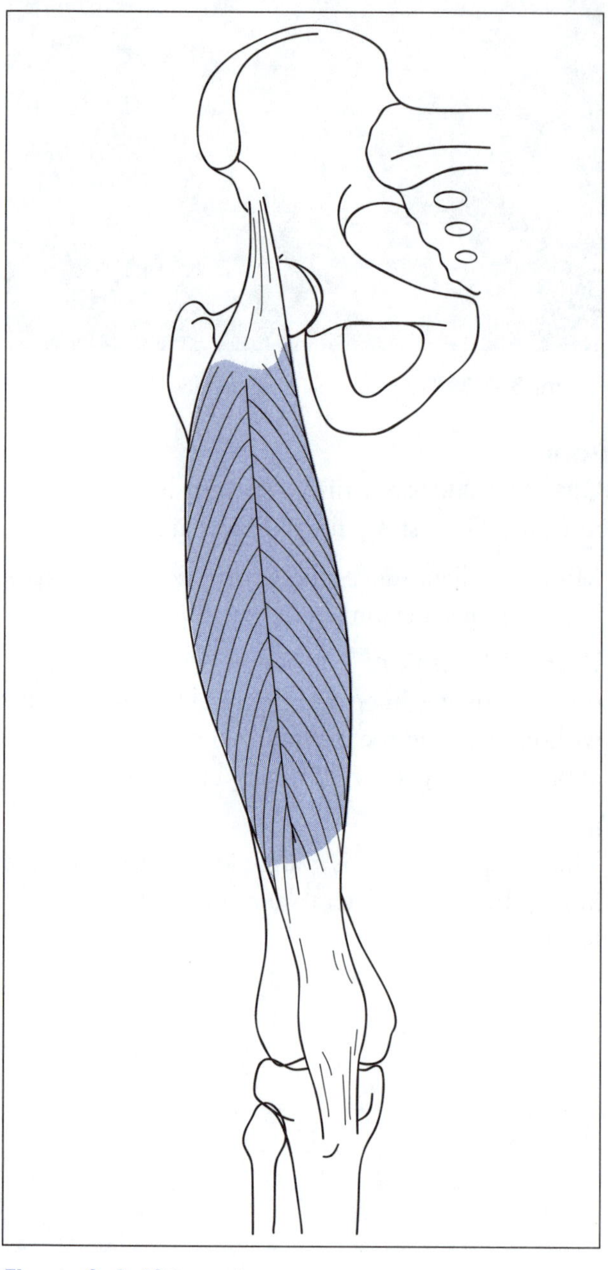

Figure 3-6-40 Rectus femoris

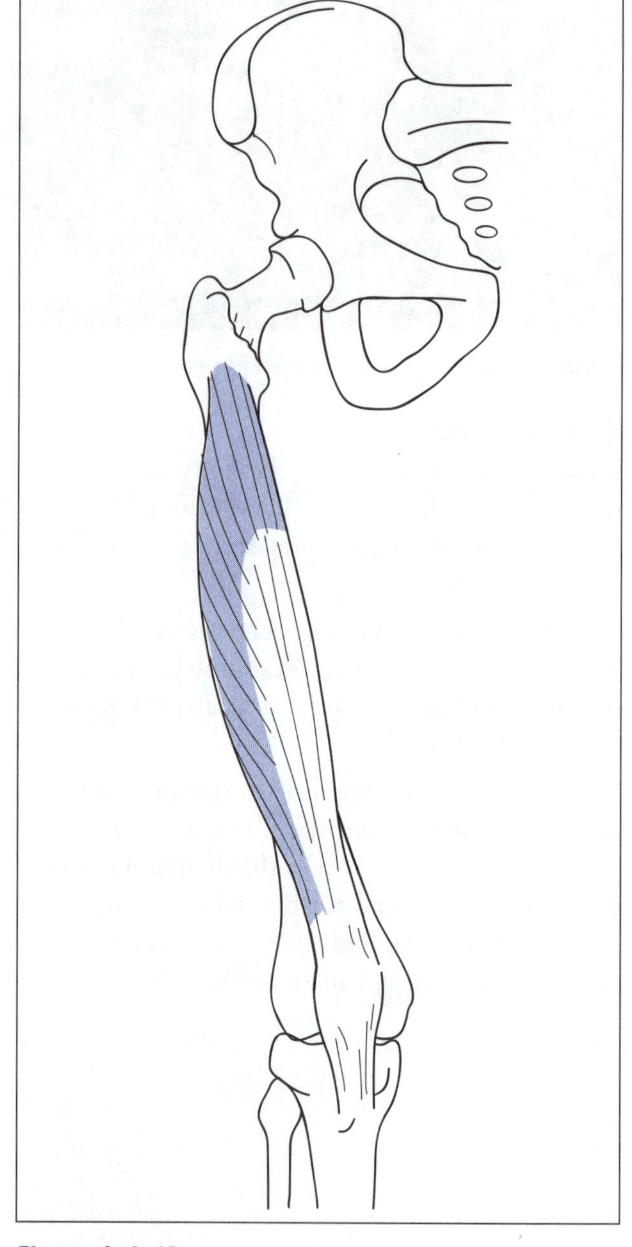

Figure 3-6-41 Vastus intermedius

Rectus femoris

Origin: Straight head—anterior aspect of the anterior inferior iliac spine. Reflected head—ilium above the acetabulum

Insertion: Base of the patella and through the patellar ligament to the tibial tuberosity

Innervation: Femoral nerve

Action: Knee extension, hip fexion

Vastus intermedius

Origin: Anterior and lateral surfaces of the femoral shaft

Insertion: Base of the patella and through the patellar ligament to the tibial tuberosity

Innervation: Femoral nerve

Action: Knee extension

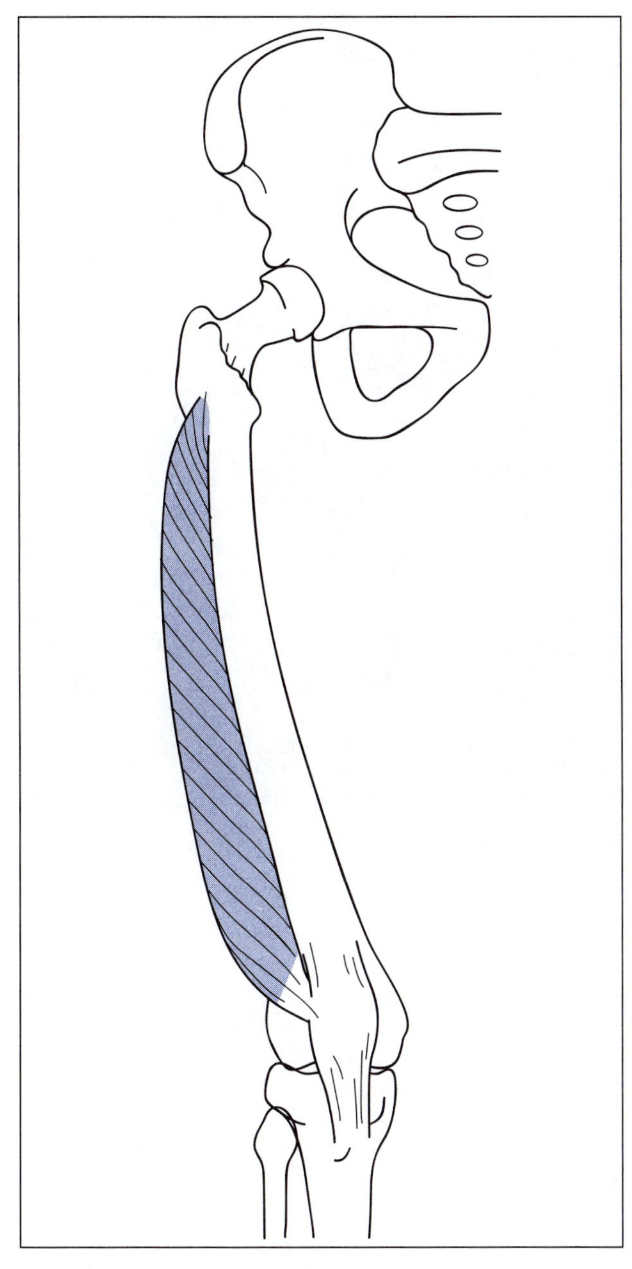

Figure 3-6-42 Vastus lateralis

Vastus lateralis

Origin: Anterior femur

Insertion: Lateral border of the patella and through the patellar ligament to the tibial tuberosity

Innervation: Femoral nerve

Action: Knee extension

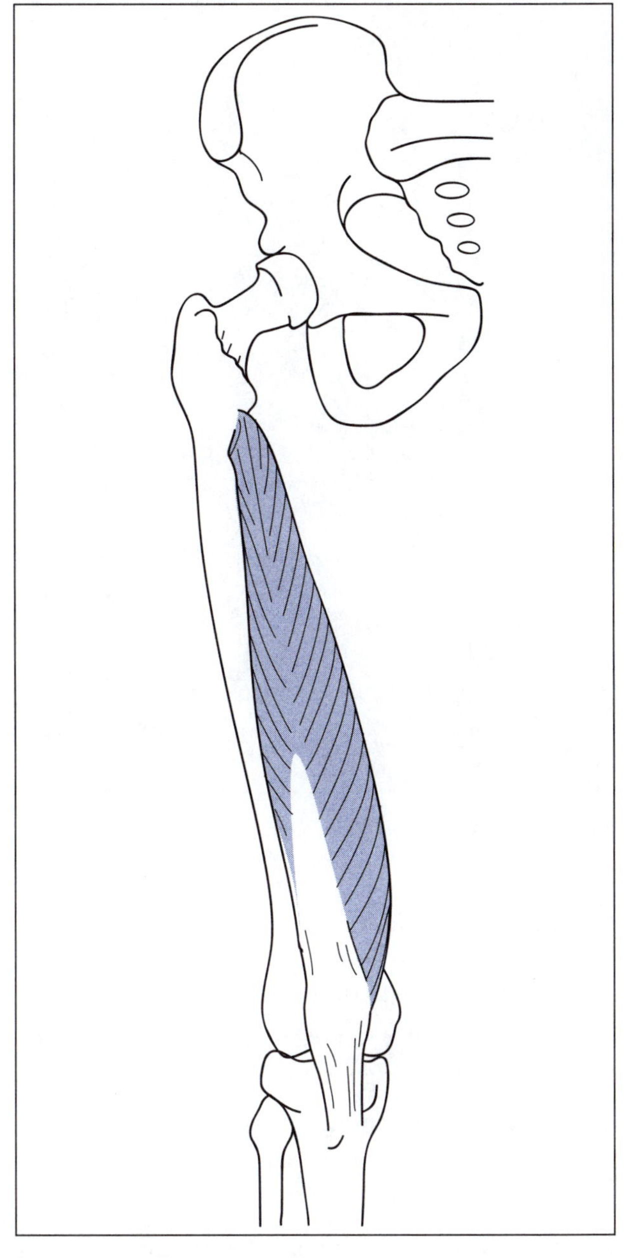

Figure 3-6-43 Vastus medialis

Vastus medialis

Origin: Inferior aspect of the intertrochanteric line, medial lip of the linea aspera, proximal aspect of the supracondylar line, and the intermuscular septum

Insertion: Medial border of the patella and through the patellar ligament to the tibial tuberosity

Innervation: Femoral nerve

Action: Knee extension

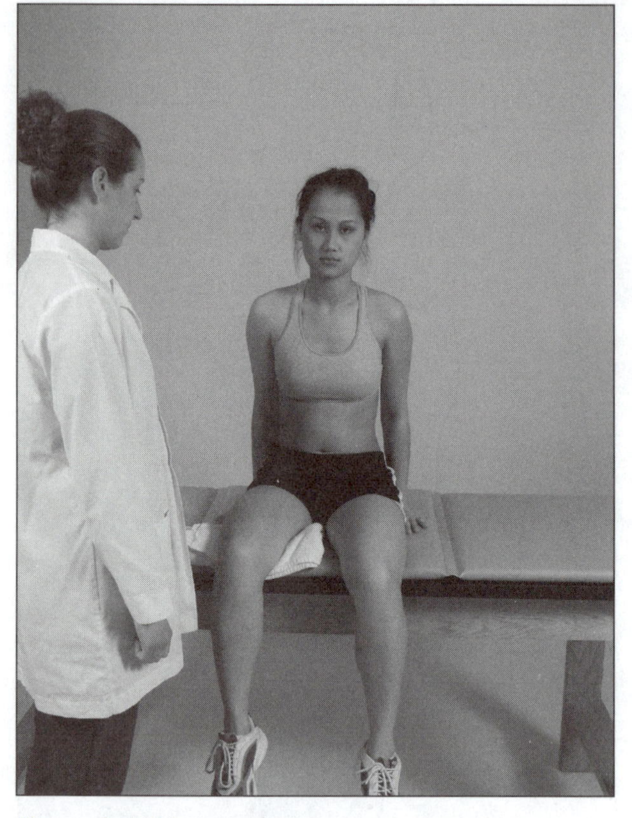

Figure 3-6-44 Start position for rectus femoris, vastus intermedius, vastus lateralis, and vastus medialis.

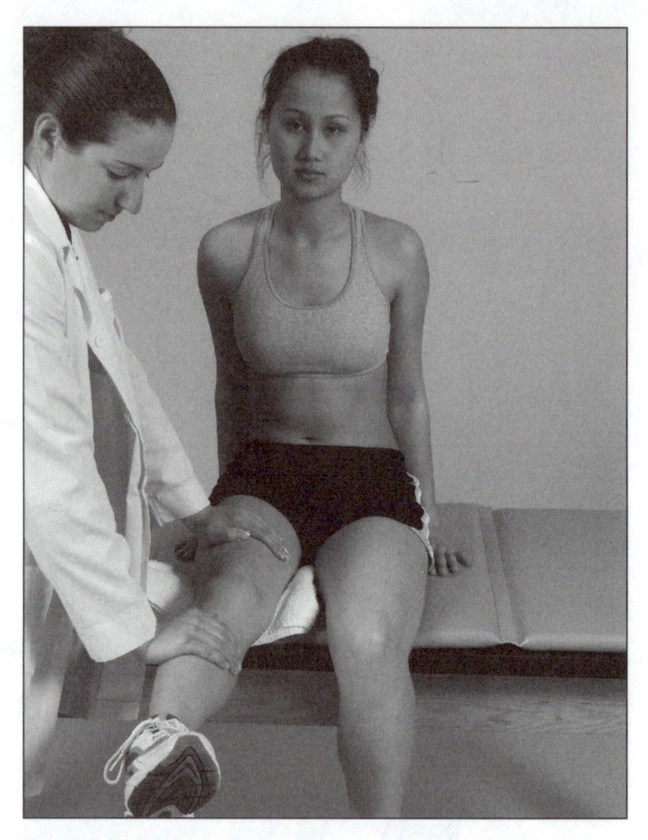

Figure 3-6-45 End position for rectus femoris, vastus intermedius, vastus lateralis, and vastus medialis.

Normal, Good, Fair

Client Position: Starting—client is sitting with a pad supported under the distal thigh. The testing knee is flexed and lower leg and feet are over edge of testing surface (Figure 3-6-44).

Motion—the client moves the testing extremity into knee extension (no hyperextension) (Figure 3-6-45).

Therapist Position: Stabilize the testing thigh. Resistance is applied on the anterior surface of the distal lower extremity in the direction of knee flexion when testing Normal or Good strengths. No resistance is applied when testing Fair strength.

Poor

Client Position: Starting—client is lying on non-test side. The testing hip is extended and the knee is flexed.

Motion—client moves the testing extremity into maximal knee extension.

Therapist Position: Stabilize the thigh. Therapist supports the testing extremity to eliminate gravity without assisting the motion. No resistance is applied in the gravity-eliminated position.

Trace

The rectus femoris is palpated on the anterior midthigh.

The vastus intermedius is too deep to be palpated.

The vastus lateralis is palpated on the lateral aspect of the midthigh.

The vastus medialis is palpated on the medial aspect of the thigh.

SECTION 3-7: Isolated Manual Muscle Testing of the Ankle and Foot

Ankle: *tibialis anterior*

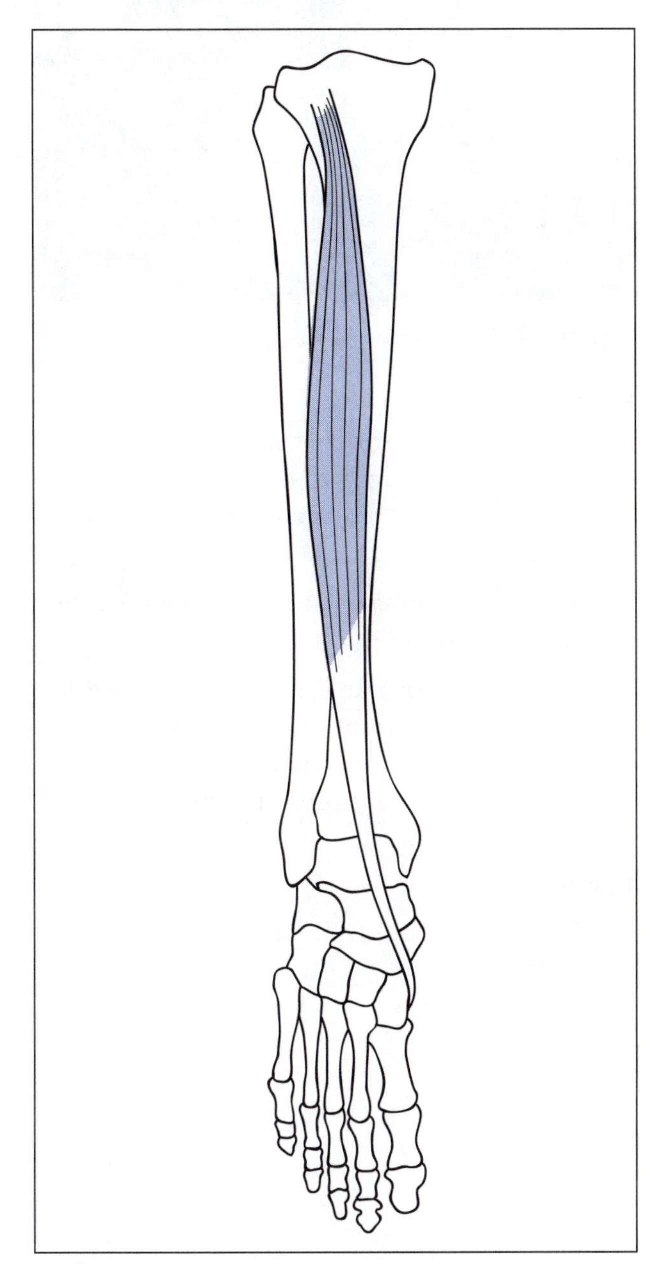

Figure 3-7-1 Tibialis anterior

Origin: Lateral condyle of the tibia, 2/3 of lateral shaft of the tibia

Insertion: Medial cuneiform bone and medial aspect of the base of first metatarsal

Innervation: Deep peroneal nerve

Action: Ankle dorsiflexion and foot inversion

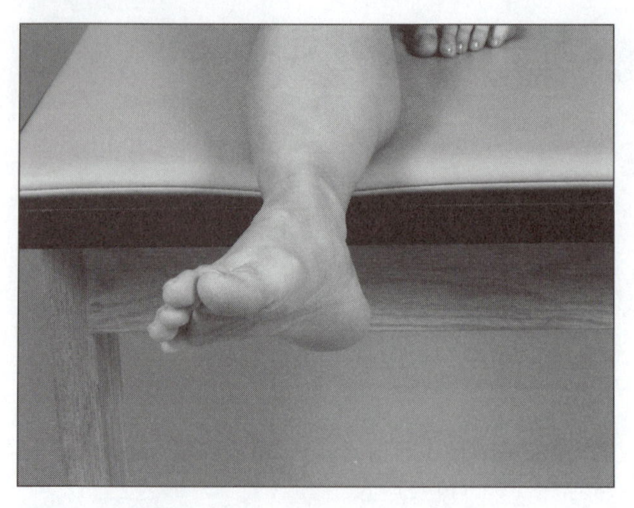

Figure 3-7-2 Start position for tibialis anterior.

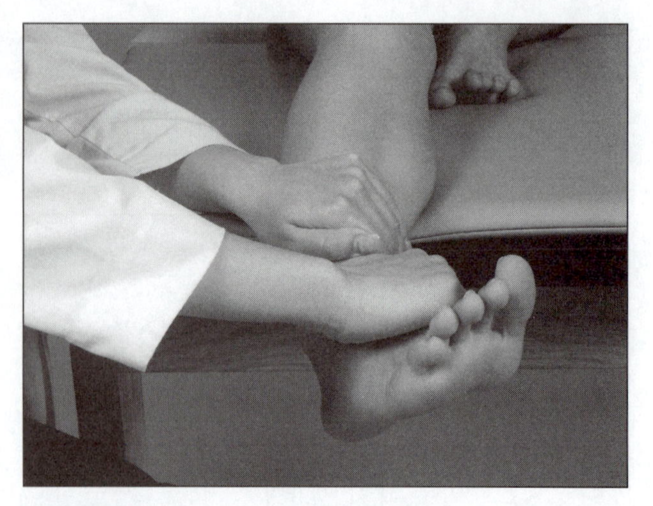

Figure 3-7-3 End position for tibialis anterior.

Normal, Good, Fair

Client Position: Starting—client is sitting with lower leg and foot over edge of testing surface. The ankle is in plantar flexion and foot in slight eversion (Figure 3-7-2).

Motion—client moves the testing extremity into dorsiflexion and foot inversion with toes relaxed (Figure 3-7-3).

Therapist Position: Stabilize the lower leg proximal to the ankle. Resistance is applied on the medial side and dorsal aspect of the forefoot in the direction of plantar flexion and foot eversion when testing Normal or Good strengths. No resistance is applied when testing Fair strength.

Poor

Client Position: Starting—client is lying on side on test side. The testing hip is extended, the knee is flexed, the ankle is in plantar flexion, and the foot in slight eversion.

Motion—client moves the testing extremity into maximal ankle dorsiflexion and foot inversion.

Therapist Position: Stabilize the lower leg proximal to the ankle. Therapist supports the testing extremity to eliminate gravity without assisting the motion. No resistance is applied in the gravity-eliminated position.

Trace

The tibialis anterior is palpated on the anterior lateral portion of the lower leg.

Ankle: *gastrocnemius*

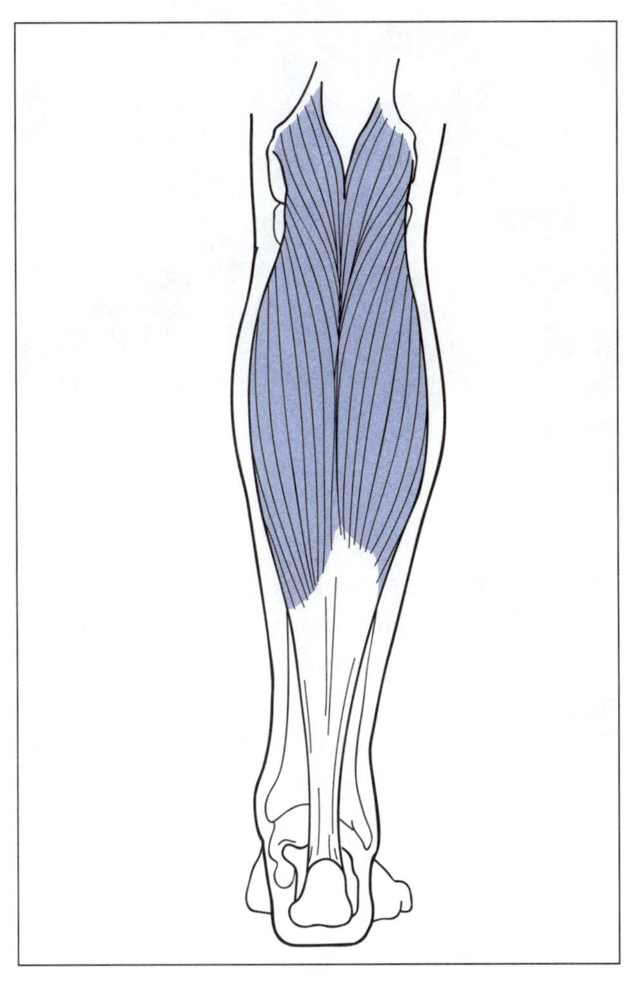

Figure 3-7-4 Gastrocnemius

Origin: Medial head—proximal and posterior aspect of the medial condyle of the femur. Lateral head—lateral and posterior aspect of the lateral condyle of the femur.

Insertion: Via the Achilles tendon into the calcaneus

Innervation: Tibial nerve

Action: Ankle plantar flexion

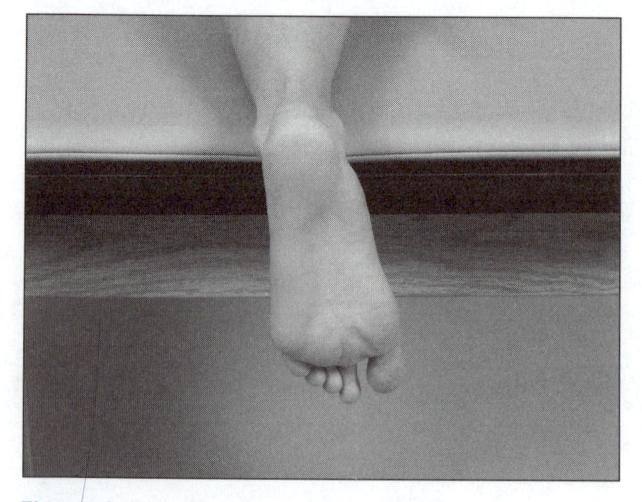

Figure 3-7-5 Start position for gastrocnemius.

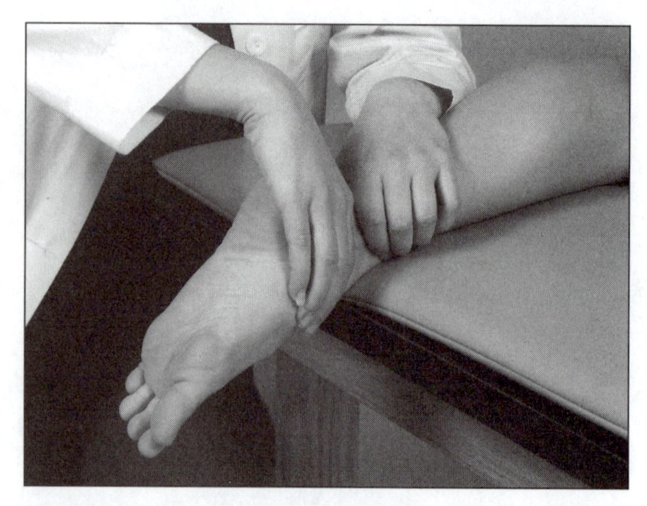

Figure 3-7-6 End position for gastrocnemius.

Normal, Good, Fair

Client Position: Starting—client is prone with knee extended and feet are over edge of testing surface. The ankle is in dorsiflexion (Figure 3-7-5).

Motion—client moves the testing extremity into plantar flexion with toes relaxed. (Figure 3-7-6).

Therapist Position: Stabilize the lower leg proximal to the ankle. Resistance is applied on the posterior aspect of the calcaneus in the direction of dorsiflexion when testing Normal or Good strengths. No resistance is applied when testing Fair strength.

Poor

Client Position: Starting—client is lying on side on test side. The nontest knee is flexed. The testing knee is extended and the ankle is in dorsiflexion.

Motion—client moves the testing extremity into maximal ankle plantar flexion.

Therapist Position: Stabilize the lower leg proximal to the ankle. No resistance is applied in the gravity-eliminated position.

Trace

The gastrocnemius is palpated at the medial and lateral margin of the popliteal fossa, distal to the knee joint.

Some references recommend isolating the gastrocnemius by completing heel raises in standing. This test is not included in this manual because of the variability of grading in the literature.

Ankle: *soleus*

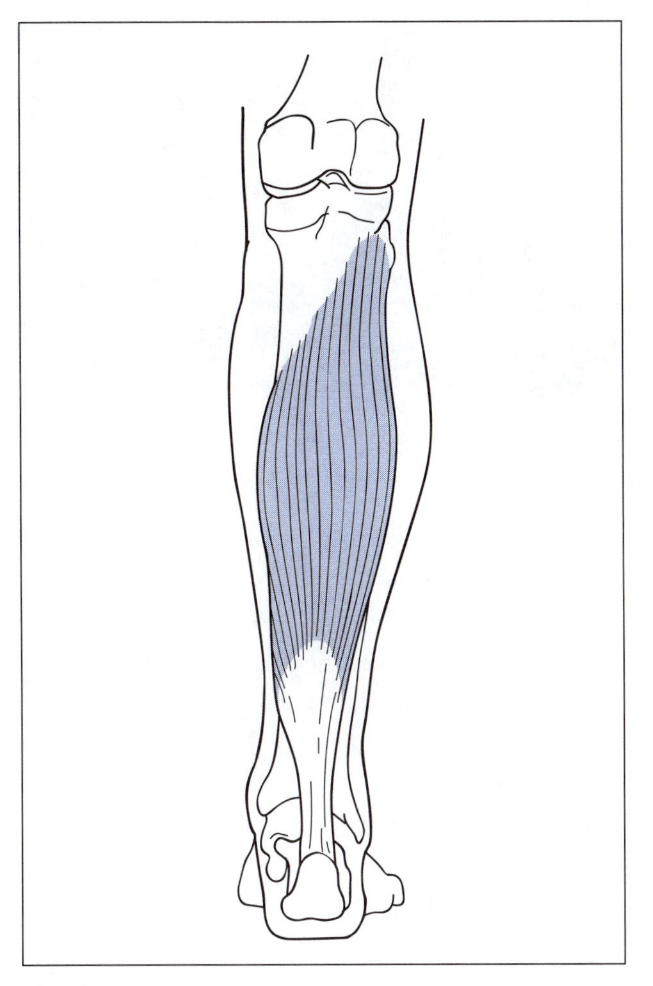

Figure 3-7-7 Soleus

Origin: Posterior aspect of the head and proximal shaft of the fibula, soleal line, and medial border of the tibia

Insertion: Via the Achilles tendon into the calcaneus

Innervation: Tibial nerve

Action: Ankle plantar flexion

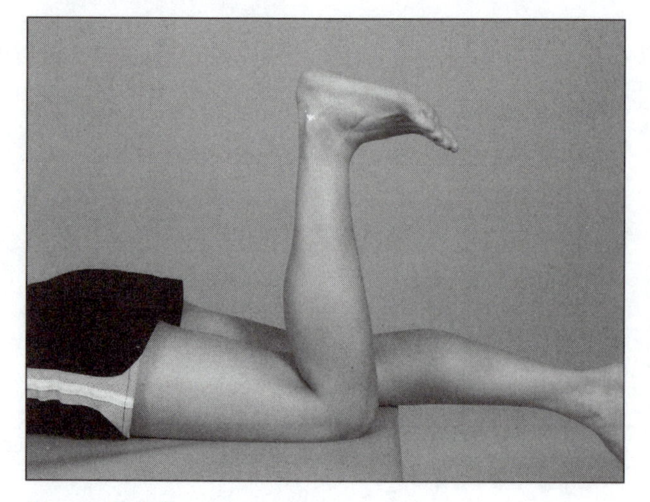

Figure 3-7-8 Start position for soleus

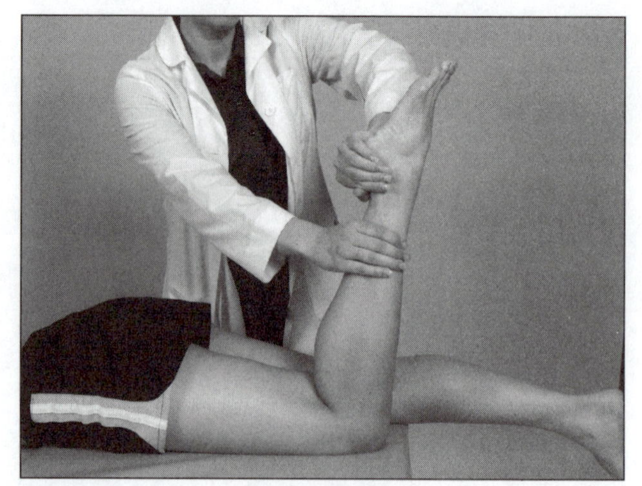

Figure 3-7-9 End position for soleus

Normal, Good, Fair

Client Position: Starting—client is prone with knee flexed. The ankle is in dorsiflexion (Figure 3-7-8).

Motion—the client moves the testing extremity into plantar flexion with toes relaxed (Figure 3-7-9).

Therapist Position: Stabilize the lower leg proximal to the ankle. Resistance is applied on the posterior aspect of the calcaneum in the direction of dorsiflexion when testing Normal or Good strengths. No resistance is applied when testing Fair strength.

Poor

Client Position: Starting—client is lying on test side. The nontest knee is flexed. The testing knee is flexed and the ankle is in dorsiflexion.

Motion—client moves the testing extremity into maximal ankle plantar flexion.

Therapist Position: Stabilize the lower leg proximal to the ankle. No resistance is applied in the gravity-eliminated position.

Trace

The soleus is palpated on either side of the gastrocnemius midway down the calf.

Foot: *tibialis posterior*

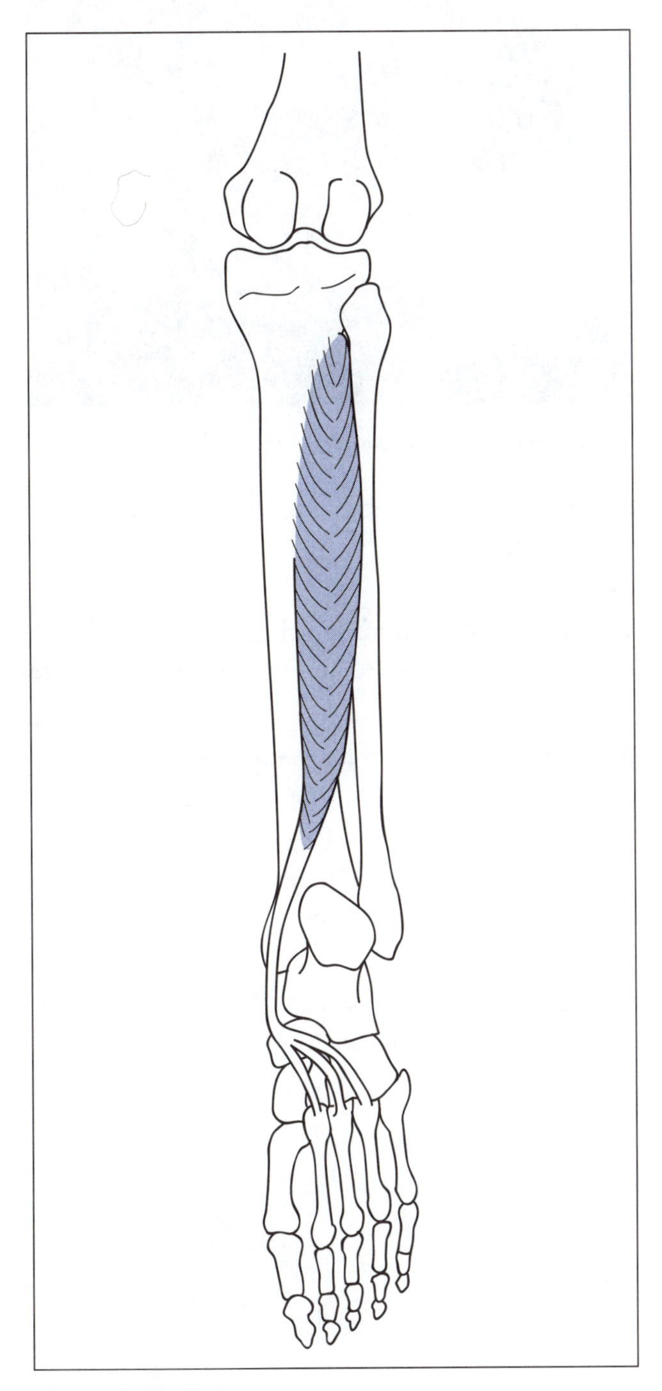

Figure 3-7-10 Tibialis posterior

Origin: Posterolateral surface of the proximal tibia and medial aspect of the proximal fibula

Insertion: Navicular, fibrous expansions to the three cuneiforms, cuboid, and the bases of the second, third, and fourth metatarsals

Innervation: Tibial nerve

Action: Foot inversion

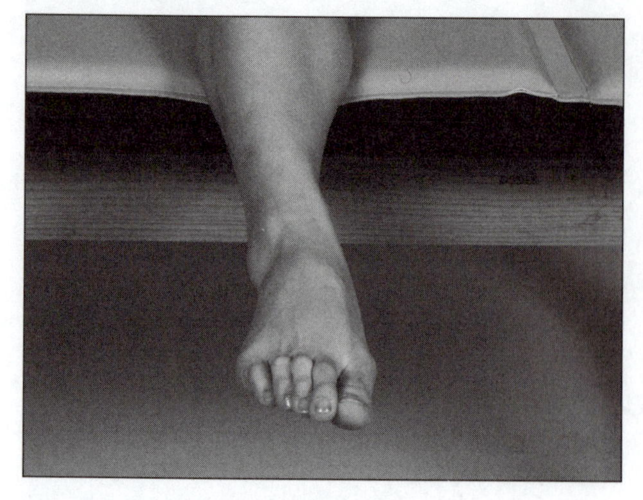

Figure 3-7-11 Start position for tibialis posterior.

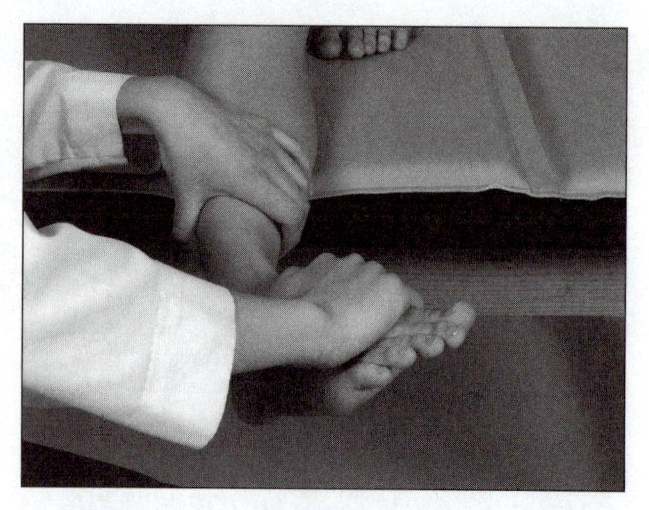

Figure 3-7-12 End position for tibialis posterior.

Normal, Good, Fair

Client Position: Starting—client is sitting with lower leg and foot over edge of testing surface. The ankle is in slight plantar flexion and foot in neutral (Figure 3-7-11).

Motion—client moves the testing extremity into inversion with toes relaxed (Figure 3-7-12).

Therapist Position: Stabilize the lower leg proximal to the ankle. Resistance is applied on the medial border of the forefoot in the direction of foot eversion when testing Normal or Good strengths. No resistance is applied when testing Fair strength.

Poor

Client Position: Starting—client is supine. The testing knee is extended and the foot and ankle are in neutral.

Motion—client moves the testing extremity into maximal foot inversion.

Therapist Position: Stabilize the lower leg proximal to the ankle. No resistance is applied in the gravity-eliminated position.

Trace

The tibialis posterior is palpated between the medial malleolus and the navicular.

Foot: *peroneus longus* and *peroneus brevis* (tested together)

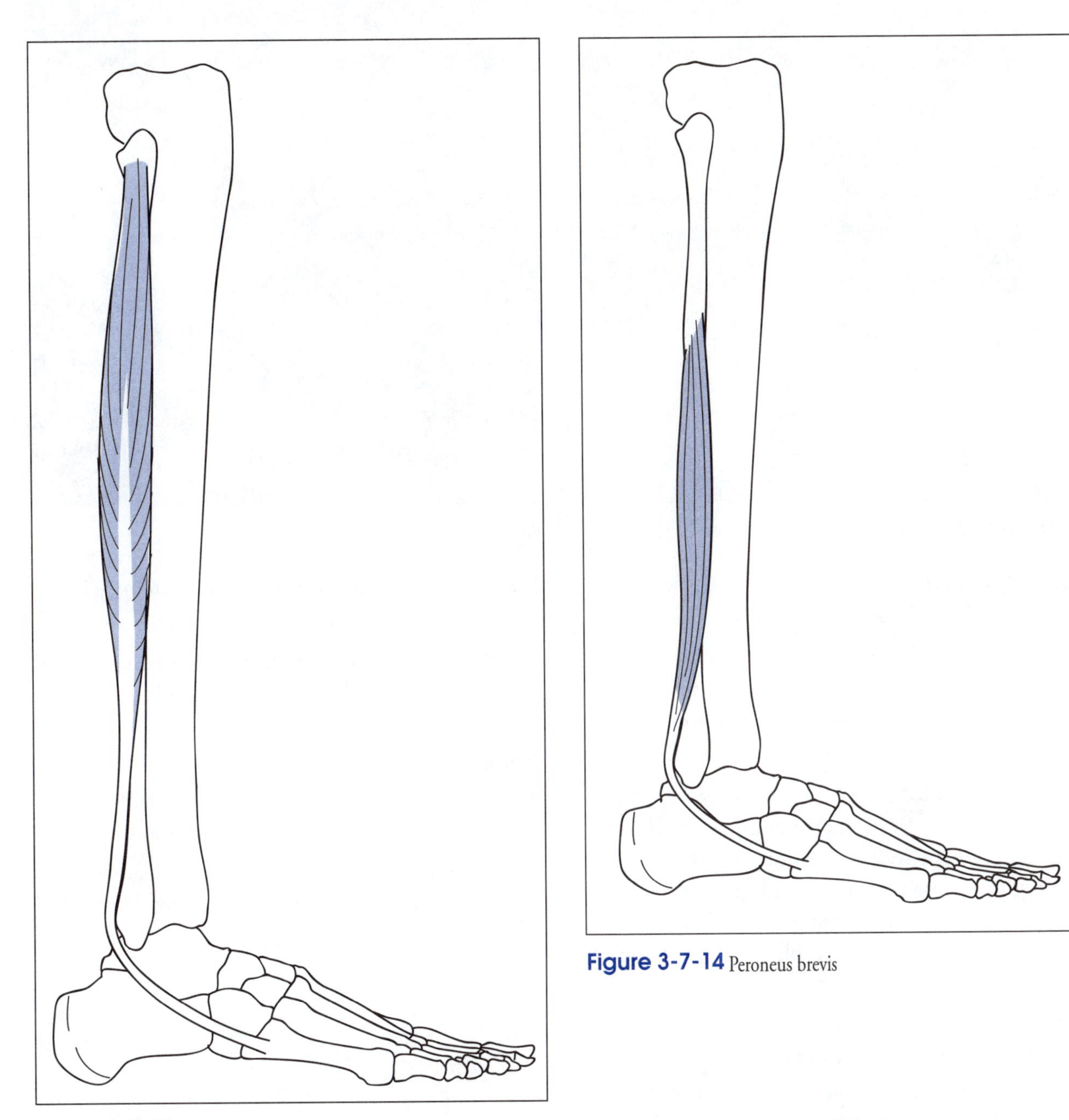

Figure 3-7-13 Peroneus longus

Figure 3-7-14 Peroneus brevis

Peroneus longus

Origin: The head and lateral surface of the fibula

Insertion: Lateral aspect of the base of the fifth metatarsal and the medial cuneiform

Innervation: Superficial peroneal nerve

Action: Foot eversion

Peroneus brevis

Origin: Lateral surface of the fibula, adjacent fascia, and intermuscular septa

Insertion: Lateral aspect of the base of the fifth metatarsal

Innervation: Superficial peroneal nerve

Action: Foot eversion

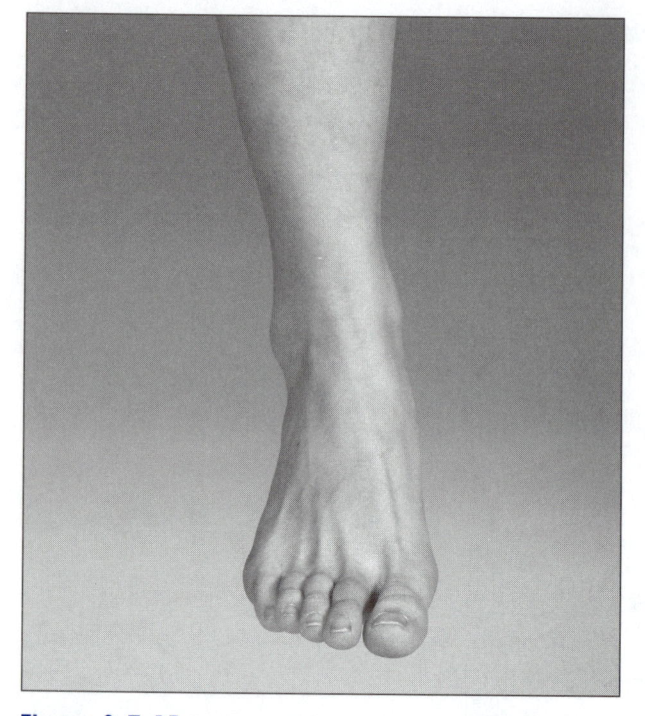

Figure 3-7-15 Start position for peroneus longus and brevis.

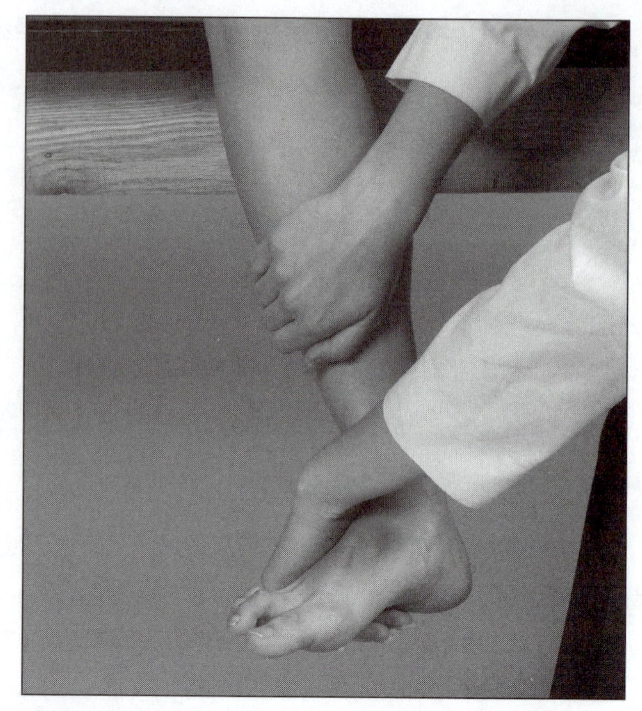

Figure 3-7-16 End position for peroneus longus and brevis.

Normal, Good, Fair

Client Position: Starting—client is sitting with lower leg and foot over edge of testing surface. The ankle and foot are in neutral (Figure 3-7-15).

Motion—client moves the testing extremity into foot eversion (Figure 3-7-16).

Therapist Position: Stabilize the lower leg proximal to the ankle. Resistance is applied on the lateral border of the foot and on the plantar surface of the head of the first metatarsal in the direction of foot inversion when testing Normal or Good strengths. No resistance is applied when testing Fair strength.

Poor

Client Position: Starting—client is supine with the testing knee extended and the heel resting over the edge of testing surface. The foot and ankle are in neutral.

Motion—client moves the testing extremity into maximal foot eversion.

Therapist Position: Stabilize the lower leg proximal to the ankle. No resistance is applied in the gravity-eliminated position.

Trace

The peroneus longus is palpated posterior to the lateral malleolus or distal to the head of the fibula.

The peroneus brevis is palpated proximal to the base of the fifth metatarsal on the lateral border of the foot.

Toes: *flexor hallucis brevis* and *lumbricales* (tested together)

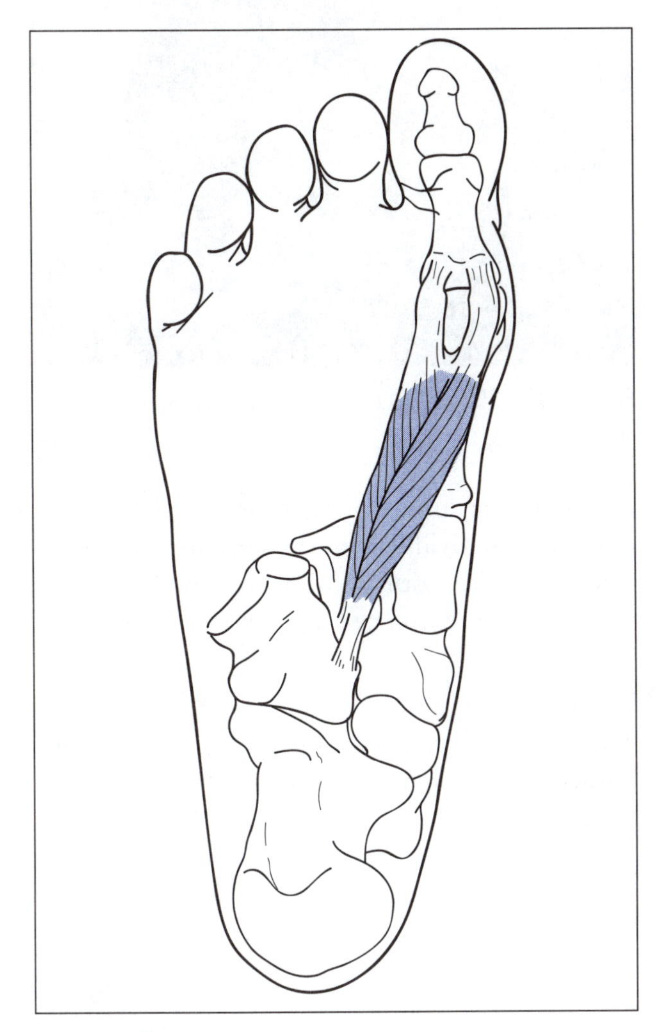

Figure 3-7-17 Flexor hallucis brevis

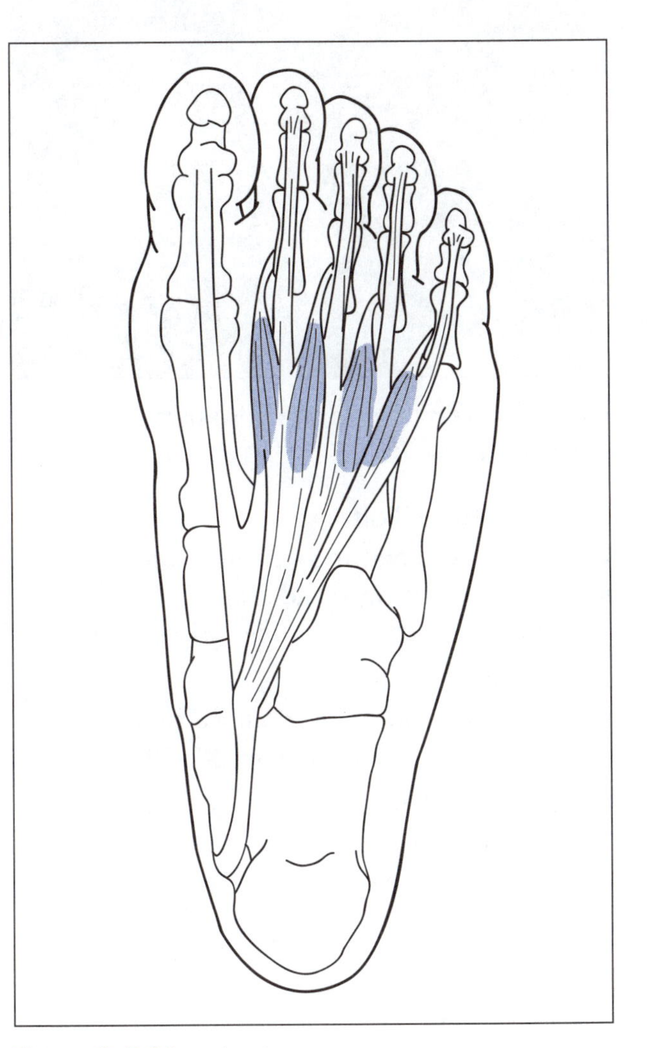

Figure 3-7-18 Lumbricales

Flexor hallucis brevis: great toe

Origin: Medial aspect of the plantar surface of the cuboid, the lateral aspect of the cuneiform, and the tendon of the tibialis posterior muscle

Insertion: Medial and lateral aspects of the base of the proximal phalanx of the great toe

Innervation: Medial plantar nerve

Action: MTP joint flexion of the great toe

Lumbricales: toes #2–5

Origin: Flexor digitorum longus

Insertion: Expansions of extensor tendons of toes #2–5

Innervation: Medial and lateral plantar nerves

Action: MTP flexion

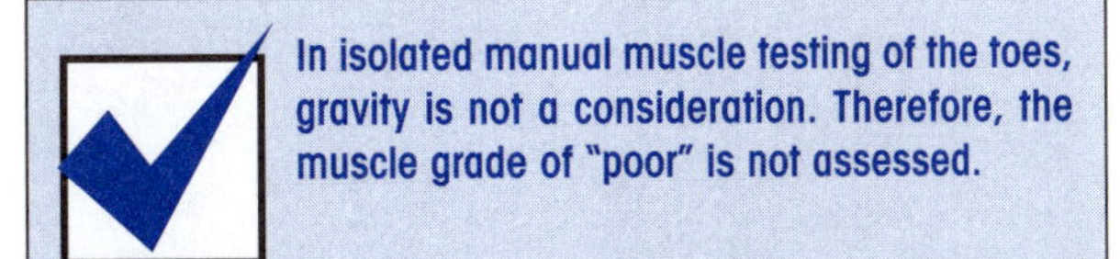

In isolated manual muscle testing of the toes, gravity is not a consideration. Therefore, the muscle grade of "poor" is not assessed.

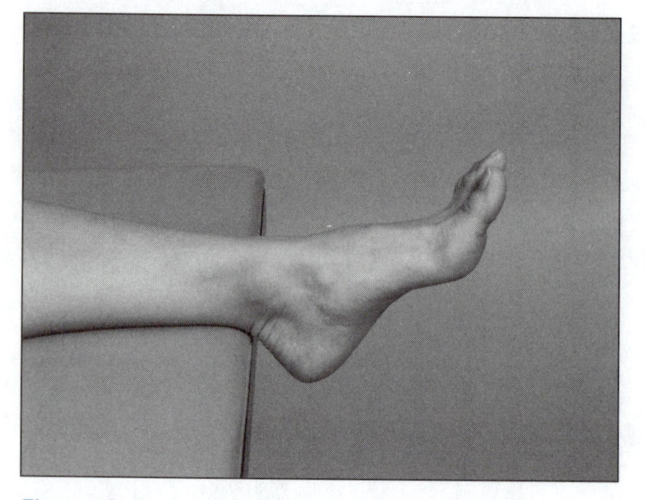

Figure 3-7-19 Start position for flexor hallucis brevis and lumbricales.

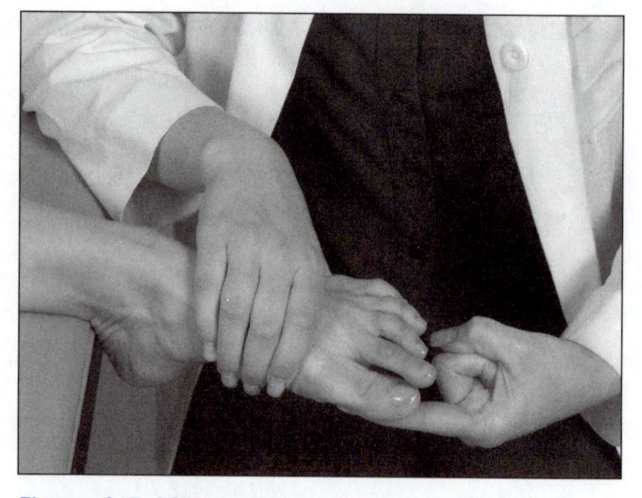

Figure 3-7-20 End position for flexor hallucis brevis and lumbricales.

Normal, Good, Fair

Client Position: Starting—client is supine. The testing knee is extended and lower leg and foot resting in neutral on the testing surface (Figure 3-7-19).

Motion—client moves the testing extremity into MTP flexion of each toe (Figure 3-7-20).

Therapist Position: Stabilize the metatarsals and maintain IP joint extension. Resistance is applied on the plantar surface of the proximal phalanges of each toe individually in the direction of MTP extension when testing Normal or Good strengths. No resistance is applied when testing Fair strength.

Trace

The flexor hallucis brevis is palpated on the medial border of the sole of the foot. The lumbricales are not palpable.

Toes: *flexor hallacis longus, flexor digitorum longus,* and *flexor digitorum brevis* (tested together)

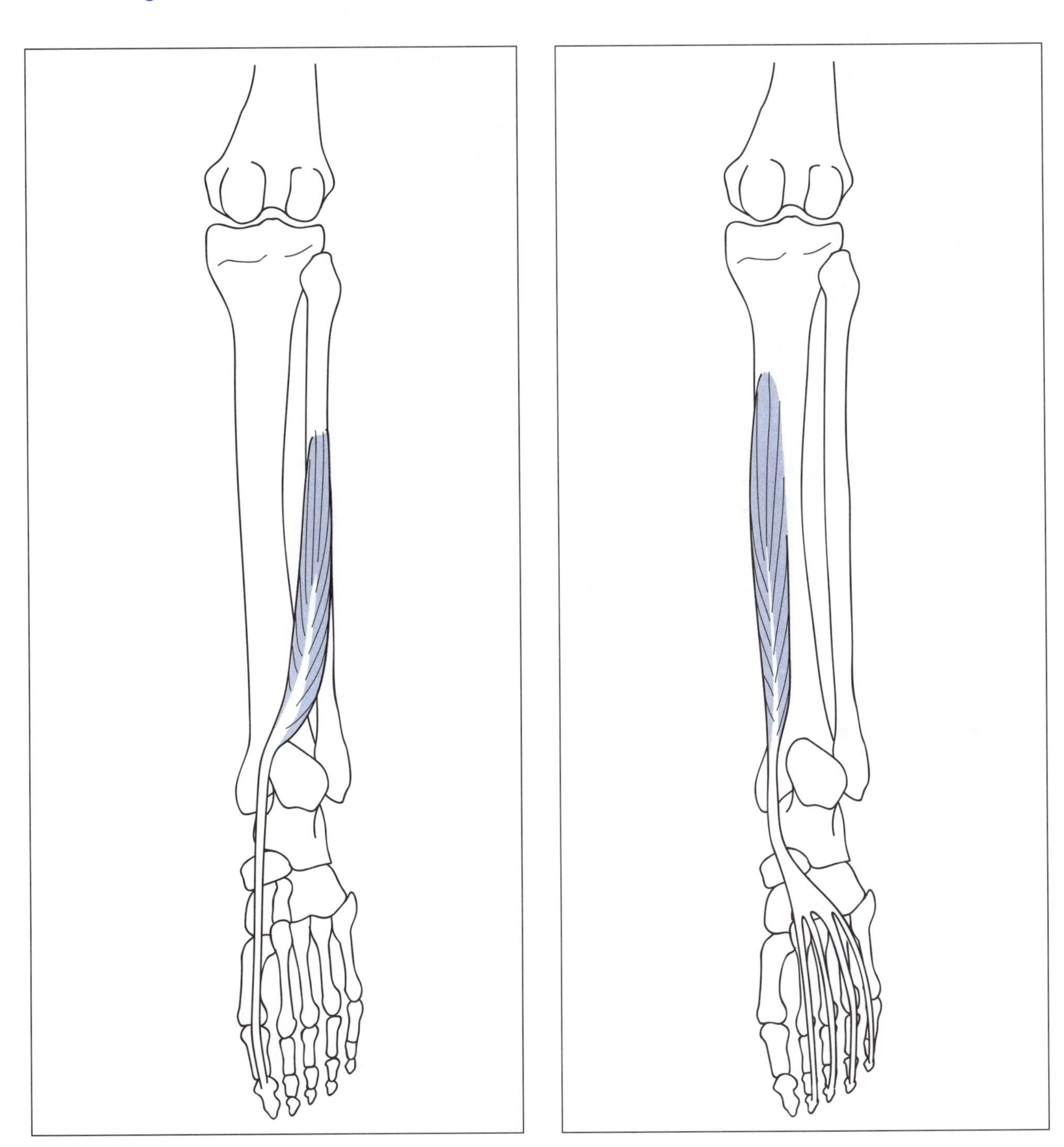

Figure 3-7-21 Flexor hallucis longus

Figure 3-7-22 Flexor digitorum longus

Flexor hallucis longus: great toe

Origin: Posterior surface of the fibula

Insertion: Plantar aspect of the base of the distal phalanx of the great toe

Innervation: Tibial nerve

Action: IP joint flexion of the great toe

Flexor digitorum longus: toes #2–5

Origin: Posterior surface of the tibia

Insertion: Plantar aspects of the bases of the distal phalanges of toes #2–5

Innervation: Medial plantar nerve

Action: DIP flexion

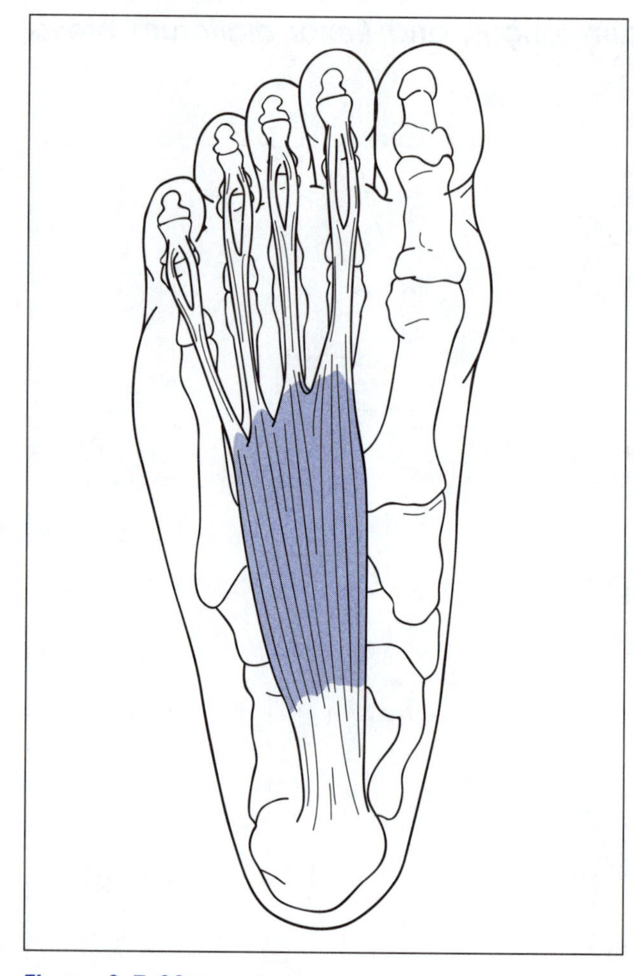

Figure 3-7-23 Flexor digitorum brevis

Flexor digitorum brevis: toes #2-5

Origin: Calcaneal tuberosity and medial and lateral intermuscular septa

Insertion: Medial and lateral aspects of the middle phalanges of toes #2–5

Innervation: Medial plantar nerve

Action: PIP flexion

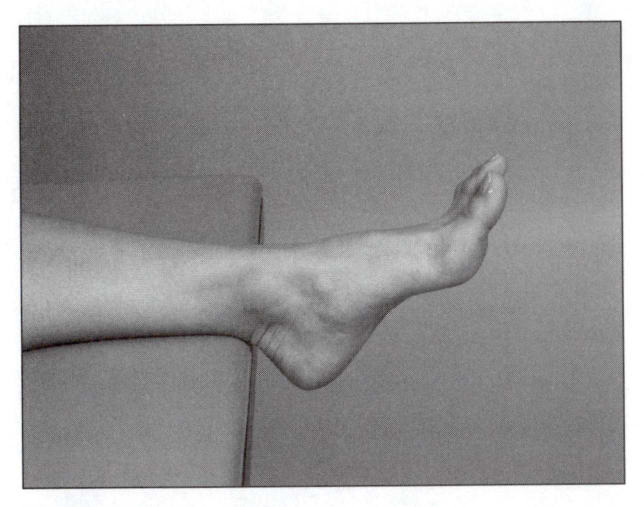

Figure 3-7-24 Start position for flexor hallucis longus, flexor digitorum longus, and flexor digitorum brevis.

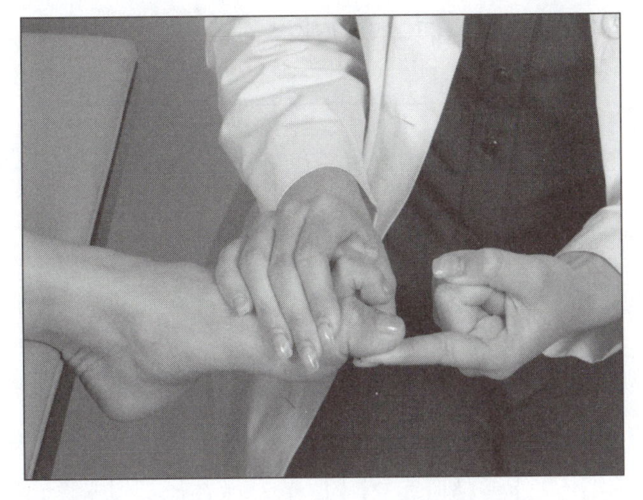

Figure 3-7-25 End position for flexor hallucis longus, flexor digitorum longus, and flexor digitorum brevis.

Normal, Good, Fair

Client Position: Starting—client is supine. The testing knee is extended and lower leg and foot resting in neutral on the testing surface (Figure 3-7-24).

Motion—client moves the testing extremity into IP flexion of each toe (Figure 3-7-25).

Therapist Position: Stabilize the MTP joint of each toe tested. Resistance is applied on the plantar surface of the distal phalanx of the great toe and the distal and middle phalanges of toes #2–5 individually in the direction of IP extension when testing Normal or Good strengths. No resistance is applied when testing Fair strength.

Trace

The flexor hallucis longus may be palpated on the plantar surface of the proximal phalanx of the great toe or inferior to the medial malleolus.

The flexor digitorum brevis is not palpable.

The flexor digitorum longus may be palpated on the plantar aspect of the proximal phalanges.

Toes: *abductor hallucis*

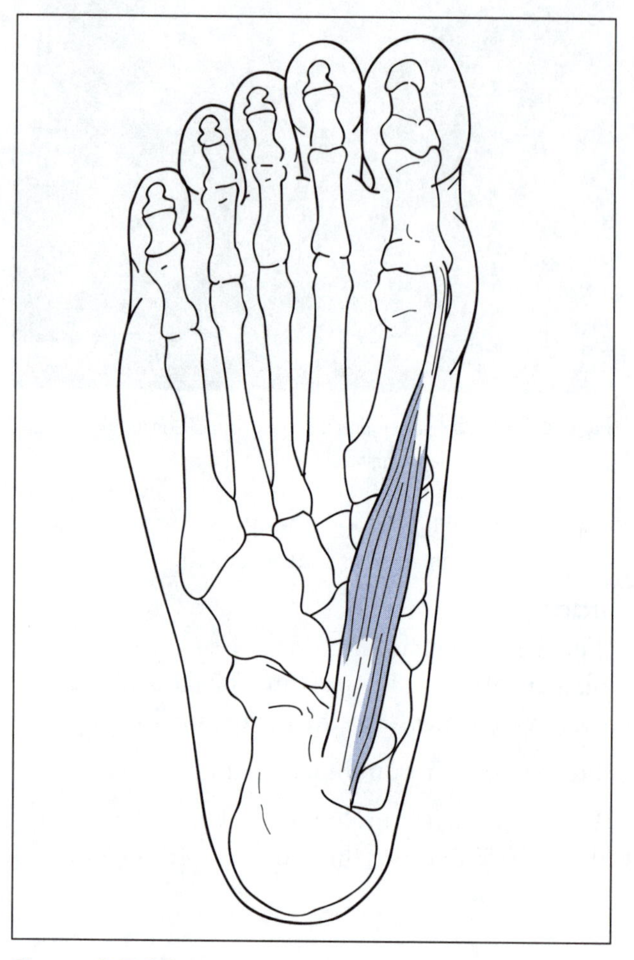

Figure 3-7-26 Abductor hallucis

Origin: Medial process of the calcaneal tuberosity, flexor retinaculum, and medial intermuscular septa

Insertion: Medial aspect of the base of the proximal phalanx of the great toe

Innervation: Medial plantar nerve

Action: Abduction of the great toe

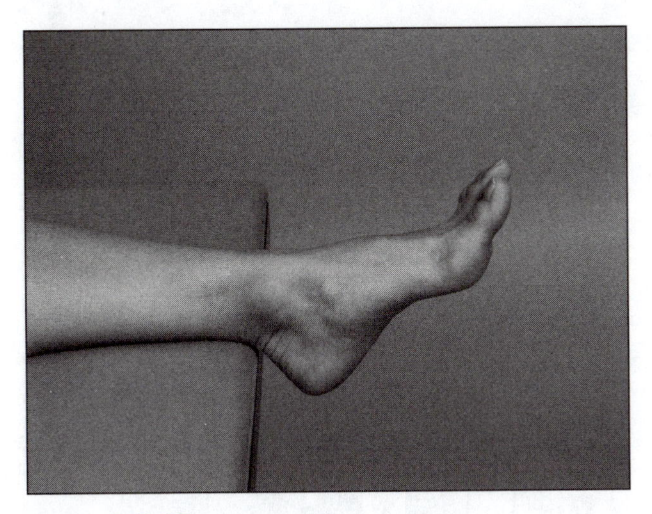

Figure 3-7-27 Start position for abductor hallucis.

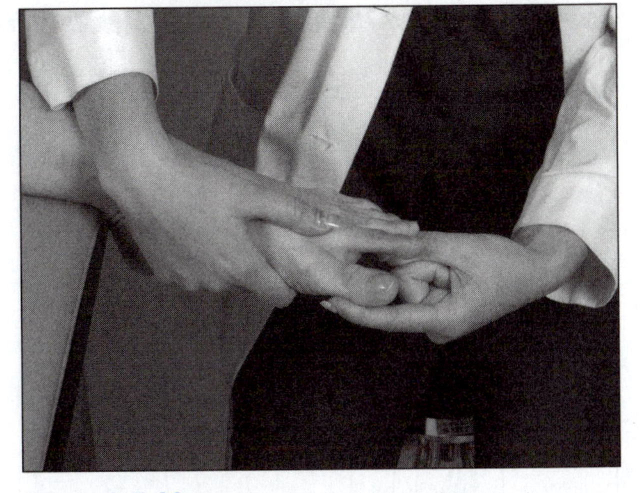

Figure 3-7-28 End position for abductor hallucis.

Normal, Good, Fair

Client Position: Starting—client is supine. The testing knee is extended and lower leg and foot resting in neutral on the testing surface. The toes are in adduction (Figure 3-7-27).

Motion—client moves the great toe into abduction (Figure 3-7-28).

Therapist Position: Stabilize the first metatarsal. Resistance is applied on the medial aspect of the proximal phalanx of the great toe in the direction of adduction when testing Normal or Good strengths. No resistance is applied when testing Fair strength.

Trace

The abductor hallucis is palpated on the medial border of the foot superficial to the first metatarsal.

Toes: *abductor digiti minimi* and *dorsal interossei* (tested together)

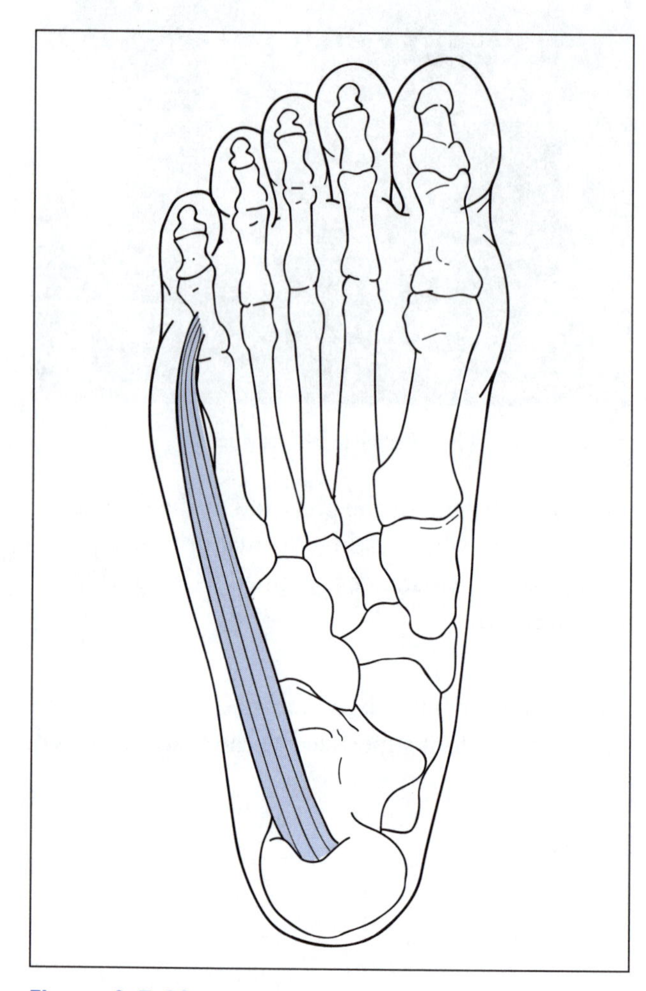

Figure 3-7-29 Abductor digiti minimi

Abductor digiti minimi

Origin: Medial and lateral process of the calcaneal tuberosity

Insertion: Lateral aspect of the base of the proximal phalanx of the fifth toe

Innervation: Lateral plantar nerve

Action: Abduction of the fifth toe

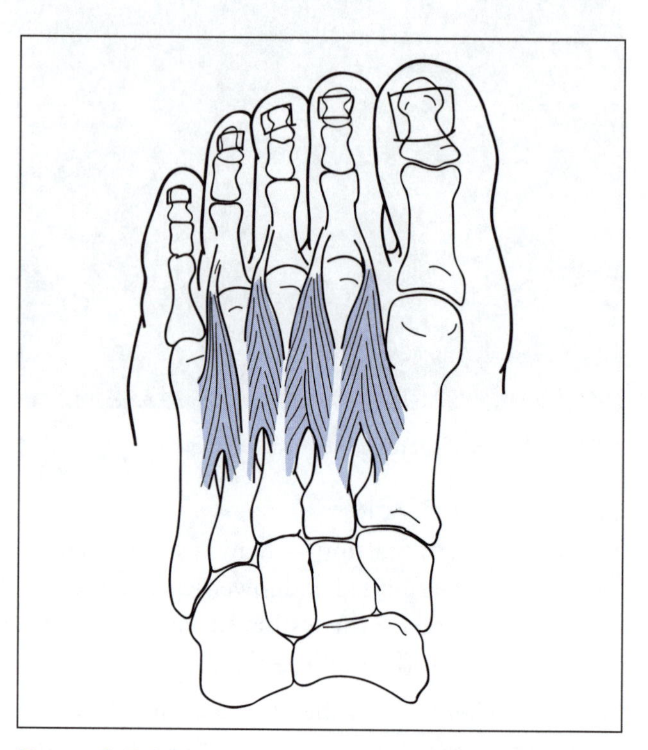

Figure 3-7-30 Dorsal interossei

Dorsal interossei

Origin: Sides of metatarsals

Insertion: Medial and lateral aspect of toe #2 and lateral aspect of toes #3 and #4

Innervation: Lateral plantar nerve

Action: Abduction of the toes #2–4

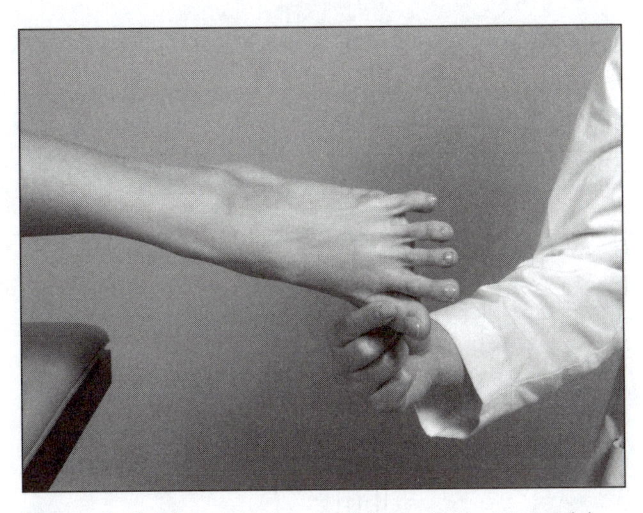

Figure 3-7-31 Functional test of abductor digiti minimi and dorsal interossei.

Manual muscle testing is not performed on these muscles. Observation of toes #2–5 provides a functional level as the tester stabilizes the great toe (Figure 3-7-31).

Toes: *extensor hallucis longus, extensor digitorum longus,* and *extensor digitorum brevis* (tested together)

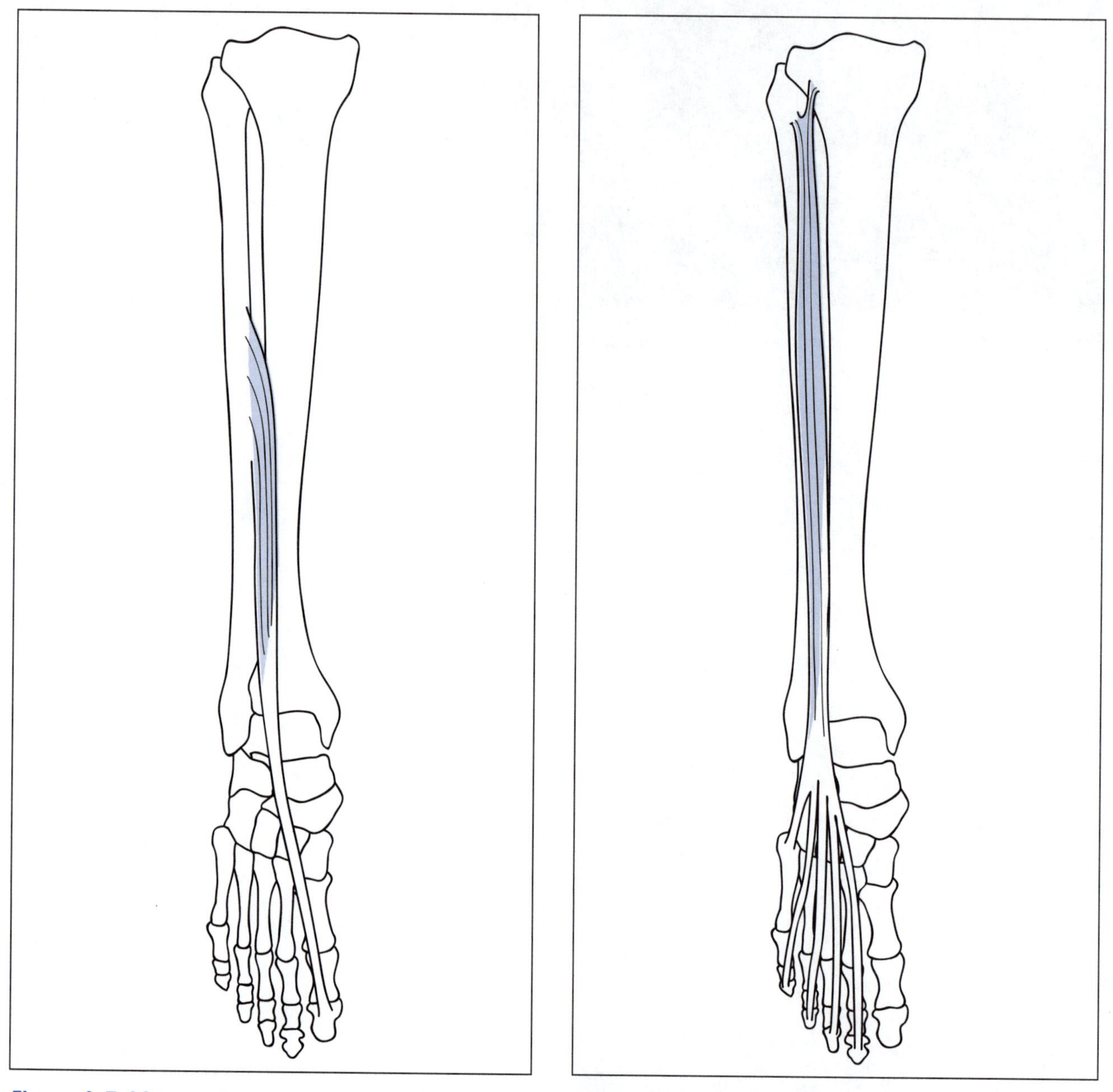

Figure 3-7-32 Extensor hallucis longus

Figure 3-7-33 Extensor digitorum longus

Extensor hallucis longus: great toe

Origin: Anterior surface of the fibula and the interosseous membrane

Insertion: Dorsal surface of the base of the distal phalanx of the great toe

Innervation: Deep peroneal nerve

Action: IP joint extension of the great toe

Extensor digitorum longus: toes #2–5

Origin: Lateral condyle of the tibia, medial surface of the fibula, anterior surface of the interosseous membrane, and crural fascia

Insertion: Dorsal aspect of the base of the middle phalanx of toes #2–5 and dorsal aspect of the base of the distal phalanx of toes #2–5

Innervation: Deep peroneal nerve

Action: DIP flexion

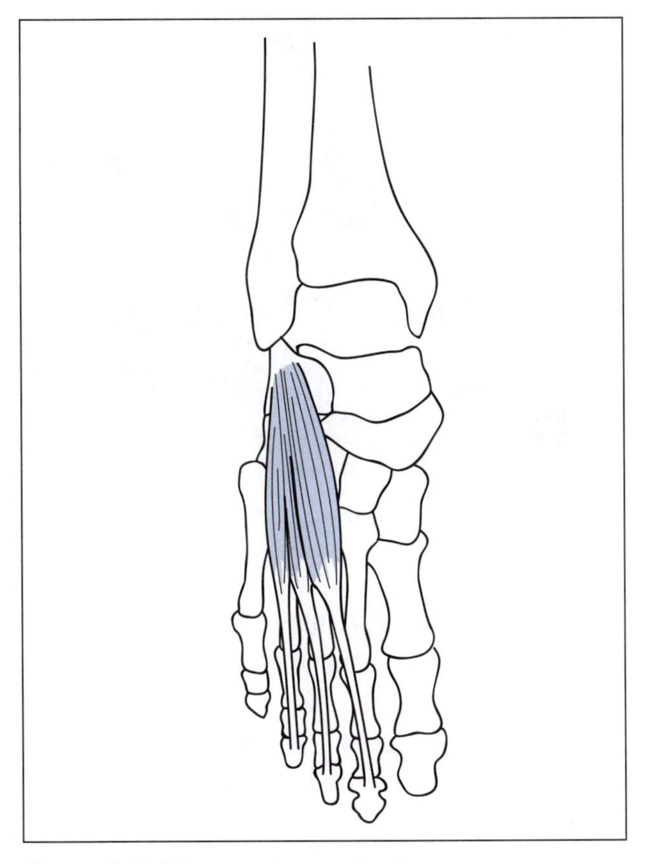

Figure 3-7-34 Extensor digitorum brevis

Extensor digitorum brevis: great toe and #2–4

Origin: Dorsal surface of the calcaneum

Insertion: Tendons to toes #2–4 of the corresponding extensor digitorum longus tendons and proximal phalanx of great toe

Innervation: Deep peroneal nerve

Action: MTP extension of the great toe and IP extension of toes #2–4

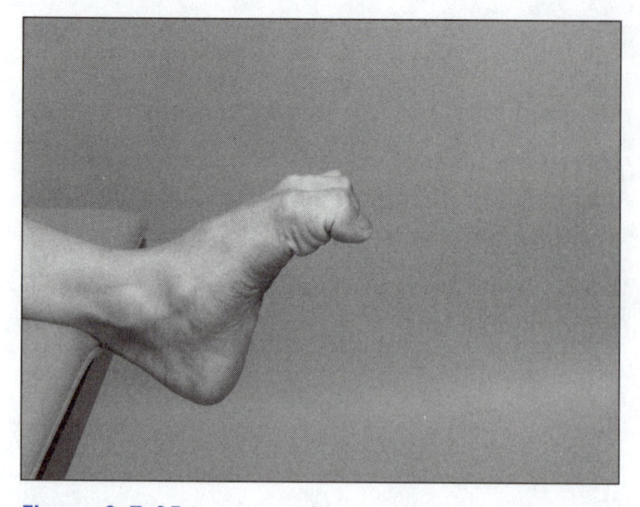

Figure 3-7-35 Start position for extensor hallucis longus, extensor digitorum longus, and extensor digitorum brevis.

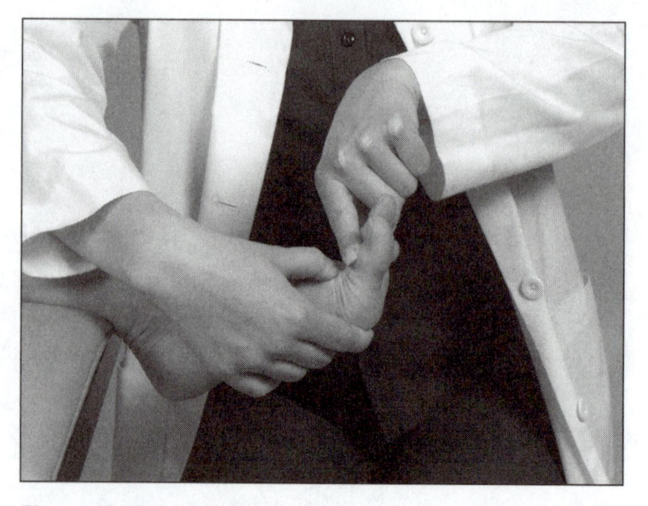

Figure 3-7-36 End position for extensor hallucis longus, extensor digitorum longus, and extensor digitorum brevis.

Normal, Good, Fair

Client Position: Starting—client is supine. The testing knee is extended and lower leg and foot resting in neutral on the testing surface. The toes are flexed (Figure 3-7-35).

Motion—client moves the great toe into MTP extension and toes #2–4 into IP extension (Figure 3-7-36). If it is too difficult for the client to extend toes in isolation, they may be tested as a group.

Therapist Position: Stabilize the metatarsals of each toe tested. Resistance is applied on the dorsal surface of the distal phalanx of the great toe and the distal surface of toes #2–5 individually (or together) in the direction of IP flexion when testing Normal or Good strengths. No resistance is applied when testing Fair strength.

Trace

The extensor hallucis longus is palpated on the dorsal aspect of the first MTP joint or on the anterior aspect of the ankle joint lateral to the tendon of the tibialis anterior.

The extensor digitorum brevis is palpated on the dorsal aspect of the foot anterior to the lateral malleolus.

The extensor digitorum longus is palpated on the dorsal aspect of the metatarsal bones of toes #2–5 or on the anterior aspect of the ankle joint lateral to the tendon of the extensor hallucis longus.

Glossary

Active range of motion—movement of the extremity by the client through the available arc of motion without the therapist's assistance

Against gravity—a position in which the client moves the extremity or body part perpendicular to the floor because the force of gravity is exerted down toward the floor

Axis of the body—the location around which movement of the body occurs

Biomechanical frame of reference—the frame of reference that defines function and dysfunction in terms of an individual's range of motion, strength, and endurance

Clinical reasoning—the decision-making process used to determine the need for further assessment, taking into account all known factors and observations

Compensation—use of alternative motions by the client to achieve the active range of motion that has been requested by the therapist

End feel—the feeling that is elicited when the joint is brought through the entire available range of motion

Frames of reference—a guide to the therapist for the evaluation and intervention process

Fulcrum—part of the goniometer that is placed over the axis of motion when measuring range of motion

Functional observation—observation of a client completing a functional activity

Goniometer—the most commonly used instrument for measuring joint motion

Goniometry—the measurement of arc of motion of a joint

Gravity-eliminated—a position in which the client moves the extremity or body part parallel to the floor

Gross manual muscle testing—a test of entire muscle groups rather than individual muscles

Isolated manual muscle testing—a test of each specific muscle within a muscle group

Movable arm—part of the goniometer that is aligned with the plane of motion but is distal to the joint being measured and follows the arc of motion

Passive range of motion—movement of the extremity by the therapist through the available arc of motion without the client's assistance

Plane of the body—the flat surface along which movement of the body occurs

Resistance—application of pressure by the therapist in order to determine which muscle strength grade a client demonstrates

Screening—an informal functional assessment to determine quickly which joints need further assessment

Stabilization—applied manually by the therapist in order to avoid compensation by the client

Stationary arm—part of the goniometer that stays fixed and aligned with the plane of motion proximal to the joint being measured

References

American Academy of Orthopedic Surgeons. (1965). *Joint motion: Method of measuring and recording.* Chicago: Author.

American Medical Association. (1988). *Guides to the evaluation of permanent impairment.* Chicago: Author.

Clarkson, H. M., & Gilewich, G. B. (1989). *Musculoskeletal assessment: Joint range of motion and manual muscle strength.* Baltimore, MD: Williams & Wilkins.

Kendall, F. P., & McCreary, E. K. (1983). *Muscles: Testing and function* (3rd ed.). Baltimore, MD: Williams & Wilkins.

Mosey, A.C. (1970). *Three frames of references for mental health.* Thorofare, NJ: Slack, Inc.

Suggested Readings

The American Society of Hand Therapists. (1992). *Clinical assessment recommendations* (2nd ed.). Chicago: Author.

Cole, M.B. (1998). *Group dynamics in occupational therapy.* Thorofare, NJ: Slack, Inc.

Daniels, L., & Worthingham, C. (1986). *Muscle testing* (5th ed.). Philadelphia, PA: W.B. Saunders Co.

Jenkins, D. B. (1998). *Hollinshead's functional anatomy of the limbs and back* (7th ed.). Philadelphia, PA: W.B. Saunders Co.

Norkin, C. C., & White, D. J. (1995). *Measurement of joint motion: A guide to goniometry* (2nd ed.). Philadelphia, PA: F.A. Davis Company.

Rockwood, C.A., & Matsen, F.M. (1990). *The shoulder* (Vol. 1). Philadelphia, PA: W.B. Saunders Co.

Appendix A: Muscle Tables

The Trunk

MUSCLE	ORIGIN	INSERTION	INNERVATION	ACTION
Rectus abdominus	Pubic crest, ligaments of the pubic symphysis	Xyphoid process, ribs 5–7	Lower intercostal nerves	Trunk flexion
Internal oblique	Iliopsoas fascia & inguinal ligament, anterior iliac crest, thoracolumbar fascia	Aponeurosis into the linea alba, lower ribs	Lower intercostal nerves, iliohypogastric & ilioinguinal nerves	Trunk flexion & trunk oblique rotation
External oblique	Lower 6 ribs	Anterior iliac crest, aponeurosis into the linea alba	Lower intercostal nerves, iliohypogastric & ilioinguinal nerves	Trunk flexion & trunk oblique rotation
Erector spinae	Common tendon of origin: posterior surface of the sacrum, iliac crest, spinous processes of lumbar & last 2 thoracic vertebrae (each specific muscle of the erector spinae group also has its own specific origin)	Each specific muscle of the erector spinae group has its own insertion	Dorsal rami of spinal nerves specific to each muscle in the erector spinae group	Trunk extension
Interspinales	Spinous processes of vertebrae	Spinous processes of vertebrae	Dorsal & ventral rami of spinal nerves	Trunk extension
Intertransversarii	Transverse processes of vertebrae	Transverse processes of vertebrae	Dorsal & ventral rami of spinal nerves	Lateral flexion
Multifidi	Sacrum & transverse processes of C4–L5	Spinous processes of lumbar through second cervical vertebrae	Dorsal rami of spinal nerves	Trunk extension & trunk oblique rotation
Semispinalis thoracis	Transverse processes of T6–T10 vertebrae	Spinous processes of C6, C7 & T1–4	Dorsal rami of cervical and thoracic spinal nerves	Trunk extension
Quadratus lumborum	Iliolumbar ligament, iliac crest	Inferior border of last rib, transverse processes of L1–4	T12, L1–4	Pelvic elevation & trunk lateral flexion

The Neck

MUSCLE	ORIGIN	INSERTION	INNERVATION	ACTION
Longus capitus	Transverse processes of C3–6	Occipital bone	Ventral rami of C1–3	Neck flexion
Longus colli	Bodies of T1–3, transverse processes of C3–5, bodies of C5–7	Transverse processes of C5–6, anterior surface of atlas, bodies of C2–4	Ventral rami of C2–6	Neck flexion
Rectus capitis anterior	Transverse processes of atlas	Occipital bone	Ventral rami of C1–2	Neck lateral flexion
Sternocleido-mastoid	Sternum, medial 1/3 of clavicle	Mastoid process of temporal bone	Accessory nerve (motor), C2–3 (sensory)	Neck flexion
Scalenus anterior	Transverse processes of C3–6	1st rib	Ventral rami of cervical spinal nerves	Neck flexion
Erector spinae	*see Trunk	*see Trunk	*see Trunk	Neck extension
Obliquus capitus	Inferior—spinous process of axis Superior—transverse process atlas	Occipital bone	Dorsal ramus of C1	Inferior—neck rotation Superior—neck extension & neck lateral flexion
Rectus capitis posterior	Spinous process of axis	Occipital bone	Dorsal ramus of C1	Neck extension & neck rotation
Splenius capitus	Ligamentum nuchae, spinous processes of C7 & T1–4	Mastoid process, occipital bone	Dorsal rami of middle cervical spinal nerves	Neck extension & neck rotation
Splenius cervicis	Spinous processes of T3–6	Transverse processes of C1–3	Dorsal rami of lower cervical spinal nerves	Neck extension & neck rotation
Semispinalis cervicis	Transverse processes of T1–6	Spinous processes of C2–5	Dorsal rami of cervical & thoracic spinal nerves	Neck extension
Semispinalis capitis	Transverse processes of T1–7, articular processes of C5–7	Occipital bone	Dorsal rami of cervical & thoracic spinal nerves	Neck extension

The Shoulder & Scapula

MUSCLE	ORIGIN	INSERTION	INNERVATION	ACTION
Posterior deltoid	Inferior lip, spine of scapula	Deltoid tuberosity of the humerus	Axillary nerve	Humeral extension, humeral horizontal abduction & humeral external rotation
Middle deltoid	Acromion process	Deltoid tuberosity of the humerus	Axillary nerve	Humeral abduction
Anterior deltoid	Lateral 1/3 of clavicle	Deltoid tuberosity of the humerus	Axillary nerve	Humeral flexion, humeral hori-ontal adduction & humeral inte-nal rotation
Coracobrachialis	Coracoid process of the scapula	Opposite the deltoid tuberosity on the medial aspect of the mid-humerus	Musculocutaneous nerve	Humeral flexion
Pectoralis major (clavicular head)	Anterior surface of sternal 1/2 of clavicle	Greater tubercle of the humerus	Lateral & medial pectoral nerves	Humeral flexion, humeral horizontal adduction & humeral adduction
Pectoralis major (sternal head)	Sternum, costal cartilage ribs 1–6	Greater tubercle of the humerus	Lateral & medial pectoral nerves	Humeral horizontal adduction & humeral extension
Latissimus dorsi	Spinous process of the last 6 thoracic vertebrae, all lumbar & sacral vertebrae, posterior iliac crest, posterior last 3 ribs, inferior angle of the scapula	Bottom of intertubercular groove of the humerus	Thoracodorsal nerves	Humeral extension, humeral adduction, humeral internal rotation & scapular depression
Subscapularis	Subscapular fossa of the scapula	Lesser tubercle of the humerus, capsule of the shoulder joint	Superior upper & inferior lower subscapular nerves	Humeral internal rotation & is one of the rotator cuff muscles
Infraspinatus	Medial 2/3 of infraspinatus fossa of the scapula	Greater tubercle of the humerus, capsule of the shoulder joint	Suprascapular nerve	Humeral external rotation, humeral horizontal abduction & is one of the rotator cuff muscles

(*continues*)

The Shoulder & Scapula (*continued*)

MUSCLE	ORIGIN	INSERTION	INNERVATION	ACTION
Teres minor	Upper 2/3 of the lateral, dorsal border of the scapula	Greater tubercle of the humerus, capsule of the shoulder joint	Axillary nerve	Humeral external rotation, humeral horizontal abduction & is one of the rotator cuff muscles
Supraspinatus	Medial 2/3 of the supraspinatus fossa	Greater tubercle of the humerus, capsule of the shoulder joint	Suprascapular nerve	Humeral abduction & is one of the rotator cuff muscles
Upper trapezius	Occipital protuberance, medial 1/3 of nuchal line of the occipital bone, ligamentum nuchae, spinous process of C7	Lateral 1/3 of clavicle, acromion process	Spinal accessory nerve	Scapular elevation & scapular upward rotation
Levator scapulae	Transverse process of C1–C4	Superior angle of the scapula	Dorsal scapular nerve	Scapular elevation
Middle trapezius	Inferior aspect of the ligamentum nuchae, C7–T5	Medial margin of the acromion process, superior spine of the scapula	Spinal accessory nerve	Scapular adduction
Lower trapezius	T6–T12	Medial aspect of the scapula, tubercle at the apex of the spine of the scapula	Spinal accessory nerve	Scapular depression & scapular upward rotation
Teres major	Dorsal surface of the inferior angle of the scapula	Below the lesser tuberosity of the humerus, posterior to the latissimus dorsi insertion	Inferior subscapular nerve	Humeral extension, humeral internal rotation & humeral adduction
Rhomboids	Spinous process of C7–T5, ligamentum nuchae	Entire medial border of the scapula	Dorsal scapular	Scapular adduction & scapular downward rotation
Servatus anterior	Ribs 1–9	Anterior medial border of the scapula	Long thoracic nerve	Scapular abduction
Pectoralis minor	Ribs 3, 4, 5	Coracoid process of the scapula, superior surface	Medial & lateral pectoral nerve	Scapular abduc- downward rotation

The Elbow and Forearm

MUSCLE	ORIGIN	INSERTION	INNERVATION	ACTION
Biceps brachii	Short head—coracoid process of the scapula Long head—supraglenoid process of the scapula	Short head—posterior aspect of the radial tuberosity Long head—bicipital aponeurosis	Musculocutaneous nerve	Elbow flexion & forearm supination
Brachialis	Distal 1/2 of the anterior aspect of the humerus, medial/lateral intermuscular septa	Tuberosity & coronoid process of the ulna	Musculocutaneous & radial nerves	Elbow flexion
Brachioradialis	Proximal 2/3 of lateral supracondylar ridge of the humerus, lateral intramuscular septa	Lateral side of the base of ulnar styloid process	Radial nerve	Elbow flexion
Triceps	Long head—infraglenoid tubercle of the scapula Lateral head—posterolateral surface of the humerus between the radial groove and the insertion of the teres minor Medial head—posterior surface of the humerus below the radial groove	Posterior surface of the olecranon process	Radial nerve	Elbow extension
Anconeus	Lateral epicondyle of the humerus	Lateral side of the olecranon process, upper 1/4 of the ulna	Radial nerve	Elbow extension
Supinator	Lateral epicondyle of the humerus	Proximal 1/3 of the radius	Posterior interosseus branch of the radial nerve	Forearm supination
Pronator teres	Humeral head—proximal to the medial epicondyle and common flexor tendon Ulnar head—medial side of the coronoid process of the ulna	Lateral surface of the radial shaft	Median nerve	Forearm pronation
Pronator quadratus	Distal 1/4 of the anterior surface of the ulnar shaft	Distal 1/4 of the anterior surface of the radial shaft	Anterior interosseous branch of the median nerve	Forearm pronation

The Wrist

MUSCLE	ORIGIN	INSERTION	INNERVATION	ACTION
Flexor carpi radialis	Medial epicondyle, common extensor tendon	Base of the 2nd metacarpal	Median nerve	Wrist flexion & wrist radial deviation
Flexor carpi ulnaris	Medial epicondyle, common flexor tendon, proximal ulna	Pisiform	Ulnar nerve	Wrist flexion & wrist ulnar deviation
Palmaris longus	Medial epicondyle, common flexor tendon	Palmar aponeurosis	Median nerve	Wrist flexion
Extensor carpi radialis longus	Lateral supracondylar ridge, lateral epi- condyle, common extensor tendon	Base of the 2nd metacarpal	Radial nerve	Wrist extension & wrist radial deviation
Extensor carpi radialis brevis	Lateral epidondyle, common extensor tendon	Base of the 3rd metacarpal	Radial nerve	Wrist extension & wrist radial deviation
Extensor carpi ulnaris	Lateral epicondyle, common extensor tendon, proximal ulna	Base of the 5th metacarpal	Radial nerve	Wrist extension & wrist ulnar deviation

The Hand

MUSCLE	ORIGIN	INSERTION	INNERVATION	ACTION
Flexor digitorum superficialis	Medial epicondyle, coronoid process, ulna, proximal radius	Lateral & medial surface of the middle phalanx of digits 2–5	Median nerve	PIP joint flexion of digits 2–5
Flexor digitorum profundus	Body of the ulna	Through the insertions of the flexor digitorum superficialis onto the distal phalanx of digits 2–5	Ulnar nerve (digits 4 & 5), Median nerve (digits 2 & 3)	DIP joint flexion of digits 2–5
Flexor digiti minimi	Hook of the hamate	Base of the 5th digit proximal phalanx, ulnar side	Ulnar nerve	MCP flexion of the 5th digit
Extensor digitorum	Lateral epicondyle	Base of the middle & distal phalanges of digits 2–5	Radial nerve	MCP extension of digits 2–5
Extensor indicis	Posterior ulna	Tendon of the extensor digitorum, dorsal aponeurosis	Radial nerve	MCP, PIP, DIP extension of the 2nd digit

The Hand (*continued*)

MUSCLE	ORIGIN	INSERTION	INNERVATION	ACTION
Extensor digiti minimi	Lateral epicondyle	Tendon of the extensor digitorum—5th digit	Radial nerve	MCP, PIP, DIP extension of the 5th digit
Lumbricals	First digit—FDP 2nd digit tendon Second digit—FDP 3rd digit tendon Third digit—FDP 3rd & 4th digit tendons Fourth digit—FDP 4th & 5th digit tendons	Radial side of dorsal aponeurosis	1st & 2nd digits—median nerve 3rd & 4th digits—ulnar nerve	MCP digit flexion with PIP/DIP extension
Palmar interosseus	First interossei—1st metacarpal, ulnar surface Second interossei—2nd metacarpal, ulnar surface Third interossei—4th metacarpal, radial surface Fourth interossei—5th metacarpal, radial side	First interossei—base of the 1st digit proximal phalanx, ulnar side Second interossei—base of the 2nd digit proximal phalanx, ulnar side Third interossei—base of the 4th digit proximal phalanx, radial side Fourth interossei—base of the 5th digit proximal phalanx, radial side	Ulnar nerve	MCP digit adduction
Dorsal interosseus	Each interossei has its origin on both of the adjacent metacarpals	First interossei—base of the 2nd digit proximal phalanx, radial side Second interossei—base of the 3rd digit proximal phalanx, radial side Third interossei—base of the 3rd digit proximal phalanx, ulnar side Fourth interossei—base base of the 4th digit proximal phalanx, ulnar side	Ulnar nerve	MCP digit abduction

(continues)

The Hand (*continued*)

MUSCLE	ORIGIN	INSERTION	INNERVATION	ACTION
Abductor digit minimi	Pisiform	Base of the 5th digit proximal phalanx, ulnar side	Ulnar nerve	MCP abduction of the 5th digit
Opponens digit minimi	Hamate	5th digit metacarpal, ulnar side	Ulnar nerve	5th digit opposition
Opponens pollicis	Trapezium	1st digit metacarpal, radial side	Median nerve	1st digit opposition
Flexor pollicis brevis	Trapezium, trapezoid	Base of the 1st digit proximal phalanx	Median & ulnar nerves	Thumb MCP flexion & assist with CMC flexion
Flexor pollicis longus	Anterior radius	Base of the 1st digit distal phalanx	Median nerve	Thumb IP flexion
Abductor pollicis brevis	Scaphoid, trapezium	Base of the 1st digit proximal phalanx, radial side	Median nerve	Thumb CMC abduction
Abductor pollicis longus	Posterior, middle radius & ulna	Base of the 1st digit metacarpal	Radial nerve	Thumb CMC abduction
Adductor pollicis	3rd digit metacarpal, capitate, trapezoid	Base of the 1st digit proximal phalanx, ulnar side	Ulnar nerve	Thumb CMC adduction
Extensor pollicis longus	Middle, posterior ulna	Base of the 1st digit distal phalanx, dorsal surface	Radial nerve	Thumb IP extension
Extensor pollicis brevis	Posterior radius	Base of the 1st digit proximal phalanx, dorsal surface	Radial nerve	MCP extension & assists with CMC extension

The Hip

MUSCLE	ORIGIN	INSERTION	INNERVATION	ACTION
Iliacus	Superior 2/3 of ilium, anterior iliac crest	Lesser trochanter of the femur	Femoral nerve	Hip flexion
Psoas major	Transverse processes of L1–L5, vertebral bodies of T12–L5	Lesser trochanter of the femur	Lumbar plexus, L2–L4	Hip flexion
Gluteus maximus	Lateral surface of the ilium at the posterior gluteal line, posterior surface of sacrum, posterior coccyx & sacrotuberous ligaments	Iliotibial tract of fascia latae, gluteal tuberosity of the femur	Inferior gluteal nerve	Hip extension
Sartorius	Anterior superior iliac spine (ASIS)	Proximal aspect of the medial surface of the tibia	Femoral nerve	Hip flexion, hip abduction& hip external rotation
Gluteus medius	Lateral surface of the ilium, anterior & posterior gluteal line	Greater trochanter of the femur	Superior gluteal nerve	Hip abduction & hip internal rotation
Gluteus minimus	Lateral surface of the ilium between the anterior & inferior gluteal lines	Greater trochanter of the femur	Superior gluteal nerve	Hip abduction & hip internal rotation
Tensor fascia latae	Iliac crest posterior to the ASIS	Iliotibial tract	Superior gluteal nerve	Hip flexion, hip abduction & hip internal rotation
Pectineus	Superior ramus of the pubis	Between the lesser trochanter & linea aspera of the posterior femur	Femoral & obturator nerves	Hip adduction
Adductor magnus	Inferior pubic ramus, ramus of the ischium, ischial tuberosity	Linea aspera, adductor tubercle on the medial condyle of the femur	Obturator and sciatic nerves	Hip adduction
Gracilis	Inferior ramus of the pubis & ischium	Proximal aspect of the tibia distal to the medial condyle	Obturator nerve	Hip adduction
Adductor longus	Pubic tubercle/anterior crest of pubis	Medial lip of the linea aspera of the femur	Obturator nerve	Hip adduction
Adductor brevis	Body & inferior ramus of the pubis	Between the lesser trochanter & linea aspera	Obturator nerve	Hip adduction

(continues)

The Hip (*continued*)

MUSCLE	ORIGIN	INSERTION	INNERVATION	ACTION
Piriformis	Anterior sacrum & sciatic notch of the ilium	Superior border of the greater trochanter of the femur	Sacral plexus	Hip external rotation
Quadratus femoris	Lateral border of the ischial tuberosity	Posterior surface of the femur between the greater & lesser trochanters	Sacral plexus	Hip external rotation
Obturator internis	Obturator membrane, margin of obturator foramin, internal surface of the pelvis	Medial surface of the greater trochanter proximal to the trochanter fossa	Sacral plexus	Hip external rotation
Obturator externus	Obturator membrane, bone around foramen on external surface of pelvis	Trochanteric fossa of the femur	Obturator nerve	Hip external rotation
Gemellus superior	Dorsal aspect of the spine of ischium	Greater trochanter of the femur	Sacral plexus	Hip external rotation
Gemellus inferior	Proximal aspect of the ischial tuberosity	Greater trochanter of the femur	Obturator nerve	Hip external rotation

The Knee

MUSCLE	ORIGIN	INSERTION	INNERVATION	ACTION
Semitendinosus	Superior aspect of the ischial tuberosity	Proximal aspect of the the medial surface of the tibia	Sciatic nerve (tibial branch)	Knee flexion & internal rotation of the tibia during flexion & hip flexion when knee is flexed
Semimembranosus	Superolateral aspect of the ischial tuberosity	Medial tibial condyle & medial condyle of the femur	Sciatic nerve (tibial branch)	Knee flexion & internal rotation of the tibia during flexion & hip flexion when knee is flexed
Biceps femoris	Long head—ischial tuberosity Short head—posterior, distal femur	Lateral head of the fibula & condyle of the tibia	Sciatic nerve (tibial & peroneal branches)	Knee flexion & external rotation of the tibia during flexion
Rectus femoris	Straight head—anterior aspect of the anterior inferior iliac spine Reflected head—ilium above the acetabulum	Base of the patella & through the patellar ligament to the tibial tuberosity	Femoral nerve	Knee extension & hip flexion
Vastus intermedius	Anterior & lateral surfaces of the femoral shaft of the femur	Base of the patella through the patellar ligament to the tibial tuberosity	Femoral nerve	Knee extension
Vastus lateralis	Anterior femur	Lateral border of the patella through the patellar ligament to the tibial tuberosity	Femoral nerve	Knee extension
Vastus medialis	Inferior aspect of the intertrochanteric line, medial lip of the linea aspera, proximal aspect of the supracondylar & intermuscular septum	Medial border of the patella through the patellar ligament to the tibial tuberosity	Femoral nerve	Knee extension

The Ankle

MUSCLE	ORIGIN	INSERTION	INNERVATION	ACTION
Tibialis anterior	Lateral condyle of the tibia, 2/3 of lateral shaft of the tibia	Medial cuneiform bone, medial aspect of the base of the 1st metatarsal	Deep peroneal nerve	Ankle dorsiflexion ¶ foot inversion
Gastrocnemius	Medial head—proximal & posterior aspect of the medial condyle of the femur Lateral head—lateral & posterior aspect of the lateral condyle of the femur	Via the Achilles tendon into the calcaneum	Tibial nerve	Ankle plantar flexion
Soleus	Posterior aspect of the head & proximal shaft of the fibula, soleal line, medial border of the tibia	Via the Achilles tendon into the calcaneum	Tibial nerve	Ankle plantar flexion
Tibialis posterior	Posterolateral surface of the tibia, medial aspect of the proximal fibula	Navicular, fibrous expansions to the 3 cuneiforms, cuboid, bases of the 2nd, 3rd & 4th metatarsals	Tibial nerve	Foot inversion

The Foot

MUSCLE	ORIGIN	INSERTION	INNERVATION	ACTION
Peroneus longus	The head & lateral surface of the fibula	Lateral aspect of the base of the 5th metatarsal, medial cuneiform bone	Superficial peroneal nerve	Foot eversion
Peroneus brevis	Lateral surface of the fibula, adjacent fascia, intermuscular septa	Lateral aspect of the base of the 5th metatarsal	Superficial peroneal nerve	Foot eversion
Flexor hallucis brevis	Medial aspect of the plantar surface of the cuboid, lateral aspect of the cuneiform, tendon of the tibialis posterior muscle	Medial & lateral aspects of the base of the proximal phalanx of the great toe	Medial plantar nerve	MTP joint flexion of the great toe
Lumbricales	Flexor digitorum longus	Expansions of extensor tendons of toes #2–5	Medial & lateral plantar nerves	MTP joint flexion of toes #2–5
Flexor hallucis longus	Posterior surface of the fibula	Plantar aspect of the base of the distal phalanx of the great toe	Tibial nerve	IP joint flexion of the great toe
Flexor digitorum longus	Posterior surface of the tibia	Plantar aspects of the bases of the distal phalanges of toes #2–5	Medial plantar nerve	DIP joint flexion of toes #2–5
Flexor digitorum brevis	Calcaneus, medial & lateral intermuscular septa	Medial & lateral aspects of the middle phalanges of toes #2–5	Medial plantar nerve	PIP joint flexion of toes #2–5
Abductor hallucis	Medial process of the calcaneal tuberosity, flexor retinaculum, medial intermuscular septa	Medial aspect of the base of the proximal phalanx of the great toe	Medial plantar nerve	Abduction of the great toe
Abductor digit minimi	Medial & lateral process of the calcaneal tuberosity	Lateral aspect of the base of the proximal phalanx of the 5th toe	Lateral plantar nerve	Abduction of the 5th toe
Dorsal interossei	Side of the metatarsals	Medial & lateral aspect of toe #2 & lateral aspect of toes #3 & 4	Lateral plantar nerve	Abduction of toes #2–4
Extensor hallucis longus	Anterior surface of the fibula & interosseous membrane	Dorsal surface of the base of the distal phalanx of the great toe	Deep peroneal nerve	IP joint extension of the great toe

(continues)

The Foot (*continued*)

MUSCLE	ORIGIN	INSERTION	INNERVATION	ACTION
Extensor digitorum longus	Lateral condyle of the tibia, medial surface of the fibula, anterior surface of the interosseous membrane, crural fascia	Dorsal aspect of the base of the middle phalanx of toes #2–5 & dorsal aspect of the base of the distal phalanx of toes #2–5	Deep peroneal nerve	DIP joint flexion of toes #2–5
Extensor digitorum brevis	Dorsal surface of the calcaneum	Tendons to toes #2–4 of the corresponding extensor digitorum longus tendons	Deep peroneal nerve	MTP joint extension of the great toe & IP joint extension of toes #2–4

Appendix B: Normal Range of Motion Tables

Norms in Degrees for Upper Extremity Ranges of Motion from Selected References

JOINT	MOTION	KENDALL & MCCREARY (1983)	CLARKSON & GILEWICH (1989)	AMERICAN ACADEMY OF ORTHOPEDIC SURGEONS (1965)	AMERICAN MEDICAL ASSOCIATION (1988)
Trunk	Flexion		0–80 (4 in)	0–80 (4 in)	0–50
	Extension		0–20–30	0–25	0–25
	Lateral flexion		0–35	0–35	0–35
	Oblique rotation		0–45	0–45	0–30
Neck	Flexion	0–45	0–45	0–45	0–60
	Extension	0–45	0–45	0–45	0–75
	Lateral flexion		0–45	0–45	0–45
	Rotation		0–60	0–60	0–80
Shoulder	Flexion	0–180	0–180	0–180	0–150
	Extension	0–45	0–60	0–60	0–50
	Abduction/ Adduction	0–180	0–180	0–180	0–180
	External rotation	0–90	0–90	0–90	0–90
	Internal rotation	0–70	0–70	0–70	0–90
	Horizontal abduction		0–45		
	Horizontal adduction		0–135		
Elbow	Flexion/Extension	0–145	0–150	0–150	0–140
Forearm	Supination	0–90	0–90	0–80	0–80
	Pronation	0–90	0–80	0–80	0–80

(continues)

Norms in Degrees for Upper Extremity Ranges of Motion from Selected References (*continued*)

JOINT	MOTION	KENDALL & MCCREARY (1983)	CLARKSON & GILEWICH (1989)	AMERICAN ACADEMY OF ORTHOPEDIC SURGEONS (1965)	AMERICAN MEDICAL ASSOCIATION (1988)
Wrist	Flexion	0–80	0–80	0–80	0–60
	Extension	0–70	0–70	0–70	0–60
	Radial deviation	0–20	0–20	0–20	0–20
	Ulnar deviation	0–35	0–30	0–30	0–30
Digits					
#2–5					
MCP	Flexion	0–90	0–90	0–90	0–90
	Hyperextension		0–45	0–45	0–20
	Abduction				0–20
PIP	Flexion		0–100	0–100	0–100
	Extension		0		0
DIP	Flexion		0–90	0–90	0–70
	Hyperextension		0	0–10	0–30
Thumb					
CMC	Flexion	0–45	0–15	0–15	
	Hyperextension	0	0–20	0–15	
	Abduction	0–80	0–70	0–20	0–8 cm
	Opposition	Pad of thumb to base or tip of 5th digit		Tip of thumb to base or tip of 5th digit	
MCP	Flexion		0–50	0–50	0–60 cm
	Extension		0		
IP	Flexion		0–80	0–80	0–80
	Extension		0–20		

Norms in Degrees for Lower Extremity Ranges of Motion from Selected References

JOINT	MOTION	CLARKSON & GILEWICH	AMERICAN ACADEMY OF ORTHOPEDIC SURGEONS	AMERICAN MEDICAL ASSOCIATION
Hip	Flexion	0–120	0–120	0–100
	Extension	0–30	0–30	0–30
	Abduction	0–45	0–45	0–40
	Adduction	0–30	0–30	0–20
	External rotation	0–45	0–45	0–40
	Internal rotation	0–45	0–45	0–50
Knee	Flexion/Extension	0–135/135–0	0–135	0–150
Ankle	Dorsiflexion	0–20	0–20	0–20
	Plantar flexion	0–50	0–50	0–40
	Eversion	0–5	0–15	0–20
	Inversion	0–5	0–35	0–30
Foot				
#1 MTP	Flexion	0–45	0–45	0–30
	Extension	0–70	0–70	0–50
IP	Flexion	0–90	0–90	0–30
	Extension	0	0	0
#2-5 MTP	Flexion	0–40	0–40	#2—0–30, #3—0–20, #4—0–10, #5—0–10
	Extension	0–40	0–40	
#2-5 PIP	Flexion	0–35	0–35	
	Extension	0	0	
#2-5 DIP	Flexion	0–60	0–60	
	Extension			

Appendix C: Sample Evaluation Forms

Assessment Report for Functional Observation of the Upper Extremity

ACTION OBSERVED	FUNCTIONAL LIMITATION	FURTHER ASSESSMENT NEEDED
Trunk:		
Neck:		
Shoulder:		
Elbow:		
Forearm:		
Wrist:		
Digits:		
Thumb:		

Assessment Report for Functional Observation of the Lower Extremity

ACTION OBSERVED	FUNCTIONAL LIMITATION	FURTHER ASSESSMENT NEEDED
Hip:		
Knee:		
Ankle:		
Foot:		

Example of Assessment Report

ACTION(S) OBSERVED	FUNCTIONAL LIMITATION(S)	POSSIBLE FURTHER ASSESSMENT(S) NEEDED
Shoulder: Humeral flexion	*Reaching into an overhead cabinet*	• *Evaluation of the scapula* • *Goniometric measurements of the shoulder* • *Gross manual muscle testing of the shoulder* • *Decision tree based on above data to determine need for iso lated manual muscle testing* • *ADL assessment*

Assessment Report for Goniometry & Gross Manual Muscle Testing of the Upper Extremity

LEFT				RIGHT		
AROM	PROM	MUSCLE GRADE		AROM	PROM	MUSCLE GRADE
			Trunk:			
			Flexion			
			Extension			
			Lateral Flexion			
			Oblique Rotation			
			Cervical:			
			Flexion			
			Extension			
			Lateral Flexion			
			Rotation			
			Scapula:			
			Elevation			
			Depression			
			Abduction			
			Adduction			
			Shoulder:			
			Flexion			
			Hyperextension			
			Abduction			
			Adduction			
			External Rotation			
			Internal Rotation			
			Horizontal Abduction			
			Horizontal Adduction			
			Elbow:			
			Flexion			
			Extension			
			Forearm:			
			Supination			
			Pronation			
			Wrist:			
			Flexion			
			Extension			

Assessment Report for Goniometry & Gross Manual Muscle Testing of the Hand

LEFT				RIGHT		
AROM	PROM	MUSCLE GRADE		AROM	PROM	MUSCLE GRADE
			Hand: Digit #2			
			MCP—Flexion			
			Extension			
			Hyperextension			
			Abduction			
			Adduction			
			PIP—Flexion			
			Extension			
			DIP—Flexion			
			Extension			
			Hand: Digit #3			
			MCP—Flexion			
			Extension			
			Hyperextension			
			Abduction			
			PIP—Flexion			
			Extension			
			DIP—Flexion			
			Extension			
			Hand: Digit #4			
			MCP—Flexion			
			Extension			
			Hyperextension			
			Abduction			
			Adduction			
			PIP—Flexion			
			Extension			
			DIP—Flexion			
			Extension			

(continues)

Assessment Report for Goniometry & Gross Manual Muscle Testing of the Hand *(continued)*

LEFT				RIGHT		
AROM	PROM	MUSCLE GRADE		AROM	PROM	MUSCLE GRADE
			Hand: Digit #5			
			MCP—Flexion			
			Extension			
			Hyperextension			
			Abduction			
			Adduction			
			PIP—Flexion			
			Extension			
			DIP—Flexion			
			Extension			
			Thumb:			
			CMC—Flexion			
			Extension			
			Abduction			
			Adduction			
			Opposition			
			MCP—Flexion			
			Extension			
			IP—Flexion			
			Extension			

Assessment Report for Goniometry & Gross Manual Muscle Testing of the Lower Extremity

LEFT				RIGHT		
AROM	PROM	MUSCLE GRADE		AROM	PROM	MUSCLE GRADE
			Hip:			
			Flexion			
			Extension			
			Abduction			
			Adduction			
			External Rotation			
			Internal Rotation			
			Knee:			
			Flexion			
			Extension			
			Ankle:			
			Dorsiflexion			
			Plantar Flexion			
			Eversion			
			Inversion			

Assessment Report for Goniometry & Gross Manual Muscle Testing of the Foot

LEFT				RIGHT		
AROM	PROM	MUSCLE GRADE		AROM	PROM	MUSCLE GRADE
			Foot: Toe #1			
			MTP—Flexion			
			Extension			
			Abduction			
			Adduction			
			Foot: Toe #2			
			MTP—Flexion			
			Extension			
			Abduction			
			Adduction			
			PIP—Flexion			
			Extension			
			DIP—Flexion			
			Extension			

(continues)

Assessment Report for Goniometry & Gross Manual Muscle Testing of the Foot *(continued)*

LEFT				RIGHT		
AROM	PROM	MUSCLE GRADE		AROM	PROM	MUSCLE GRADE
			Foot: Toe #3			
			MTP—Flexion			
			Extension			
			Abduction			
			Adduction			
			PIP—Flexion			
			Extension			
			DIP—Flexion			
			Extension			
			Foot: Toe #4			
			MCP—Flexion			
			Extension			
			Abduction			
			Adduction			
			PIP—Flexion			
			Extension			
			DIP—Flexion			
			Extension			
			Foot: Toe #5			
			MCP—Flexion			
			Extension			
			Abduction			
			Adduction			
			PIP—Flexion			
			Extension			
			DIP—Flexion			
			Extension			

Assessment Report for Isolated Manual Muscle Testing of the Upper Extremity

LEFT MUSCLE GRADE		RIGHT MUSCLE GRADE
	Trunk:	
	Flexor group	
	Extensor group	
	Lateral flexion group	
	Rotator group	
	Quadratus lumborum	
	Cervical:	
	Flexor group	
	Extensor group	
	Lateral Flexion group	
	Rotator group	
	Scapula:	
	Rhomboids	
	Serratus anterior	
	Pectoralis minor	
	Shoulder:	
	Posterior deltoid	
	Middle deltoid	
	Anterior deltoid	
	Coracobrachialis	
	Pectoralis major (clavicular head)	
	Pectoralis major (sternal head)	
	Teres major	
	Latissimus dorsi	
	Subscapularis	
	Infraspinatus	
	Teres minor	
	Supraspinatus	
	Trapezius (Upper)	
	Levator Scapulae	
	Trapezius (Middle)	
	Trapezius (Lower)	

(continues)

Assessment Report for Isolated Manual Muscle Testing of the Upper Extremity (*continued*)

LEFT MUSCLE GRADE		RIGHT MUSCLE GRADE
	Elbow:	
	Biceps brachii	
	Brachialis	
	Brachioradialis	
	Triceps	
	Aconeus	
	Forearm:	
	Pronator Teres	
	Pronator Quadratus	
	Supinator	
	Wrist:	
	Flexor carpi radialis	
	Flexor carpi ulnaris	
	Palmaris longus	
	Extensor carpi radialis longus	
	Extensor carpi radialis brevis	
	Extensor carpi ulnaris	

Assessment Report for Isolated Manual Muscle Testing of the Hand

HAND:	GRADE							
	LEFT				RIGHT			
DIGIT #	2	3	4	5	2	3	4	5
Flexor digitorum superficialis								
Flexor digitorum profundus								
Flexor digiti minimi								
Extensor digitorum								
Extensor indicis								
Extensor digiti minimi								
Lumbricals								
Palmar interosseous								
Dorsal interosseous								
Abductor digiti minimi								

HAND/THUMB:	GRADE	
	LEFT	RIGHT
Opponens digiti minimi		
Opponens pollicis		
THUMB:		
Flexor pollicis brevis		
Flexor pollicis longus		
Abductor pollicis brevis		
Abductor pollicis longus		
Adductor pollicis		
Extensor pollicis longus		
Extensor pollicis brevis		

Assessment Report for Isolated Manual Muscle Testing of the Lower Extremity

LEFT MUSCLE GRADE		RIGHT MUSCLE GRADE
	Hip:	
	Iliacus	
	Psoas major	
	Gluteus maximus	
	Sartorius	
	Gluteus medius	
	Gluteus minimus	
	Tensor fascia latae	
	Pectineus	
	Adductor magnus	
	Gracilis	
	Adductor longus	
	Adductor brevis	
	Piriformis	
	Quadratus femoris	
	Obturator internis	
	Obturator externus	
	Gemellus superior	
	Gemellus inferior	
	Knee:	
	Semitendinosus	
	Semimembranosus	
	Biceps femoris	
	Rectus femoris	
	Vastus intermedius	
	Vastus lateralis	
	Vastus medialis	
	Ankle:	
	Tibialis anterior	
	Gastrocnemius	
	Soleus	
	Tibialis posterior	
	Peroneus longus	
	Peroneus brevis	

Assessment Report for Isolated Manual Muscle Testing of the Foot

FOOT:	GRADE							
	LEFT				RIGHT			
DIGIT #	2	3	4	5	2	3	4	5
Lumbricales								
Flexor digitorum longus								
Flexor digitorum brevis								
Abductor digiti minimi								
Dorsal interossei								
Extensor digitorum longus								
Extensor digitorum brevis								

GREAT TOE:	GRADE	
	LEFT	RIGHT
Flexor hallucis brevis		
Flexor hallucis longus		
Abductor hallucis		
Extensor hallucis longus		
Extensor digitorum brevis		

Index

D

E

I

K

L

M

T

U

V

W